D1593110

Roy Adaptation
Model-Based Research
25 Years of Contributions to Nursing Science
Boston Based Adaptation Research in Nursing Society (BBARNS)

Sigma Theta Tau International
Center Nursing Press
Peer-reviewed Publications

For other Center Nursing Press publications and videos contact:

Sigma Theta Tau International
550 West North Street
Indianapolis, IN 46202
1.888.634.7575
FAX: 317.634.8188
www.stti.iupui.edu

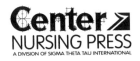

ISBN: 0-9656391-8-5

Printed in the United States of America.

Boston Based Adaptation Research in Nursing Society (BBARNS)

Sr. Callista Roy, RN, PhD, FAAN
Professor & Nurse Theorist
School of Nursing
Boston College

Susan E. Pollock, RN, PhD, FAAN
Professor & Associate Dean
School of Nursing
Texas Tech University

Veta H. Massey, RN, PhD
Dean, Division of Nursing
Baptist Memorial College of Health Sciences

Kathy Lauchner, RN, PhD
Coordinator of Non-traditional Nursing Education, Division of Nursing
Austin Community College

Martha Velasco-Whetsell, RN, PhD
Associate Professor
Florida International University

Keville Frederickson, RN, EdD, FAAN
Professor & Director, Graduate Nursing Program
Lehman College, The City University of New York

Stacey H. Barone, RN, PhD, CRRN
Lecturer, College of Nursing
University of Massachusetts, Boston

Margaret Anne Carson, RN, PhD
Clinical Researcher
V.A. Research Service, Manchester, New Hampshire

TABLE OF CONTENTS

Preface

In the *Roy Adaptation Model-Based Research: 25 Years of Contributions to Nursing Science*, we do a critical analysis and synthesis of 163 studies based on the Roy Adaptation Model. The purposes of the research synthesis project were (a) to critically analyze research based on the Roy Adaptation Model, (b) to evaluate the relationships of the research to the Roy Adaptation Model, and (c) to synthesize the contributions of the research findings to nursing, including implications for nursing practice and for future research and theory development. The team of investigators are committed to advancing nursing knowledge through research. In particular, we believe that nursing models can play a key role in guiding research for clinical knowledge development. We have used and continue to use the Roy Adaptation Model for individual programs of research and have carried out collaborative projects for the past 8 years.

Our group, known as The Boston Based Adaptation Research in Nursing Society (BBARNS) began the project with the conviction that the Roy Adaptation Model (RAM) has the breadth, scope, and flexibility to be useful across patient populations. Further, we believe that research questions derived from the model can be answered by both qualitative and quantitative approaches. The close connection of the model to nursing practice in its derivation and development has set up the link that makes the derived knowledge particularly significant for nursing practice. However, the investigators were keenly aware that the possibilities of such knowledge affecting high-quality practice were limited by the lack of a critical appraisal and integrated synthesis of such research. Thus together we chose to seize the opportunity of the 25th anniversary of the first publication of the RAM (March 1970) to conduct and publish a thorough critique and integration of RAM Research from March 1970 through January 1, 1995. Given their mutual commitments to scholarship, the authors also remained open to questions of the quality and comprehensiveness of the body of research. The group was eager to identify areas in need of further study and directions for future model and theory development.

Common beliefs about nursing research and practice, and use of a nursing model in particular, sustained the group through an intense 5-year commitment to the demands of organizing the project, developing strategies for identifying and reporting the research, establishing guidelines for critical analysis and processes to evaluate the relationships of the research to the model, conducting pilot studies to establish inter-rater reliability, and finally conducting the review and writing up the design and findings to accomplish the specific purposes of the project. Each of the 163 studies has been described and critically analyzed, evaluated for its relationship to the RAM, and synthesized for knowledge related to model-based practice and research.

The monograph is divided into 13 Chapters. The first two chapters are introductory; in Chapter One, the historical development of the RAM is described and in Chapter Two the methods for critical analysis and synthesis of the research are described. In Chapters 3 through 9 are descriptions of major portions of the work for critical analysis and synthesis of the research studies. The research is reported in the following categories: Physiologic mode adaptation ($n=21$); self concept mode adaptation ($n=19$); role function mode adaptation ($n=10$); interdependence mode adaptation ($n=21$); adaptive modes and processes ($n=36$); studies focusing on stimuli ($n=19$); and nursing intervention studies ($n=28$). In additional chapters, we address measurement of the model concepts (Chapter 10) and findings from Chapters 3 through 9 to identify contributions to nursing science, testing model propositions (Chapter 11), applications to nursing practice (Chapter 12), and directions for future theory development and research (Chapter 13).

We hope that this monograph can enhance efforts to make theory more relevant for the practice of nursing and stimulate further development of nursing science by leading the way to critical analysis and synthesis of research based on other nursing models. The monograph differs from other nursing theory and research sources in that it is a comprehensive review of research based on a given model and moves beyond description of the literature to critique, synthesis, and direction setting. Nurses studying models at the undergraduate and graduate levels will benefit from the many examples of use of the RAM that are provided. The monograph will be of interest to nurses in all areas of practice including nurse educators and nurse administrators because the research synthesis includes multiple specialty areas.

The members of BBARNS are indebted to all who have encouraged and assisted with the development of the project. Our first debt of gratitude is to the investigators who conducted and reported the 163 studies based on the RAM that provided the data for the analysis and synthesis. In addition, BBARNS members gratefully acknowledge contributions of the librarians at Boston College, Anne F. Lippman and Marilyn A. Grant, who provided professional services for the literature searches and we thank undergraduate research fellow, Kimberly Jonas, who prepared copies of journal articles for review. The BBARNS investigators are also indebted to colleagues and staff of the several schools of nursing, health care and research facilities represented in the project for support and assistance with the many aspects of the project. Monograph acquisitions editor, Jacqui Fawcett, merits particular thanks for her generously provided expertise throughout all phases of the project. Finally, each BBARNS member is grateful for the support of family and friends during the last 5 years, and Dr. Roy has a special word of appreciation to Susan Pollock, and the other members of the group, who kept the project going while she was away unexpectedly during the early months of 1996. All BBARNS members appreciate the efforts of Dr. Pollock and Estelle Beaumont, RN, PhD, copy editor for Sigma Theta Tau International, on many details of the production of the monograph.

Sr. Callista Roy
Chestnut Hill, Massachusetts

Susan E. Pollock
Lubbock, Texas

Chapter 1

The Roy Adaptation Model and Nursing Science

The Roy Adaptation Model (RAM) for nursing practice provides a basis for developing the science of nursing. The first publication on the model (Roy, 1970) outlined its basic elements. Major theoretic developments and refinement of the model have been published since that time by theorist, Sr. Callista Roy. Primary source publications, as well as numerous secondary sources, have directed nurses in applications of the RAM in nursing practice, education, and research, during the past 25 years. In addition, groups of nurse scholars have developed several major nursing science projects based on the RAM. One of these projects is the topic of this monograph, a project to critically analyze, synthesize, and publish 25 years of research based on the Roy Adaptation Model of nursing.

In this chapter, we provide an overview of the model by highlighting its development, refinement, major concepts, and propositions. In this chapter we also review approaches to major Roy model-based contributions to nursing science, including the founding of the Boston Based Adaptation in Nursing Research Society (BBARNS). Finally, we introduce the BBARNS project of synthesizing research based on the RAM from 1970 through 1994.

Overview of Roy Adaptation Model

The development and refinement of the Roy Adaptation Model of Nursing encompasses many stages. Initial development of the RAM when Roy was a master's student in pediatric nursing at the University of California, Los Angeles, is well documented (Roy & Andrews, 1991; Roy, 1992). Roy (1997a) summarized the key factors influencing the inception of the model: commitment to describe the goal of nursing; clinical insights into pediatric nursing; systems theory; and belief in human potential. Recent refinements of the basic definition of adaptation and of the scientific and philosophic assumptions of the model (Roy, 1997b; Roy & Andrews, 1999) also have implications for developing nursing knowledge.

Theoretic Development and Refinement

In essence, the model focuses on the goal of nursing to enhance interaction of people with the environment to promote adaptation. Roy outlined the assumptions of the model in the first textbook on conceptual models for nursing practice (Riehl & Roy, 1974). The assumptions were based on the theorist's approach to the concept of person, as a unified whole coping with a changing environment, and to the process of adaptation. Adaptation was initially defined as a function of the stimuli to which people or groups respond and their adaptation level. This definition relied on the work of Helson (1964) whose systematic approach was assumed to provide a useful description of behavior encountered by nurses. Adaptive or ineffective behavior was based on the strength of the focal, or confronting stimulus; the contextual or environmental stimuli; and other residual or nonspecific stimuli. The nursing model's developer considered that nurses could make an important contribution to health by promoting adaptation thus making more of a patient's energy available for healing. Nurses are also concerned with the person as a total being in areas of health and illness.

Theory refinement in the 1970s and 1980s involved scientific and philosophic assumptions of the RAM model. Roy summarized a set of assumptions based on systems theory and Helson's Adaptation Level Theory. Emphasis was placed on holism, interdependence, control processes, information feedback, and complexity of living systems. Behavior was viewed as adaptive; adaptation, as a function of stimuli and adaptation level. The individual and dynamic nature of adaptation levels, and positive and active processes of responding were also emphasized (see summary in Roy & Corliss, 1993). Philosophic assumptions of humanism were explicated along with introduction of the principle of veritivity (Roy, 1988a). The focus was on creativity, purposefulness, holism, interpersonal processes, purposefulness of human existence, unity of purpose, activity, creativity, and value and meaning of life.

Theory development of the RAM model in the early decades was influenced further by use of the model as a basis of nursing curriculum and by Roy's doctoral work in sociology and post-doctoral work in neuroscience nursing. Given that the model focused on promoting adaptation, the person or group was viewed as an adaptive system. Addition of the concept of adaptive modes to the core concept of the person as an adaptive system was an effort to delineate content for nursing curriculum and to describe assessment factors for the nursing process. Derivation of the four modes—physiologic, self concept, role function, and interdependence—from an inductive content analysis of 500 samples of patient behavior is described elsewhere (Roy, 1971).

Recognizing the need for theory construction in nursing, Roy and Roberts (1981) designed a taxonomy for theory development based on the model. A theory of the adaptive person and theories related to the adaptive modes were derived. Further, conceptual work on the cognator subsystem led to Roy's (1988b) proposal of a nursing model of cognitive processing. Roy used the cognitive processing model to derive and test hypotheses for recovery from mild and moderate head injury (Roy, 1990).

Theory developments in viewing groups as adaptive systems were published by Roy in relation to the family (1983a), the community (1984a), and nursing administration (Roy & Anway,1989).

Refinements of the Roy Adaptation Model in the 1990s include redefinition of the concept of adaptation for the 21st century. Roy (1997b) has described the challenge posed by both the promise and limitations of her work in neuroscience nursing and in the review of Roy model-based research as the impetus for the urgency to expand her conceptual work. Rooted in the original scientific and philosophic assumptions of the RAM, the theorist's development of a concept of adaptation addresses a cosmic scientific perspective of the potential for human creativity and well-being in a new epoch of the earth's biosystems. The redefinition also takes into account the contemporary influences of earth science, cosmology, and creation spirituality. Adaptation is redefined (Roy, 1997b) as the process and outcome by which the thinking and feeling person uses conscious awareness and choice to create human and environment integration. Roy used characteristics of the new definition of adaptation to restate the scientific and philosophic assumptions and thus offered an "enriched understanding of the adapting person with immense capabilities and responsibilities" (p. 47).

Major Concepts and Propositions

Fawcett (1995) describes a conceptual framework as a set of general concepts and the propositions that integrate the concepts into a meaningful configuration. The major concepts of the RAM can be reviewed by describing how the theorist views nursing's metaparadigm concepts of person, environment, health, and nursing. As noted above people—as individuals and groups—are viewed as holistic adaptive systems. A system has internal control processes, inputs, outputs, and feedback. For the individual, the control processes are the regulator and cognator subsystems. The regulator is a subsystem that processes automatically through neural, chemical, and endocrine coping channels. The cognator uses four cognitive-emotive channels—perceptual information processing, learning, judgment, and emotion—to promote adaptation. For the group as an adaptive system, the comparable central control processes are known as the stabilizer and the innovator. The responses, or behaviors, created by the regulator and cognator, or stabilizer and innovator, are the output of the adaptive system. Ways of adapting are categorized into four modes: physiologic-physical, self concept-group identity, role function, and interdependence (Roy & Andrews, 1999). Adaptive behaviors are those that promote survival, growth, reproduction, mastery, and person and environment transformation. Ineffective behaviors are those that do not lead to the goals of adaptation. Behavior, both adaptive and ineffective, acts as feedback, or further information to be processed by the system.

The environment forms the input for the individual or group adaptive system. Environment includes both internal and external inputs. Roy has relied on the work of Helson (1964) to identify three classes of stimuli useful for analyzing clinical situations. The focal stimulus is the internal or external stimulus most immediately in the awareness of the human system, that is, the object, event, or feeling most present in consciousness. Contextual stimuli are all other stimuli present in the situation that contribute to the effect of the focal stimulus. These environmental factors are present to the human system, but are not the focus of attention or energy, though they may affect how the system deals with the focal stimulus. The residual stimuli are environmental factors inside or outside human adaptive systems, the effects of which are unclear in the current situation. An important internal stimulus is the adaptation level, currently defined as integrated processes, compensatory processes, or compromised processes (Roy & Andrews, 1999).

Within the RAM, understanding of health is rooted in understanding both the human adaptive system and the environment, and in scientific and philosophic assumptions fundamental to the model. Individuals and groups are adaptive systems that are constantly growing and developing within changing environments. Health is a reflection of interactions of the adaptive person and the environment. Adaptive responses promote integrity and wholeness relative to human goals. Health is viewed within the context of the purposefulness of human existence and thus the goals of the person or group are significant in defining health in each situation. On a general level, according to the model, health is a state and a process of being and becoming integrated and whole. Lack of being integrated represents lack of health for an individual or group.

According to the RAM, nursing is a science and a practice discipline. As a practice discipline, the goal of nursing is to promote adaptation by enhancing the interaction of human systems with the environment, thereby contributing to health. Nursing activities, according to the model, involve assessment of adaptive behavior and of the stimuli that influence adaptive behavior. Nursing judgments are based on assessments, and nursing interventions are planned to manage stimuli and to enhance the coping processes of the individual or group.

As reviewed here, and further described in several publications (Andrews & Roy, 1986; Roy & Andrews, 1991, 1999; Roy & Roberts, 1981), the major concepts of the RAM are used to develop propositions that provide an integrated view of nursing. A simplified version of the relationships among the major concepts was published by Roy (1983b). Two general propositions can be stated to link all the concepts: (a) people or adaptive systems interact with the environment and move toward the goal of adaptation and health and (b) the nursing process based on the model influences that movement.

Based on the concepts of the RAM, the theory construction by Roy and Roberts (1981) took a major step in identifying specific propositions derived from the model. In particular, the theory of the person as an adaptive system was developed in detail and 40 propositions were derived related to the regulator and cognator processes. In addition, theory construction with each of the adaptive modes provided the basis for deriving sample propositions in each mode. Work on the physiologic mode included 11 sample propositions; self concept, eight; role function, eight; and interdependence, seven sample propositions. In all, 74 propositions were included in an integrated view of nursing based on the adaptation model.

Developing Nursing Science Based on the Roy Adaptation Model

Roy has often noted that her professional work aims to develop knowledge for nursing and that the Roy Adaptation Model is one way of developing such knowledge. In several seminal papers, Roy has outlined her evolving view of the structure of nursing knowledge. Through the years, in several different formats, Sr. Roy has been joined by groups of scholars in the work of building the science of nursing based on the RAM. As a context for the current project, briefly examining Roy's thinking related to the structure for nursing knowledge that provides guidelines for model-based research will be useful. In addition, samples of the approaches used by groups of nurse scholars in this endeavor are highlighted.

Structure for Knowledge Development

Nearly two decades ago, Roy focused on the significance of theory construction as essential to the development of nursing science. She viewed the text by Roy and Roberts (1981) as providing direction to develop and validate the science of nursing, and stated, "Ultimately, we want to demonstrate that the practice of nursing, based on the science of nursing, makes a difference in the health status of the population"(p. xv). Roy suggested that testing theory based on the RAM, as outlined in the text, provided a sense of direction in working toward that goal. The structure of knowledge, then, was based on the core concepts of the model and their use in theorizing and deriving propositions for empiric testing.

In 1983, Roy also published a proposal for direction of theory development in nursing. In this work, she used a concept of "person" from a nursing model as key to developing a basic science theory for nursing, or knowledge of order. Similarly, Roy stated that the goal of nursing directs theorizing about nursing practice, or knowledge of control. Theory about knowledge of disorder or problems encountered in nursing practice were derived from both the description of person in the model and the goal of nursing. Roy (1983b) credits unpublished ideas from Dorothy E. Johnson as the basis for her distinctions among knowledge of order, disorder, and control.

From 1983 to 1987, Roy conducted postdoctoral research in neuroscience nursing with Connie R. Robinson at the University of California at San Francisco. During this time, Roy continued holistic scientific and philosophic inquiry into the nature of the person. The resulting development of her thinking on the nature of nursing knowledge was published in one paper that described an integrated metaparadigm of nursing (Roy, 1988a), and another that looked at the metaparadigm's implications for physiological research in nursing (Breslin, Roy, & Robinson, 1992).

Roy then referred to two branches of nursing knowledge—basic nursing science and clinical nursing science. Basic nursing science includes understanding life processes that promote health, derived from the earlier understanding of knowledge of order. The clinical science of nursing involves understanding how people cope with health and illness and what can be done to enhance coping. Terms such as disorder and control did not seem useful in this later description, given the published explication of the philosophic assumptions of the RAM (Roy, 1988a).

More recently, Roy specifically addressed application of the model in nursing research and outlined the structure of knowledge based on the RAM (Roy & Andrews, 1991; 1999). The focus of knowledge of basic nursing science is the person or group as an adaptive system. Categories of basic nursing science knowledge include: (a) adaptive processes—that is, cognator-regulator activity, stabilizer-innovator activity, stability of adaptive patterns, and dynamics of evolving adaptive patterns; (b) adaptive modes, their development, interrelatedness, and cultural and other influences; and (c) adaptation related to health from the perspective of person-environment interaction and including integration within and among the adaptive modes.

The clinical science of nursing includes: (a) changes in cognator-regulator or stabilizer-innovator effectiveness; (b) changes within and among adaptive modes; and (c) nursing care to promote adaptive processes in times of transition, during environmental changes, and during acute and chronic illness, injury, treatment, and technologic threats. With increased emphasis on processes and patterns in the structure of knowledge, Roy (1991) noted that flexibility is increasing for the expansion of new knowledge to meet the changing needs of practice in the next century.

A specific blueprint for the use of the RAM in nursing research was described in the application of model-based research to rehabilitation nursing (Roy & Barone, 1996). Knowledge for nursing in the future treats people as co-extensive with their physical and social environment; takes a values-based stance; and believes in people as creators of the future (Roy, 1997c).

Efforts of Groups of Nurse Scholars

Since the publication of the first article on the RAM more than 25 years ago, other nurse scholars have contributed to development of nursing science based on the model. A few key groups are mentioned here. Nurse faculty at Mount St. Mary's College in Los Angeles conducted the conceptual development of the four adaptive modes. Their individual and collective contributions are recognized in two editions of the basic textbook on the model (Roy, 1976, 1984b).

Sr. Roy and other faculty members consulted extensively about curriculum based upon the model throughout the United States and Canada in the 1970s, and conducted summer workshops on the RAM on the home campus where the model was developed. International conferences on the model were sponsored throughout the 1970s and 1980s by Alverno College in Milwaukee, Mount St. Mary's College in Los Angeles, and William Patterson College in Wayne, New Jersey, with scholarly developments presented in both theory and research. A group of nurse researchers, now called the University of Montreal Research Team in Nursing Science has worked on a program of research based on the RAM to test a theoretic longitudinal model of psychosocial determinants of adaption in different populations (Lévesque, Ricard, Ducharme, Duquette, & Bonin, 1998; Ducharme, Ricard, Duquette, Levasque, & Lachance, 1998).

Use of the model in nursing practice is a constant source of stimulation for further development of nursing science based on the model. Many nurse scholars worked in groups that included both educators and practitioners to develop research-based implementation projects concerning the RAM. Among scholars in practice, Gray (1984, 1991) is noted for publishing one of the first implementation projects and for her later experiences as a consultant for four implementation projects. Two other implementation projects carried out collaboratively with educators and practitioners are at St. Joseph's Regional Medical Center, Lewiston, Idaho (Connerly, Ristau, Lindberg, & McFarland, 1999) and the Institute Philippe Pinel de Montreal in Hull, Quebec, Canada.

Founding of the Boston Based Adaptation Research in Nursing Society (BBARNS).

Notable among the groups of scholars who have worked on developing nursing science based on the RAM are members of the Boston Based Adaptation in Nursing Research Society. The group began in 1991 with a small group of scholars presenting their research and publishing joint papers. Each investigator had been using the RAM to guide her individual work. The investigators believed that a synthesis of findings of several authors using the same model would be particularly productive (Pollock, Frederickson, Carson, Massey, & Roy, 1994). When the studies were viewed collectively, new insights about theoretic and empiric relationships emerged.

Purposes of the BBARNS group were broadly stated as: (a) to advance nursing practice by developing basic and clinical nursing knowledge based on the model; (b) to provide the scholarly collegiality needed for knowledge development and research; (c) to enhance networks of dissemination of research for practice; and (d) to encourage scholars in the field and facilitate related programs of research. Recognizing the benefits that could be derived from multiple studies based on the model, the group took the next logical step and planned a project to critically analyze and synthesize research based on the RAM.

RAM Research Project

Since publication of the first article on the RAM in 1970, numerous investigators have used the model to derive and test research questions to contribute to nursing knowledge. However, the scope of the literature on Roy model-based research and its contribution to nursing knowledge were unclear. The BBARNS group of researchers shared the conviction that theory and research are interrelated (Fawcett & Downs, 1992; Moody, 1990; Polit & Hungler, 1994; Woods & Catanzaro, 1988), a theme of nursing literature in recent decades. Theory provides the basis for proposing hypotheses for testing in research; similarly, new theories or revised theories result from both qualitative and quantitative research (Chinn & Kramer, 1999).

In discussing aggregate analysis of qualitative research, Kearney (1998) proposes that techniques of linking findings of multiple studies among geographic, cultural, and historic settings are worthy of pursuit and refinement. Instead of research that focuses on a specific topic and reflects several different, often implicit, conceptual models, research that focuses on a specific conceptual model has a unique usefulness in developing nursing science. The variables of several studies based on one model can be compared because they derive from common concepts.

Basically, studies designed in relation to the same nursing model have a common understanding of person, environment, health, nursing, and the interrelationship of the concepts. A nursing conceptual model provides researchers with a common reference point and encourages critical inquiry and conceptual clarity. Further, a given nursing model provides a basis for organizing findings from different content areas into a structure of knowledge.

Most important, synthesizing model-based research allows for generalizations at higher levels of abstraction than the variables or phenomena of a given study allow. With a belief in these advantages, the BBARNS research team committed themselves to undertake the research synthesis project of doing an integrated review of known research on a given nursing model.

The first step was to identify and locate the extant literature of nursing research based on the RAM in the English language. Second, since the particular task had not been undertaken before, the BBARNS group developed the methods for critical analysis and synthesis of research based on the RAM. The presentation of findings of the project are the subject of this monograph.

The purposes of this monograph are: (a) to critically analyze research based on the Roy Adaptation Model; (b) to evaluate the relationships of the research to the RAM; and (c) to synthesize the contributions of the research findings to nursing science, determining implications for nursing practice and directions for future research and theory development.

In Chapter 2, the methods for the research review that were derived and pilot tested are described. Findings of the research review project are presented in the remaining chapters.

References

Andrews, H., & Roy, C. (1986). *Essentials of the Roy Adaptation Model.* Norwalk, CT: Appleton-Century-Crofts.

Breslin, E., Roy, C., & Robinson, C. (1992). Physiological nursing research in dyspnea: A paradigm shift and a metaparadigm exemplar. *Scholarly Inquiry for Nursing Practice, 6,* 81-104.

Chinn, P., & Kramer, M. (1999). *Theory and nursing.* St. Louis: Mosby.

Connerly, K., Ristav, S. Lindberg, C., & McFarland, M. (1999). The Roy model in nursing practice. In C. Roy & H. Andrews. The Roy Adaptation Model (pp. 515-534). Stamford, CT: Appleton & Lange.

Ducharme, F., Ricard N., Duquette, A., Lévesque, L. & Lachance, L. (1998). Empirical Testing of a longitudinal model derived from the Roy Adaptation Model. Nursing Science Quarterly, 11, 149-159.

Fawcett, J. (1995). *Analysis and evaluation of conceptual models of nursing.* (3rd ed.). Philadelphia: F.A. Davis.

Fawcett, J., & Downs, F.S. (1992). *The relationship of theory and research* (2nd ed.). Philadelphia: F.A. Davis.

Gray, J. (1984). The implementation of a conceptual model of nursing into practice. Unpublished Master's Thesis, Los Angeles: California State University.

Gray, J. (1991). The Roy Adaptation Model in nursing practice. In C. Roy, & H. Andrews (Eds.) *The Roy Adaptation Model: The definitive statement* (pp. 429-443). Norwalk, CT: Appleton & Lange.

Helson, H. (1964). *Adaptation level theory.* New York: Harper & Row.

Kearney, M. (1998) Ready to wear: Discovering grounded formal theory. *Research in Nursing & Health, 21,* 179-186.

Lévesque, L., Ricard, N., Ducharme, F., Duquette, A., & Bonin, J. (1998). Empirical verfication on a theoretical model derived from the Roy Adaption Model: Findings from five studies. *Nursing Science Quarterly, 11,* 31-39.

Moody, L. (1990). *Advancing nursing science through research.* (Vol. 1). Newbury Park, CA: Sage.

Polit, D.F., & Hungler, B.P. (1994). *Nursing research: Principles and methods* (5th ed.). Philadelphia: J.B. Lippincott.

Pollock, S., Frederickson, K., Carson, M., Massey, V., & Roy, C. (1994). Contributions to nursing science: Synthesis of findings from adaptation model research. *Scholarly Inquiry for Nursing Practice, 8,* 361-372.

Riehl, J.P., & Roy, C. (1974). Conceptual models for nursing practice. New York: Appleton-Century-Crofts.

Roy, C. (1970). Adaptation: A conceptual framework for nursing. *Nursing Outlook, 18,* 43-45.

Roy, C. (1971). Adaptation: A basis for nursing practice. *Nursing Outlook, 19,* 254-257.

Roy, C. (1976). *Introduction to nursing: An adaptation model.* Englewood Cliffs, NJ: Prentice Hall.

Roy, C. (1983a). Roy Adaptation Model and analysis and application to the expectant family and the family in primary care. In L. Clements, & F. Roberts, *Family health: A theoretical approach to nursing care* (pp. 255-278; 298-303; 375-378). NY: Wiley & Sons.

Roy, C. (1983b). Theory development in nursing: Proposal for direction. In Chaska, N. *The nursing profession: A time to speak* (pp. 453-467). NY: McGraw Hill.

Roy, C. (1984a). The Roy Adaptation Model in nursing: Applications in community health nursing. In M. K. Assoy & C. C. Ossler (Eds.), *Proceedings of the Eighth Annual Community Nursing Conference* University of North Carolina: Chapel Hill.

Roy, C. (1984b). *Introduction to nursing: An adaptation model* (2nd ed.). Englewood Cliffs, NJ: Prentice Hall.

Roy, C. (1988a). An explication of the philosophical assumptions of the Roy Adaptation Model. *Nursing Science Quarterly, 1,* 26-34.

Roy, C. (1988b). Altered cognition: An information processing approach. In P. Mitchell, L. Hodges, M. Muwaswes, & C. Walleck, (Eds.), *Neuroscience nursing: Phenomena and practice* (pp.185-211). Norwalk, CT: Appleton & Lange.

Roy, C. (1990). Nursing care in theory and practice: Early interventions in brain injury. In R. Harris, R. Burns, & R. Rees (Eds.), *Recovery from brain injury* (pp. 95-110). Adelaide, So. Australia: Flinders University, Institute for Learning Difficulties.

Roy, C. (1991). Structure of knowledge: Paradigm, model and research specifications for differentiated practice. In American Academy of Nursing Proceedings of eighteenth annual meeting. *Differentiating nursing practice into the twenty-first century* (pp. 31-40). Kansas City, MO: American Academy of Nursing.

Roy, C. (1992). Vigor, variables, and vision: Commentary on Florence Nightingale. In F. Nightingale, *Notes on nursing: What it is and what it is not* (Commemorative Ed., pp. 63-71). Philadelphia: Lippincott.

Roy, C. (1997a).Overview of the Roy Adaptation Model (RAM) and The Integrated Review Project. Paper presentation at *Roy Adaptation Model: 25 years of Research*. Conference at Gainesville, GA: Brenau University Department of Nursing.

Roy, C. (1997b). Future of the Roy Model: Challenge to redefine adaptation. *Nursing Science Quarterly, 10*, 42-48.

Roy, C. (1997c). Knowledge as universal cosmic imperative. In D. Jones & C. Roy (Eds.), Proceedings of Knowledge Impact Conference 1996-*Developing Knowledge for Nursing Practice: Three Philosophical Modes for Linking Theory and Practice* (pp. 95-117). Chestnut Hill, MA: Boston College.

Roy, C. , & Andrews, H. (1991). *The Roy Adaptation Model: The definitive statement.* E. Norwalk, CT: Appleton & Lange.

Roy, C., & Andrews, H. (1999). *The Roy Adaptation Model* (2nd ed.). Stamford, CT: Appleton & Lange.

Roy, C., & Anway, J. (1989). Roy's adaptation model: Theories and propositions for administration. In B. Henry, C. Arndt, M. DiVicenti, & G. Marriner-Toomy (Eds.), *Dimensions and issues in nursing administration* (pp. 75-88). St. Louis, MO: Mosby.

Roy , C., & Barone, S. (1996). The Roy Adaptation Model in research: Rehabilitation nursing. In P. Walker & B. Neuman, *Blueprint for use of nursing models: Education, research, practice, and administration* (pp. 64-87). NY: National League for Nursing.

Roy, C., & Corliss, C. (1993). The Roy Adaptation Model: Theoretical update and knowledge for practice. In M. Parker (Ed.), *Patterns of nursing theories in practice* (pp. 215-229). NY: National League for Nursing.

Roy, C., & Roberts, S. (1981). *Theory construction in nursing: An adaptation model.* Englewood Cliffs, NJ: Prentice Hall.

Woods, N., & Catanzaro, M. (1988). *Nursing research: Theory and practice.* St. Louis: Mosby.

Chapter 2

Methods for Critical Analysis and Synthesis of Research Based on the Roy Adaptation Model

In this chapter, we describe methods used to design and implement a project for reviewing research based on the Roy Adaptation Model (RAM) from 1970 through 1994. The purposes of the research review were to develop (a) strategies to identify and organize research based on the RAM; (b) guidelines for description and critical analyses of the studies; (c) processes to evaluate the relationship of the research to the RAM; and (d) approaches for synthesis of knowledge from the model-based research and contributions to nursing science.

The literature on integrated research reviews provided guidance for the methods of this project. However, the unique focus of the review, nursing model-based studies, required a derivation of specific methods. Literature from nursing and other fields that described methods relevant to the project was reviewed. Methods appropriate for this research review were developed considering those methods. The research review was conducted by eight investigators including the theorist–referred to collectively as the Boston Based Adaptation Research in Nursing Society (BBARNS).

Review of Literature

The use of integrated research reviews has been described in the education and social science literature as a strategy for knowledge development. Further insights into this approach were gained from discussions about application of this strategy in nursing research. A third segment of literature relevant to the methods of this project was the literature on model-based research in nursing.

Integrative Research Reviews in Education and Social Science

Seminal work in methods for integrative reviews of research was contributed by Jackson (1980) and Cooper (1982, 1989). Jackson was a pioneer in describing integrated research reviews that were published in the education literature. He emphasized inferring generalizations about substantive issues from a set of studies that had direct bearing on a single topic. Jackson identified a systematic procedure of six tasks for conducting an integrative review. The tasks included selecting the questions or hypotheses, sampling, representing characteristics of the primary studies, analyzing the primary studies, interpreting the results, and reporting the review.

Cooper (1982, 1989) focused on developing an operational process for Jackson's six tasks for integrated reviews of research. The process was explicated as five steps or stages: (a) problem formulation, (b) data collection, (c) data evaluation, (d) analysis and interpretation, and (e) presentation of results. Recognizing the increasing role of research reviews in developing knowledge, Cooper aimed to standardize the process and make it more rigorous. He expanded the scientific guidelines for evaluating integrative reviews and identified methodological choices at each stage of the process that represented threats to the validity of the review.

Applications of Integrative Reviews in the Nursing Literature

Ganong (1987) analyzed 17 integrative reviews from the nursing research literature from 1979 through 1983. He pointed out that most reviews demonstrated little adherence to the guidelines published by Jackson (1980) and Cooper (1982, 1989). Ganong's review began 1 year after Jackson's publication and ended 1 year after Cooper's (1982) first publication. Usual lag time may account for Ganong's observation that these guidelines were not used in the integrated reviews studied.

However, Ganong's evaluation of the early research reviews was useful in improving the quality of research reported. For example, a particular deficiency of the reviews Ganong analyzed was lack of information about the findings concerning the hypothesized direction and magnitude of the results. A further contribution was that Ganong recommended extensive use of tables because of the complex nature of the data to be reported.

A noteworthy application of the methods of integrated research reviews in nursing was the initiation of the *Annual Review of Nursing Research* (Werley & Fitzpatrick, 1983). The editors recommended that contributing authors use Cooper's (1982) process for conducting integrated reviews. To date, 16 volumes of the annual review have been published, each containing approximately 10 reviews of research in such areas as nursing practice, health care delivery, and international nursing inquiry. Although the volumes have made a significant contribution to organizing knowledge from the nursing research literature, the quality of the integrated research reviews varies throughout each volume. A formal evaluation of the project was not found in the literature.

Nursing scholars have contributed to the methods of integrated reviews by their writings on meta-analysis. Smith and Stullenbarger (1991) recommended research synthesis, reporting it was an increasingly common way to manage large bodies of information within disciplines. They presented an adaptation of Cooper's (1989) integrative research review and of Hedges and Olkin's (1985) work in meta-analysis. Their prototype is particularly useful because they derived substantive study characteristics from the nursing literature.

For example, research was analyzed according to human responses, self-care requisites, nursing situation, and nursing orientation—categories identified by the American Nurses Association Social Policy Statement (1980). In addition, Smith and Stullenbarger provided an inclusive master coding form. They listed methodologic characteristics, substantive characteristics, and quality-of-instrument elements in a format appropriate for a computer software program.

Brown (1991) highlighted the importance of meta-analysis for building a body of knowledge applicable to clinical practice. She noted that, whereas the quality of meta-analysis had improved, persistent issues, which had been identified by Cooper (1989), were the quality of the original studies and their integration into findings. Brown reviewed the issue of research quality and of effects on research outcomes and then proposed a method for measuring quality specifically for meta-analysis. She provided a research quality scoring method that allocated points for various aspects of research studies. Brown also correctly noted that no perfect studies of the complexities of human behavior in natural environments exist. She recommended continued work on methods to assess the quality of primary studies that are included in meta-analysis.

Review of Nursing Model-Based Research

Nurse authors, both metatheorists and research methodologists, argue strongly for model-based nursing research (Burns & Grove, 1997; Fawcett & Downs,1992; Moody, 1990; Polit & Hungler, 1994; Woods & Catanzaro, 1988). Reviews of nursing research literature have revealed increased use of concepts from nursing models and theories as a basis for asking significant research questions (Louis, 1995). Model-based research studies often are reported as single published articles. However, publications of multiple studies with one nursing model are very limited. Most reports of multiple studies based on a given nursing model have been presented at professional conferences (Leininger, 1981, 1984) or selected by editors for publication (Barrett, 1990; Malinski, 1986). More recently, one general survey of research on the Neuman model was published (Louis, 1995). Louis used two computerized data bases and Dr. Neuman's personal contact list to identify nearly 100 studies for which the Neuman Systems Model served as the organizing framework.

The previous report of Neuman model-based research, as well as other individual and multiple model-based research reports, were beneficial in identifying and conducting an initial assessment of research based on a given model. However, no model-based research reports reviewed, in primary or secondary sources (Fawcett, 1993, 1995; Marriner-Tomey & Aligood, 1999), used the process of an integrated research review. A paper analyzing studies based on Orem's work was listed in proceedings of the

Workgroup of European Nurse Researchers Conference (Mieke, 1992), but the study has not been available for assessment.

A complete review of research based on a given nursing model has not been reported. The members of BBARNS believe that the project presented in this monograph is the first to use a systematic methodology for the purpose of inferring generalizations from all reported research based on one conceptual model of nursing.

Processes for Identifying and Organizing Roy Model-Based Research

Criteria were established for inclusion of research to be reviewed. Strategies were developed to identify research meeting the inclusion criteria. Research was organized and assigned to various categories based on the RAM. Modifications of methods were made in keeping with the fact that all of the studies were based on one nursing model, rather than having a common subject matter. The development and use of these strategies is summarized in the following sections.

Criteria for Inclusion of Research

Three criteria for inclusion of studies were established by consensus of the BBARNS members. The first criterion was that the empiric work explicitly identify the RAM as the conceptual underpinning of the research project. The second was that the work be a primary research report. The third was that the research report be a journal publication, thesis, or dissertation.

The rationale for including theses and dissertations was that the model-based review of identified research over time had to be inclusive. Further, given the educational intent of dissertations and theses, they were more likely to include explicit information regarding conceptual frameworks.

Strategies for Identification of Research

A literature search was conducted to identify research publications where the RAM was used as the conceptual foundation of the work. A comprehensive computerized search was conducted for all publications from January, 1970 through December, 1994, and included the following eight data bases: Cancer, Cumulative Index of Nursing and Allied Health Literature (Cinahl), Dissertation Abstracts International (DAI), Educational Resources Index Citations (ERIC), Health Planning, Medline, Psychological Abstracts (Psyc Lit), and Social Science Citation Index (SSCI). The key words used to access the publications were research and adaptation, Roy Adaptation Theory, Adaptation Model, and Roy. In addition to the computerized search, studies were identified from the personal communication files of the BBARNS members.

Although members of BBARNS used every means available to make the review as complete as possible, several limitations were recognized. First, only literature in the English language was reviewed. Second, the citation indices were accepted as the best available approach to identify research reports, but their constraints were recognized. For example, nursing models were not referenced in citations of earlier years. Dissertation Abstracts International (DAI) receives entries from individual students and from institutions on a voluntary basis. In addition, abstracts from European institutions were not included in DAI until 1976. Based on these constraints, the investigators recognized that an unknown number of studies based on the RAM were not identified and, therefore, were not included in the review.

Organization of Research for Review

The studies identified from the literature searches were organized by substantive content of the model. Seven of the major concepts from the model were used for organization of the research, including the four adaptive modes, stimuli, intervention, and adaptive processes. Definitions and descriptions of the seven concepts by Roy and Andrews (1991) were used to aid in assigning the studies to content areas.

Studies were organized according to the various content areas by agreement of two of the BBARNS members. Each member evaluated the studies in one content area using the criteria for inclusion and the appropriate definition and description. All members then met to review, clarify, and make any required changes in the organization of studies. At that time, three studies did not meet the criteria for inclusion and were deleted. The preceding process was related to the first rule for conceptual model-based research, that is, identification of the phenomena to be studied (Fawcett, 1995). The initial organization of research facilitated the description, analysis, and evaluation of all reported research using the RAM. In addition, the work provided the basis for developing criteria for assignment of studies to chapters in this monograph.

Processes for Developing Guidelines for Description and Critical Analysis

Criteria for description and critical analysis of research based on the RAM were developed by the BBARNS members. It was necessary to present a brief description and analysis of the studies before evaluating the relationships of the studies to the model and synthesizing contributions to nursing science from the findings of research based on the RAM. In particular, the research needed to meet established scientific criteria for findings to be considered meaningful.

Description of reported research

Categories used for description of the research were based on those frequently used for integrative reviews (Cooper, 1989; Ganong, 1987). The categories were: author(s) and date, purpose, sample, design, and findings. Numbering of studies on the description tables was used throughout each chapter for identification in subsequent sections.

Studies were described as using a quantitative design, a qualitative design or, in the case of instrument development, a methodological design. When a researcher used more than one design, the primary focus of the study was used for descriptive purposes. The design typology used to describe the studies included the following categories for quantitative research: descriptive, correlational, quasi-experimental, and experimental. The categories used for describing qualitative research designs included: descriptive, historical, ethnographic, phenomenological, grounded theory, or case study.

Categories for description of studies were first used on a subset of studies from each content area. Results of the preliminary work supported the usefulness of the categories. There was 100% agreement among the BBARNS members that the categories were appropriate for all content areas and would provide an adequate summary of the research for the project.

Critical analysis of reported research

Similar to the derived method of description for each study, specific guidelines for a common critical analysis of the studies were developed. Critical analysis was the process by which the reviewer made inferences from the selected studies. The analytical task examined methodologic strengths and weaknesses of the research. A number of outlines for evaluating the methods, data analysis, and results of research studies (Brown, 1991; Smith & Stullenbarger, 1991) were consulted to develop the guidelines for this project.

All members of BBARNS were involved in developing guidelines for critical analysis. Five major categories were selected for use in the guidelines: (a) internal validity, (b) external validity, (c) measurement, (d) data analysis, and (e) interpretation of results. The categories were considered relevant for use in critical analysis of research reports (Burns & Grove, 1997). Tables were constructed to display the results of the critical analysis of studies assigned to all content areas for consistency of reporting throughout the chapters.

The categories were further clarified and criteria for evaluation of each were identified. Criteria for validity focused on efforts to control for threats to internal and external validity. Internal validity criteria related to history, maturation, instrumentation, mortality, and sample. External validity criteria addressed attempts to control the environment, representativeness of subjects, consistency of treatment, control of measurement, and control of extraneous variables. The method of summating the evaluation based on five criteria was similar to scoring used by Beck (1995). Basically, the method used for evaluating both internal and external validity was "Yes" if there were three or more "Yesses" for the criteria, "Partial" if there were three or more "Partials," and "No" if there were two or more "Nos."

Measurement concerns included addressing the reliability and validity of instruments used in the research. Data analysis was evaluated for its appropriateness to the design and purposes of the research. Interpretation of the results was analyzed on the basis of consistency of the conclusions with the findings.

Criteria used for critical analysis of all quantitative studies were essentially the same, except when an experimental or quasi-experimental design was used. In those cases, stricter criteria were used for evaluating efforts to exercise control for threats to internal and external validity. The criteria emphasized the need to rule out other factors or threats as rival explanations for the relationships among the variables. For external validity, the effects of subject selection, reactive effects, and effects of testing also were considered.

The guidelines for critical analysis of quantitative research were used by four of the BBARNS members in a pilot group of 21 studies that focused on the physiological mode. Based on the established criteria, 210 judgments were chosen for internal and external validity of the 21 studies. In all but six cases, the four judges independently agreed on the ratings. The criteria were then discussed among the judges until 100% agreement was reached. Use of interrater reliability to validate conclusions was used throughout the research project.

Using the same process, the BBARNS team identified categories for critical analysis of qualitative research. A rating similar to the one used for quantitative studies was modified for internal and external validity of qualitative studies. Characteristics of validity included descriptive vividness, methodologic congruence, analytic preciseness, theoretic connectedness, and heuristic relevance (Burns & Grove, 1997). Criteria related to reliability of qualitative research included research position, participant selection, contextual conditions, and procedural stages (Woods & Catanzaro, 1988). The last two categories were data analysis and interpretation of the findings and guidelines were the same as used for studies with quantitative designs.

Studies that focused on development of instruments to measure components of the RAM were also evaluated in the appropriate content chapter. Guidelines were used to summarize reported reliability and validity of the instruments. The following were used to evaluate reliability: stability, such as test-retest; equivalence, such as alternate or parallel forms and inter-rater reliability; homogeneity, such as split-half reliability; internal consistency, including Cronbach's alpha, Kruder-Richardson, and Cohen's Kappa statistic. Validity measures used included content-related validity such as the literature, adequacy and representativeness of sample, and use of content experts; factor analysis; contrasting groups; convergent validity; divergent validity; discriminate analysis; predictive validity; and concurrent validity. Finally studies were evaluated for whether data analyses were appropriate and whether findings were consistent with conclusions.

BBARNS members developed guidelines for critical analysis in order to provide a summary of the strengths and limitations of the reported research. Criteria were modified for quantitative and qualitative studies and for studies about development of instruments. A scoring system was adopted to provide a summated rating of criteria used for internal and external validity. The BBARNS members were mindful that, although evaluation of the research quality was a necessary beginning, it was only the first of three stages. Use of the criteria for critical analysis was intended to screen for the scientific merit of the studies. It is hoped that the evaluation will prove useful to those interested in pursuing a more in-depth review of research based on the RAM.

Processes Used to Evaluate the Relationship of Research to the RAM

Criteria for evaluation of relationships between research and the Roy Adaptation Model were focused on linkages of the research to the model and on propositions derived from the model.

Evaluation of Linkages to the RAM

In this critical review of research, specific linkages based on the use of the RAM were the additional substantive study characteristics that needed to be examined (Smith & Stullenbarger, 1991). Linkages discussed frequently in the nursing literature (Fawcett, 1993; Moody, 1990) were used to construct tables for evaluation of linkages of the research to the model. The linkages between the concepts of the RAM and research variables, between the model and the empiric measures, and between the findings and the model were evaluated as either explicit, implied, or absent. To be included in the synthesis, linkages between the RAM and the variables and empiric measures had to be explicit or implicit. Studies were not, however, excluded if findings were not linked back to the RAM.

Use of these ratings was reviewed by all BBARNS members. Each member conducted a pilot study with a subset of studies (n=10). Interrater reliabilities ranged from 90% to 100% agreement for all pilot work. The only point of disagreement was determining whether a linkage was implicit rather than absent. Based on these results, the criteria were determined to be useful and comprehensive, and therefore served as the basis for evaluating the relationship of all studies to the model. The BBARNS members further agreed to continue use of an external reviewer when needed to verify conclusions.

Testing of Propositions from the RAM

Testing of propositions derived from the RAM reflects the empiric adequacy of theories derived from the model. The logic of scientific inference is: if the empiric data conform to the hypothesized expectations, there is additional support for the credibility of the model propositions. Conversely, lack of support for the propositions would be an appropriate conclusion when the empiric data does not conform to the hypothesized expectations (Fawcett & Downs, 1992). Furthermore, Walker and Avant (1995) describe the relationship between and among levels of theory development that is useful in describing linkages among levels of propositions derived from the RAM. The generic propositions guide the derivation of ancillary propositions which direct practice-level propositions. Practice-level propositions in turn provide evidence for ancillary propositions that refine generic propositions.

The process of testing propositions from the model was a major step in the synthesis of the knowledge from the research based on the RAM. Twelve propositions derived from the nursing model (Roy & Andrews, 1991; Roy & Roberts, 1981) were selected by the research team as relevant for all studies in all content areas (Table 2.1). Studies used to test the propositions had met the criteria for critical analysis, and had been evaluated as having explicit or implicit linkages to the RAM.

For all studies in each content area, tables were constructed listing the 12 propositions derived from the model. Findings from each set of studies that tested a given proposition were evaluated consistently. For findings of a study related to a given proposition, the ancillary and practice-level propositions were described, then a judgment was made as to whether the findings were supportive or not supportive of the propositions. Results of that process were integrated to derive contributions to nursing science from RAM research. The results of testing the propositions of the model also were used to identify directions for theory and model development.

Approaches for Synthesis of Knowledge and Contributions to Nursing Science

Methods developed for the research project concluded with identification of the contributions to nursing science. Support for the propositions

Figures 2.1 – Linkages among levels of proposition derived from the RAM

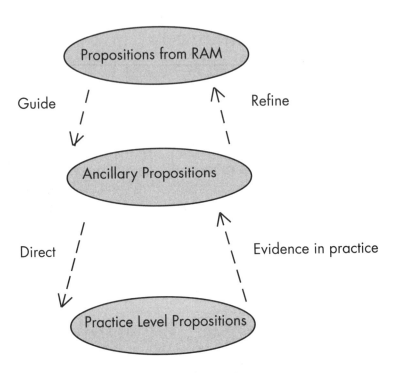

from the conceptual model were integrated to derive applications for nursing practice. Meleis (1995) discusses theory support as an alternative to theory testing. Contributions to nursing science were viewed in this broader sense of applications to practice and theory support.

Applications to Nursing Practice

Each set of studies was summarized according to the strengths and weaknesses of the design and methods, relationships to the RAM, and support for the propositions derived from the model, as they applied to practice. Clinical applications were derived from testing of the concepts and their relationships to the RAM (Pollock, Frederickson, Carson, Massey, & Roy, 1994). Applications to nursing practice then were evaluated as having high potential for implementation (category one), needing further clinical evaluation before implementation (category two), or warranting further research before implementation (category three).

Recommendations for Model-Based Research

Recommendations for RAM based research were made from the studies reviewed, but were most obvious in category three, where further testing was indicated. A rationale was provided for future work, including emphasis on measurement of the model, adaptation for use with various populations, and intervention studies that focused on client outcomes.

Directions for Theory and RAM Development

Directions for theory and model development were identified from the research project. For example, theoretical statements need to be developed that clarify relationships among the model concepts in order for hypotheses to be generated that can be tested. Relationships that need futher development include: adaptive processes related to modes; interactions between the regulator and cognator subsystems; the pooled effect of focal, contextual, and residual stimuli on adaptation level; the effect of time and perception on adaptation; management of input to adaptive systems both at the individual and group levels. The proposed work will refine the knowledge needed for nursing actions and support the efficacy of the RAM in guiding clinical practice.

Results of Selection and Evaluation of RAM Research

Results of the identification, selection, and organization of research based on the RAM are presented here.

Description of Sample

The period studied was 25 years from inception of the model (1970) through completion of the review (1994). Sources of research included journal articles, dissertations, and theses.

Number of studies identified. The initial list of publications retrieved from the computerized literature searches included 434 titles related to the RAM. Duplicate entries and papers not empirically based were eliminated by a hand search. From this list, 189 research reports were retrieved. After review by members of BBARNS, the final sample was 163 publications—87 research articles, 51 dissertations, and 25 theses.

Publications reviewed spanned a 25 year period with a marked annual increase in the number of reports noted over time (see Figure 2.2). The first publication on the RAM was in 1970 by Sr. Callista Roy, and in the 4-year time block, 1975 through 1978, the number of research-based publications was 11. Progressive increases were noted in each time block, and in the most recent 4 years, 1991 through 1994, 112 publications were identified.

Types of journals identified. The sample of RAM-based research reports appeared in 44 journals plus *Dissertation Abstracts International* and *Masters Abstracts International*. An alphabetical list of the journals is shown in Table 2.2.

Table 2.1 – Propositions Derived from the RAM

1. At the individual level, regulator and cognator processes affect innate and acquired ways of adapting.
2. At the group level, stabilizer and innovator processes affect adaptation.
3. The characteristics of the internal and external stimuli influence adaptive responses.
4. The characteristics of the internal and external stimuli influence the adequacy of cognitive and emotional processes.
5. The adequacy of cognator and regulator processes will affect adaptive responses.
6. Adaptation in one mode is affected by adaptation in other modes through the cognator and regulator as connectives.
7. The pooled effect of focal, contextual, and residual stimuli determines the adaptation level.
8. Adaptation is influenced by the integration of the person with the environment.
9. The variable of time influences the process of adaptation.
10. The variable of perception influences the process of adaptation.
11. Perception influences adaptation through linking the regulator and cognator subsystems.
12. Nursing assessment and interventions relate to identifying and managing input to adaptive systems.

The types of journals were identified based on descriptions by Swanson, McCloskey, and Bodensteiner (1991). First, general types of journals were identified; then within the category of specialty practice, specific areas of practice were designated. In some cases, categories used by Swanson and colleagues were combined for presentation due to the small number of studies in a given category. Based on the sample obtained, two categories were added; journals published outside of the United States and state professional publications.

Of the 86 research articles, those in specialty journals had the highest representation (59%). Research journals were next—16% of the total. Eleven percent of the articles were in journals published outside the United States. See Figure 2.3.

The category of specialty practice journals was then further divided into categories that best represented the RAM studies reported (see Figure 2.4). The highest percentage of specialty journal articles was identified in maternal and child health and women's health journals (44%). Critical care and oncology journals accounted for 15% and 11% of the articles, respectively. The category of "other" included neuroscience, rehabilitation, orthopedic, and mental health publications.

Figure 2.2 – Number of Research Publications Based on the RAM by Years

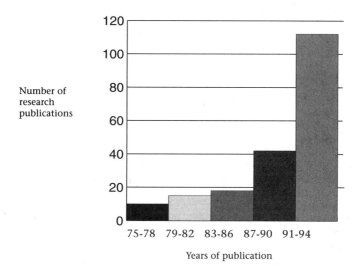

Number of research publications

Years of publication

Table 2.2 – Journals with Reports of Research Based on the RAM 1970-1994 (*N*=44)

Adolescence
American Association of Occupational
    Health Nurses Journal
Association Journal of Critical Care
Canadian Journal of Nursing Administration
Cancer Nursing
Cardiovascular Nursing
Critical Care Nursing Quarterly
Curationis: South African Journal of Nursing
Geriatric Nursing
Heart & Lung
Home Health Care Nursing
Image: Journal of Nursing Scholarship
International Journal of Nursing Studies
Issues in Comprehensive Pediatric Nursing
Issues in Mental Health Nursing
Journal of Advanced Nursing
Journal of Cardiovascular Nursing
Journal of Obstetric, Gynecologic &
    Neonatal Nursing (JOGNN)
Journal of Neuroscience Nursing
Journal of Nursing Midwifery
Journal of Pediatric Nursing

Journal of Pediatric Oncology
Journal of Post Anesthesia Nursing
Journal of Psychosocial Nursing
Journal of the New York State
    Nurses Association
Maternal Child Nursing Journal
Neonatal Network
Nursing Management
Nursing Research
Nursing Science Quarterly
Nursing Standard
Oncology Nursing Forum
Orthopaedic Nursing
Patient Education and Counseling
Psychology & Aging
Public Health Nursing
Rehabilitation Nursing
Research in Nursing and Health
Scholarly Inquiry for Nursing
    Practice
Virginia Nurse
Western Journal of Nursing Research

Figure 2.3 – Percentage of RAM-based Research Articles by Type of Journal

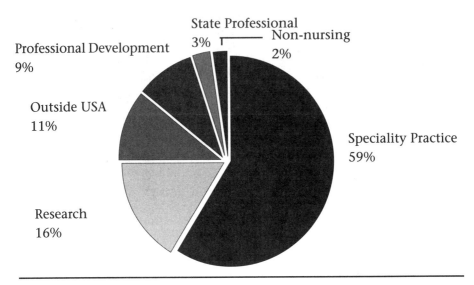

Research based on the RAM during the 25 year time period also was identified in *Dissertation Abstracts International* and *Masters Abstracts International*. The 25 theses and 51 dissertations were from a total of 35 colleges and universities. An alphabetical list of schools with dissertations or theses based on the RAM is shown in Table 2.3.

Assignment of Studies to Chapters

Definitions of model concepts were used to assign the 163 studies to seven content chapters. Based on the initial work to organize the research, BBARNS members clarified and approved the Criteria for Assignment of Research Studies to Content Chapters (see Table 2.4). Six criteria were approved by the members of BBARNS. At that time, 11 publications were reassigned to different content areas. The reassignments were accounted for mainly by a clarification in one criterion. The third criterion stated, if investigators studied two or more of the following areas: adaptive modes, regulator and cognator, the study would be assigned to the chapter on the adaptation modes and processes. Clarification of the criterion made possible mutually exclusive assignments, whereas in the first sort some research reports had been cross-referenced to more than one chapter. Final inclusion of studies for review and assignment of studies to content areas were made based on consensus among all members of BBARNS.

Figure 2.4 – Percentage of RAM-based Research Articles in Specialty Practice Journals

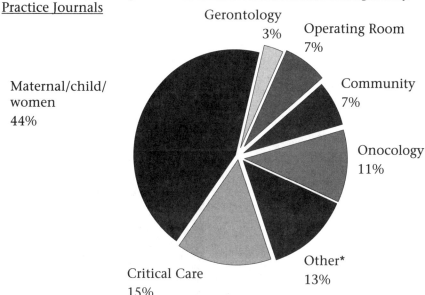

Gerontology 3%

Operating Room 7%

Maternal/child/women 44%

Community 7%

Onocology 11%

Critical Care 15%

Other* 13%

*Other includes neuroscience, rehabilitation, orthopedic, and mental health publications.

Table 2.3 – Sources of Dissertations or Theses Based on RAM (N=34)

Doctoral Dissertations:

Boston College, Massachusetts
Boston University, Massachusetts
Catholic University of America, District of Columbia
Columbia University Teachers College, New York
Temple University, Philadelphia
Texas Woman's University, Denton
University of Alberta, Canada
University of Alabama, Birmingham
University of Florida, Gainesville
University of Georgia
University of Illinois at Chicago, Health Sciences Center
University of Pennsylvania, Philadelphia
University of Rochester, New York
University of San Diego, California
University of South Carolina, Columbia
University of Tennessee, Knoxville
University of Texas at Austin
Wayne State University, Michigan

Master's Theses:

Bellarmine College, Louisville, Kentucky
California State University, Los Angeles
D'Youville College, Buffalo, New York
Florida State University, Tallahassee
Grand Valley State University, Allendale, Michigan
Madonna College, Livonia, Michigan
Michigan State University, East Lansing
San Diego State University, California
San Jose State University, California
Southern Connecticut State University, New Haven
Temple University, Philadelphia
Texas Woman's University, Denton
University of Arizona, Tucson
University of Hawaii, Honolulu
University of Lowell, Massachusetts
University of Nevada, Reno

The BBARNS members acknowledge inherent limitations in the methods used to organize the reported research and, therefore, to the assignment of studies to individual chapters. For example, although researchers examined adaptation in more than one mode, in many cases the study was assigned to the primary area of focus.

Conclusion

The methods described were developed and tested over 2 years by members of BBARNS. During this time the members met as a whole eight times at various locations throughout the United States. Smaller groups convened when necessary to clarify and revise. The results of that work are presented in the remaining chapters.

Table 2.4 – Criteria for Assignment of Research Studies to Content Chapters

1. Verify that author of study stated that the research was based on the Roy Adaptation Model.
2. Research assigned to area of primary focus of adaptation based on descriptions of key concepts. According to the descriptions, studies that focused on parenting were assigned to role function adaptive mode, and studies that focused on social support or caregiver were assigned to interdependence adaptive mode.
3. If the study involved two or more of the following areas: adaptive modes, regulator and cognator, the study was assigned to Chapter 7, Adaptive Modes and Processes.
4. Instrument development articles were assigned to chapter of primary focus such as a specific mode or stimuli.
5. If the research focused primarily on the effects of focal stimuli, contextual stimuli, or adaptation level, the study was assigned to Chapter 8, Studies Focusing on Stimuli.
6. Experimental and quasi-experimental studies that focused on the effects of interventions on adaptation in one or more modes were assigned to Chapter 9, Intervention Research.

References

American Nurses Association. (1980). *Nursing: A social policy statement.* Kansas City, MO: Author.

Barrett, E.A.M. (1990). *Visions of Rogers' science based nursing education.* New York: National League for Nursing.

Beck, C.T. (1995). The effects of postpartum depression on maternal-infant interaction: A meta-analysis. *Nursing Research, 44,* 298-304.

Brown, S.A. (1991). Measurement of quality of primary studies for meta-analysis. *Nursing Research, 40,* 352-355.

Burns, N., & Grove, S.K. (1997). *The practice of Nursing Research: Conduct, critique and utilization* (3rd ed.). Philadelphia: W. B. Saunders.

Cooper, H.M. (1982). Scientific guidelines for conducting integrative research review. *Review of Educational Research, 52,* 291-302.

Cooper, H.M. (1989). *Integrating research: A guide for literature reviews* (2nd ed.). Newbury Park, CA: Sage Publication.

Fawcett, J. (1993). *Analysis and evaluation of nursing theories.* Philadelphia: F. A. Davis.

Fawcett, J. (1995). *Analysis and evaluation of conceptual models of nursing* (3rd ed.). Philadelphia: F. A. Davis.

Fawcett, J., & Downs, F.S. (1992). *The relationship of theory and research* (2nd ed.). Philadelphia: F. A. Davis.

Ganong, L.H. (1987). Integrative reviews of Nursing Research. *Research in Nursing and Health, 10,* 1-11.

Hedges, L.V., & Olkin I. (1985). *Statistical methods for meta-analysis.* Orlando, FL: Academic Press.

Jackson, G.B. (1980). Methods for integrative reviews. *Review of Educational Research, 50,* 438-460.

Leininger, M. (1981). *Caring: An essential human need.* Thorofare, NJ: Charles B. Slack, Inc.

Leininger, M. (1984). *Care: The essence of nursing and health.* Thorofare, NJ: Charles B. Slack, Inc.

Louis, M. (1995). The Neuman Model in nursing research: An update. In B. Neuman (Ed.), *The Neuman Systems Model* (3rd ed., pp. 473-480). Norwalk, CT: Appleton & Lange.

Malinski, V.M. (1986). *Explorations on Martha Rogers' Science of Unitary Human Beings.* New York: Appleton-Century-Crofts.

Marriner-Tomey, A. (1994). *Nursing theorists and their work* (3rd ed.). St. Louis: Mosby.

Meleis, A.I. (1995). Theory testing and theory support. In B. Neuman (Ed.), *The Neuman Systems Model* (3rd ed., pp. 447-457). Norwalk, CT: Appleton & Lange.

Mieke, G. (1992, June). Critique of theory: Review of research based on the Orem Model. Paper presented at the Workgroup of European Nurse Researchers. Madrid, Spain.

Moody, L. (1990). *Advancing nursing science through research.* (Vol. 1). Newbury Park, CA: Sage.

Neuman, B. (1995). *The Neuman Systems Model* (3rd ed.). Norwalk, CT: Appleton & Lange.

Polit, D.F., & Hungler, B.P. (1994). *Nursing Research: Principles and methods* (5th ed.). Philadelphia: J. B. Lippincott.

Pollock, S.E., Frederickson, K., Carson, M.A., Massey, V.H., & Roy, C. (1994). Contributions to nursing science: Synthesis of findings from Adaptation Model Research. *Scholarly Inquiry for Nursing Practice, 8*(4), 361-372.

Roy, C. (1970). Adaptation: A conceptual framework in nursing. *Nursing Outlook, 18* (5), 42-45.

Roy C., & Andrews, H. (1991). *The Roy adaptation model: The definitive statement.* Norwalk, CT: Appleton & Lange.

Roy, C., & Roberts, S., (1981). *Theory construction in nursing: An adaptation model.* Englewood Cliffs, NJ: Prentice Hall.

Smith, M.C., & Stullenbarger, E. (1991). A prototype for integrative review and meta-analysis of nursing research. *Journal of Advanced Nursing, 16,* 1272-1283.

Swanson, E.A., McCloskey, J.C., & Bodensteiner, A. (1991). Publishing opportunities for nurses: A comparison of 92 U. S. journals. *Image: Journal of Nursing Scholarship, 23,* 33-38.

Walker, L., & Avant, K. (1995). *Strategies for theory construction in nursing.* Norwalk, CT: Appleton & Lange.

Werley, H.H., & Fitzpatrick, J.J. (Eds.). (1983). *Annual review of nursing research.* (Vol. 1). New York: Springer.

Woods, N., & Catanzaro, M. (1988). *Nursing Research: Theory and Practice.* St. Louis: Mosby.

Chapter 3

Physiologic Mode Research

In this chapter, we include research reported from 1970 through 1994 which focused primarily on the physiologic adaptive mode of the Roy Adaptation Model (RAM). Twenty-one studies based on the RAM, including dissertations and theses, were categorized as physiologic mode research. Studies of the physiologic mode in which either an experimental or quasi-experimental design was used are included in Chapter 9, while studies that investigated adaptation in more than one mode are included in Chapter 7.

Purposes

The purposes of this chapter are to (a) critically analyze research in the physiologic adaptive mode, (b) evaluate the relationship of physiologic mode research to the RAM, and (c) synthesize contributions of reported studies to nursing science. Contributions to nursing science include applications for nursing practice, recommendations for model-based physiologic research, and directions for further theory and RAM development of the physiologic mode.

Background

Physiologic adaptation refers to the way a person responds physically to stimuli from the environment. Behavior in this mode is manifested in physiologic activity of the human body (Roy & Andrews, 1991). The person is viewed holistically with stimuli affecting each mode, and each mode affecting other modes. Coping mechanisms associated with physiologic function act primarily through the regulator subsystem. Knowledge of the components of physiologic adaptation is found primarily in the basic life sciences such as anatomy, physiology, pathophysiology, physics, and chemistry. The basic need underlying the mode is physiologic integrity.

The physiologic mode of the RAM includes five basic needs—oxygenation, nutrition, elimination, activity and rest, and protection; and four complex associated processes—sensory function, fluid and electrolyte balance, neurologic function, and endocrine function. These needs and processes promote physiologic integrity of the body. Integrity has been defined as the degree of wholeness achieved by adapting to changes in needs, in this case the body's physiologic needs (Roy, 1976). The term components refers to these nine areas of the physiologic mode. Physiologic adaptation, as part of the whole person, is also influenced by processes conceptually based in psychology, sociology, anthropology, and the humanities.

The theoretic background for the physiologic mode applies propositions from the regulator subsystem to each of the physiologic components of the RAM. The physiologic adaptive mode, therefore, refers to adaptive and ineffective regulatory responses related to the needs and associated processes of the nine content components of the mode. (See Chapter 1 for explanation of adaptive and ineffective regulatory responses.)

Critical Analysis of Physiologic Mode Research

Critical analysis includes a brief description of reported research according to components of the physiologic mode, followed by evaluation of all studies based on established guidelines developed for the project. The criteria and the processes used for critical analysis and synthesis of the studies are explained in Chapter 2.

Description of Reported Research

In 21 studies, researchers investigated seven of the nine components of the physiologic mode of the RAM. The studies were focused on five of the body's basic needs: oxygenation ($n=4$), nutrition ($n=1$), elimination ($n=1$), protection ($n=2$), activity and rest ($n=5$); and two of the associated processes: the senses ($n=5$), and neurologic function, specifically the regulation of temperature ($n=3$). No investigator studied the processes of fluid and electrolyte balance or endocrine function.

Oxygenation studies. In the four studies in which oxygenation need was investigated (Table 3.1), researchers examined the effects of contextual stimuli on maintaining adequate arterial oxygen levels in preterm infants. Measured as specific interventions or activities managed by the nurse, contextual stimuli included the number of hand held ventilations (Cheng & Williams, 1989), parental touch (Harrison, Leeper, & Yoon, 1990), three nursing procedures (Norris, Campbell, & Brenkert, 1981), and environmental illumination (Shogan & Schumann, 1993).

Researchers for all the oxygenation studies identified focal and contextual stimuli according to the RAM, with oxygenation as the dependent variable. Significant differences were found in arterial oxygen saturation rates with hand held ventilations (Cheng & Williams, 1989) and two of the three nursing procedures (Norris et al., 1981), but not with parental touch (Harrison et al., 1990) or after decreasing illumination (Shogan & Schumann, 1993). Additionally, in two of the studies (Cheng & Williams, 1989; Norris et al., 1981), variability in oxygenation levels was found within the sample given the same stimuli.

Nutrition, elimination, and protection studies. Four studies focused on the physiologic needs of nutrition, elimination, and protection in adult

Table 3.1 – Description of Studies About Oxygenation in the Physiologic Adaptive Mode of the RAM (*N*=4)

Author(s) & Date	Purpose	Sample	Design	Findings
1.Cheng & Williams (1989)	To describe relationships between fraction of inspired transcutaneous oxygen pressure ($TcPO_2$) in VLBW infants receiving chest physiotherapy (CPT)	Intubated VLBW *N*=13)	Correlational	Hand ventilations and FiO_2 levels significantly accounted for variability in $TcPO_2$ levels during CPT.
2. Harrison, Leeper, & Yoon (1990)	To examine the effects of early parental touch on heart rates and arterial oxygen (O_2) saturation levels	Preterm infants, 27-33 wks ges. (*N*=36)	Descriptive	There were no significant differences in mean heart rates and O_2 levels across three parental touch classification periods.
3. Norris, Campbell, & Brenkert (1981)	To evaluate effects of three nursing procedures (suctioning, repositioning, performing a heel stick) on blood oxygen levels ($TcPO_2$) in premature infants	Infants<34 wks ges.,>1,900 gm. with RDS (*N*=25)	Correlational	$TcPO_2$ was decreased significantly during suctioning and repositioning but not during heel stick.
4. Shogan & Shumann (1993)	To determine relationship between immediate changes in environmental illumination and O_2 saturation	Sleeping infants, 26-37 wks ges., 2 or more days old (*N*=27)	Correlational	There were no significant differences in O_2 saturations after decreasing environmental illumination.

subjects (Table 3.2). The nutrition study identified the incidence of couvade syndrome in expectant Thai fathers (Khanobdee, Sukratanachaiyakul, & Gay, 1993), while development of a tool to assess incontinence in men after prostatectomies was the focus of the one elimination study (Joseph, 1994). Two investigators examined the process of protection: Gervasini (1994) who used profiles of trauma patients to develop a classification system to predict sepsis and nonsepsis, and Rustic (1992/1993) who explored physical symptoms of graduate students relocated to the United States.

Two or more symptoms suggestive of couvade syndrome appeared in 61% of Thai fathers (Khanobdee et al., 1993); the majority experienced symptoms in the first trimester. Of the fathers who reported symptoms, no significant differences were found between those who were "more happy" compared with those who were "more sad," nor were there any significant differences found according to number of children, family income, or educational level. The finding was consistent with studies that reported couvade syndrome in Western European and North American fathers. The presence of physiologic somatic symptoms was viewed as the fathers' attempts to adapt to the focal stimulus of their partner's pregnancy.

The Joseph Continence Assessment Tool (JCAT) was developed to holistically assess postprostatectomy patients—before any bladder behavior interventions for urinary incontinence. The assessment focused on identifying biopsychosocial factors, based on Roy's adaptive modes, that influenced the patients' return to continence. The purpose of this study was to establish content validity of the JCAT (Joseph, 1994) so the sample consisted of a panel of experts.

The JCAT consists of open-ended statements to assess one physiologic and all three psychosocial adaptive modes of the RAM. The tool has undergone many revisions in response to the need for a systematic method to evaluate these patients holistically and quickly. The study questioned whether the JCAT identified biopsychosocial factors that influenced a postprostatectomy patient's return to continence. A panel of experts established content validity and reliability and raised some theoretic and practical concerns about the JCAT (Joseph, 1994).

Gervasini (1994) asserted that adaptation of the critically ill trauma patient was evident in physiologic variables that could be used to determine the success or failure of therapies. The author generated a list of variables to develop a classification process to predict sepsis or non-sepsis in trauma patients. The predictive process succeeded in more correctly classifying non-septic than septic patients.

The types, frequency, and severity of physical symptoms reported by international graduate students were compared with nationality, length

Table 3.2 – Description of Studies About Nutrition, Elimination, and Protection in the Physiologic Adaptive Mode of the RAM (N=4)

Author(s) & Date	Purpose	Sample	Design	Findings
5. Khanodbee, Sukratanachaiyakul, & Gay (1993)	To describe the incidence of couvade syndrome in Thai fathers	Expectant Thai fathers whose partners were in 3rd trimester of pregnancy (N=172)	Descriptive	Symptoms suggestive of couvade syndrome appeared in 61% of the Thai males.
6. Joseph (1994)	To ascertain content validity of the Joseph Continence Assessment Tool (JCAT)	Panel of experts; urologic practitioners (9) and theoretical experts (9) (N=18)	Instrument development	Content validity and reliability by all experts was 77.5% (agreement on item means) and .88 (Winer's interclass correlation). Concerns of experts were theoretical and clinical application.
7. Gervasini (1994)	To generate a statistically significant list of variables that predict sepsis or non-sepsis in critically ill trauma patients	Adult trauma patients admitted to ICU (N=75)	Correlational	Classification process using predictor variables successfully classified 47.6% of septic patients and 81.5% of non-septic patients.
8. Rustic (1992/1993)	To describe common physical symptoms of international graduate students based on length of stay in the United States, nationality, and living arrangements	International graduate students at one state university (N=153)	Descriptive	Adaptation to the focal stimulus, relocation to the United States, had little effect on development of physical symptoms of the international graduate students.

Table 3.3 – Description of Studies About the Need for Activity and Rest in the Physiologic Adaptive Mode of the RAM (N=5)

Author(s) & Date	Purpose	Sample	Design	Findings
9. Huber, Medhat, & Carter (1988)	To develop a reliable and valid instrument to identify problem areas in the use of prostheses by lower extremity amputees	Content validity (N=36); Factor analysis (N=131) adults with prostheses	Instrument Development	Development of Prosthetic Problem Inventory Scale: 46 item, Likert-type scale measuring four dimensions of activity performance: activities of daily living, social participation, sexual activity and athletic participation. Reliability supported by Cronbach alpha co-efficients and construct validity supported by results of factor analyses techniques.
10. Medhat, Huber, & Medhat (1990)	To explore the differences in four dimensions of activity between adults with below-the-knee amputation with those with above-the-knee amputations	Adults with lower extremity amputation (N=131)	Descriptive	There were no significant differences in adults with below the knee amputations compared to adults with above the knee amputations on three of the four dimensions of activity, but persons with above the knee amputations had significantly more problems in the social participation dimension.

Citation	Aim/Purpose	Sample	Design	Findings
11. O'Leary (1990/1991)	To describe adaptive and ineffective behaviors of persons with Alzheimer's Disease (AD) as reported by family caregivers	Family caregivers of AD patients (N=32)	Descriptive	Family caregivers identified a variety of adaptive and ineffective behaviors related to sleep and activity. Sleep behaviors were mainly adaptive. Major adaptive activity behaviors were leisure behaviors and the major ineffective activity behaviors were physical repetitive behaviors.
12. O'Leary, Haley, & Paul (1993)	To develop a 24-Hour Behavioral Assessment Log, that could be completed by caregivers of Alzheimer's (AD) patients, to assess patients' adaptive and ineffective behaviors.	Family caregivers of AD patients (N=32)	Instrument development	Daily log provided data about common behavioral problems of AD, specifically severity and duration of problems. Results supported convergent validity of the daily log.
13. Cheng (1990/1991)	To examine the relationship between social support and adaptation to sleep	Southern Taiwanese hospitalized adults (N=61)	Descriptive	There were no significant differences in sleep characteristics in patients with supportive persons compared to patients without. Only items measuring daytime sleep were significantly different between supported and unsupported groups.

of stay in the United States, and living arrangements, using the RAM (Rustic, 1992/1993). While some significant differences existed between two physiologic symptoms and living arrangements, and between two physiologic symptoms and some nationalities, the researcher concluded that adaptation to the focal stimulus, relocation to the United States had little effect on the development of physical symptoms.

Activity and rest studies. Research related to the need for activity and rest in adults was reported in five studies. Two of these studies examined problems of activity in adults using prostheses, two focused on development and use of a behavioral log to assess the sleep and activity patterns of people with Alzheimer's Disease (AD), and one explored the effects of social support on adaptation to sleep in hospitalized adults (Table 3.3).

The differences in four dimensions of activity among people with below- or above-the-knee amputations were measured by the Prosthetic Problem Scale (Huber, Medhat, & Carter, 1988). The scale was developed to measure the interactive process between needs fulfillment and adaptation, based on Maslow's hierarchy of needs and the RAM. No significant differences were found between the two groups on three of the four dimensions of activity–activities of daily living, sexual functioning, and athletic participation. However, people with above-the-knee amputations had significantly more problems in social participation (Medhat, Huber, & Medhat, 1990).

O'Leary (1990/1991) described sleep and activity behaviors of patients with AD over a 2-day period. Both adaptive and ineffective behaviors occurred primarily during the day; the majority of adaptive behaviors focused on relaxation. The most common ineffective behaviors were physically repetitive behaviors.

Guided by the first level of assessment of the RAM, a 24-hour log was developed by O'Leary, Haley, and Paul (1993) to record sleep and activity behaviors of these patients. Behaviors recorded by family caregivers were used by researchers to determine physiologic adaptation to the focal stimulus of the disease. The authors reported that severity and duration of problems were easily identified by using the 24-hour log.

Cheng (1990/1991) viewed social support as a contextual factor promoting adaptation to sleep in hospitalized adults. Hospitalization was conceptualized as the focal stimulus. However, no significant differences were found in sleep characteristics and patterns between patients who had supportive people staying with them and those who did not.

Sensory function studies. Three studies investigated pain, an important dimension of sensory function, and two reports focused on visual impairment (Table 3.4). Calvillo (1991/1992) compared the effect of culture on postoperative pain, while Calvillo and Flaskerud (1993) examined the adequacy and scope of the RAM and the Gate Control Theory to guide

Table 3.4 – Description of Studies About Sensory Function in the Physiologic Adaptive Mode of the RAM (N=5)

Author(s) & Date	Purpose	Sample	Design	Findings
14. Calvillo (1991/1992)	(1) To describe and compare the effect of culture on postoperative experiences of Mexican-American and Anglo–American women, and, (2) To describe and compare patient and nurse perceptions of pain	Mexican-American (n=22) and Anglo-American women (n=38) who had elective cholecystectomy (n=60), nurses (n=30)	Correlational	There were no significant differences between the two ethnic patient groups on any measures of pain. However, nurses perceived patients' pain to differ by ethnicity and by social class. Nurses and patients differed in their evaluation of patients' pain in that patients assessed their pain as more severe than nurses assessed the patients' pain.
15. Calvillo & Flaskerud (1993)	To examine the adequacy and scope of the Roy Adaptation Model and Gate Control Theory to guide cross-cultural study of pain	Mexican-American (n=22) and Anglo-American women (n=38) who had elective cholecystectomy (n=60 women)	Descriptive	Operational adequacy was met in that all instruments had acceptable levels of reliability and validity, and were considered appropriate according to the Roy model. Empirical adequacy could not be established because some of the model-theory concepts could not be supported. Pragmatic adequacy was considered met and scope was considered adequate in the current stage of the model's development. *(continued)*

Table 3.4 *(continued)*

Author(s) & Date	Purpose	Sample	Design	Findings
16. Gujol (1994)	To explore the relationship between length of time after surgery and ventilator status with medication decisions made by critical care nurses	Critical care nurses (*N*=71)	Correlational	Length of time after surgery and patients' ventilator status had significant bearings on medication decisions made by critical care nurses. Nurses' concerns in giving medications included respiratory depression, addiction, tolerance, and physical dependence.
17. Kelly (1993/1994)	(1) To identify the incidence of visual impairment in the elderly; and (2) To identify consequences of decreased vision in elderly persons' daily lives	Adults, aged 60-89 (*N*=88)	Descriptive	Less than one-fifth of sample had visual acuity of 20/100 or less, majority of sample had moderate visual acuity. Also, the majority of sample reported minimal, if any, effects on daily life.
18. Zungu (1993)	To assess how visual impairment influenced the experiences of daily living of adults in a rural community in Kwazulu	Adults with visual impairment (*N*=16)	Qualitative-descriptive	Researcher described reactions to loss of vision wherein the grieving process varied among individuals. Findings reported for total sample included four major problems with mobility viewed as the most serious, four coping strategies that contributed to adjustment, and six factors that hindered their coping.

Table 3.5 – Description of Studies About Neurological Function in the Physiologic Adaptive Mode of the RAM (*N*=3)

Author(s) & Date	Purpose	Sample	Design	Findings
19. Hunter (1991)	To determine the clinically acceptable time in minutes at which axillary temperature of healthy newborn s remained stable	Healthy term newborns (*N*=40)	Descriptive	A three-minute axillary temperature is clinically appropriate length of time to measure temperatures of healthy newborns.
20. Pontious, Kennedy, Shelly, & Mittrucker (1994)	(1) To determine which of three thermometers was the most accurate and reliable in measuring children's temperature at axillary, oral, and rectal sites; and (2) To compare intra- and inter-rater reliability of temperature readings obtained by staff nurses with three levels of inservice education: none, moderate, or intensive	A random sample of 1,673 temperature readings obtained on 502 randomly selected children, aged 3 mos.-18 years, by experienced pediatric nurses with one of three levels of in-service education	Descriptive	The most clinically useful measuring instrument with children was TempaDOT. The oral site was found to be the most accurate and reliable. Inservice education level of nurses significantly affected all temperature readings obtained at any site and by any measurement.
21. Hart (1988/1989)	To describe how rural parents perceive and manage fever in their school-age children	Rural parents of well school-age children (*N*=50)	Descriptive	Misconceptions of rural parents included under-standing the course of untreated fever, harmful effects of fever, and the belief that all fevers must be treated. Mismanagement of fever included giving medications for all fevers.

cross-cultural study of pain. Through the use of vignettes, Gujol (1994) studied critical care nurses' decision making in administering pain medications. Research on visual impairment included a comparison between actual and perceived visual impairments in the elderly (Kelly, 1993/1994) and an assessment of how visual impairment influenced the experiences of daily living for adults in a rural community in Kwazulu (Zungu, 1993).

In all three pain studies, postoperative pain was identified as the focal stimulus. Calvillo (1991/1992) used empiric indicators from the RAM to measure patients' and nurses' perceptions of postoperative pain. Calvillo and Flaskerud (1993) concluded that operational adequacy had been met, but empiric adequacy could not be established at that time. Gujol (1994) used the RAM to demonstrate that inadequate postoperative pain management contributed to ineffective adaptation, hindering recovery from surgery. The researcher selected two variables—number of postoperative days and ventilator status—as probable influences on nurses' assessment and management of postoperative pain.

Kelly (1993/1994) and Zungu (1993) identified visual impairment as the focal stimulus requiring adaptation and both reports had a similar purpose: To assess the effect of visual impairment on daily living of older adults. Results of structured interviews conducted by Zungu identified needing help with mobility, shopping, meal preparation, and taking medications as some of the most common problems encountered in adjusting to loss of vision. Although Kelly found that the majority of her sample reported less extreme effects on daily life, the problems she identified were similar to those reported by Zungu.

Neurologic function studies. In all three studies in the category of neurologic function some aspect of temperature regulation was examined (Table 3.5). Hunter (1991) compared methods of temperature measurement in healthy newborns. Similarly, Pontious, Kennedy, Shelly, and Mittrucker, (1994) examined three types of thermometers to determine the most accurate and reliable measure for children's temperatures. In the third study, Hart (1988/1989) described how rural parents perceive and manage fever in their school age children.

The findings of the studies related to taking temperature helped specify effective procedures to use in temperature assessment. For healthy newborns, Hunter (1991) demonstrated that 3 minutes is the clinically appropriate length of time for an axillary temperature. Pontious and colleagues (1994) found that oral temperatures were most accurate and reliable for children, and that the TempaDOT is the most useful instrument of the three tested. These authors found that the level of the nurse's in-service education greatly influenced readings, regardless of the site or instrument used for measurement. Looking at parents' reports of assessment and management of fever, Hart (1988/1989) found misconceptions and misman-

Table 3.6 –Critical Analysis of Quantitative Physiologic Adaptive Research (*N*=17 studies)

Criteria	Evaluation		
	Yes	*Partially*	*No*
Design			
Efforts to control for threats to internal validity	1,4,7,19,20	2,3,5,10,11,13,14, 17,21	8,15,16
Efforts to control for threats to external validity	7,19,20	1,2,3,4,10,11,13,14, 15,16,17,21	5,8
Measurement			
Reliability of instruments addressed	1,2,3,4,5,7,11,13, 14,15,19, 20	10,17,21	8,16
Validity of instruments addressed	1,2,3,4,5,7,11,13,14, 15,17, 19,20	10,21	8,16
Data Analysis			
Appropriate	1,2,3,4,5,7,8 10,11,13,14, 15,17,19,20, 21		16
Interpretation of Results			
Consistency of findings with conclusions	1,2,4,5,7,10 11,13,14,15, 16,17,19,20, 21	3,8	

Key: 1=Cheng & Williams (1989); 2=Harrison, Leeper, & Yoon (1990); 3=Norris, Campbell, & Brenkert (1981); 4=Shogan & Schumann (1993); 5=Khanobdee, Sukratanachaiyakul, & Gay (1993); 7=Gervasini (1994); 8=Rustic (1992/1993); 10=Medhat, Huber, & Medhat (1990); 11=O'Leary (1990/1991); 13=Cheng (1990/1991); 14=Calvillo (1991/1992); 15=Calvillo & Flaskerud (1993); 16=Gujol (1994); 17=Kelly (1993/1994); 19=Hunter (1991); 20=Pontious, Kennedy, Shelly, & Mittrucker (1994); 21=Hart (1988/1989)

---

agement. Interviews with 50 rural parents of well school-aged children revealed that the parents had misconceptions, such as when fever begins, what the harmful effects of fever are, how high an untreated fever can go, and whether all fevers must be treated. Management difficulties included the temperature at which to give medication and whether to give medications for all fevers.

Based on the description of the 21 studies reviewed here, clinical research in the physiologic mode of the RAM was critically analyzed with respect to the quality of the studies. Material may have been deleted in editing individual manuscripts for publication, and if this was the case, the analyses may not reflect the author's original intent.

Critical Analysis of Reported Research

The majority of physiologic adaptive mode studies (21) were either descriptive or correlational, one was a qualitative descriptive inquiry, and three focused on instrument development. Critical analyses are presented separately for the quantitative, qualitative, and methodologic studies.

Critical analyses of quantitative research. Critical analyses of the 17 quantitative studies are presented in Table 3.6. In approximately one-fourth of the studies, adequate measures were taken to control for the threats to internal and external validity, whereas more than two-thirds of the researchers reported instrument reliability and validity data. In most of the studies, data was analyzed appropriately, results were interpreted accurately, and there was consistency between the findings and conclusions.

Authors of the oxygenation studies reported more efforts to control for threats to internal than for threats to external validity. History was not a problem while mortality, loss of subjects from one data point to another, was an issue in two of the studies. The investigators established well-defined selection criteria for the inclusion of subjects, and the procedures were described clearly enough for replication. In two studies, the need for consistency of measurement was not addressed.

All of the oxygenation studies used convenience samples, and the authors acknowledged that their samples were homogeneous, thereby limiting the generalizability of the findings. Reliability and validity of the instruments were adequately addressed in these studies. In general, the results were clearly presented and there was consistency between the findings and the conclusions.

Two researchers examined the process of protection. Due to the sample and setting, Gervasini (1994), who studied trauma patients in the intensive care unit, was better able to control for factors such as instrumentation, equivalence of subjects, and extraneous variables than did Rustic (1992/1993), who studied international graduate students at a state university. Both of these studies used appropriate methods for data analyses and demonstrated consistency between the findings and conclusions. While the descriptive study of expectant Thai fathers (Khanobdee et al., 1993) did not control for many of the threats to internal validity and, therefore, cannot be generalized to other populations, the criteria of measurement, data analysis, and interpretation of results were appropriately met.

The investigation by O'Leary (1990/1991) was the only descriptive activity and rest study that partially controlled for threats to internal validity. Specifically, a detailed procedure was followed to establish interrater reliability for the sleep/activity behavior log. In studying sleep patterns, Cheng (1990/1991) partially controlled for threats to external validity by requiring subjects to spend one night in the hospital unit before data collection to eliminate other possible sleep deprivation factors and accustom the subjects to the setting. Both of these authors adequately addressed the issues of measurement. All three investigators who examined activity and rest used appropriate data analyses techniques and made accurate interpretations of the results.

The four quantitative studies that examined sensory function were limited in controlling for threats to internal and external validity, because each used either a correlational or descriptive design. Calvillo's (1991/1992) correlational investigation of the effect of culture on pain was a good example of the researcher using reasonable efforts to control for these threats. The investigator clearly identified the possible threats to internal validity such as pain from causes other than pain associated with the surgical incision. She also addressed all the measurement issues and used appropriate statistics and analyses for the data.

The descriptive study of visual impairment in the elderly (Kelly, 1993/1994) was a good example of considerable effort being made to control for threats to internal and external validity. The instrument to measure the independent variable was sensitive to a range of visual impairments and the instrument measuring the dependent variable, functional visual status, was valid, reliable, and clinically relevant. Analysis of the four studies included accurate interpretation of the results and consistency between the findings and conclusions.

In general, the three quantitative studies that examined neurologic function met most of the scientific criteria used for analyses. In a descriptive study of the clinically acceptable time to measure axillary temperatures in healthy newborns, Hunter (1991) controlled for most threats to internal and external validity. She clearly described the temperature measurement instruments and methods, including digital display of tissue contact to assure proper placement of the temperature probe in the axillae. Another study that examined various dimensions of measuring children's temperature (Pontious et al., 1994) demonstrated efforts to control for all threats to internal validity, except history, and all possible threats to external validity. In addition, these authors clearly reported the reliability and validity of all measures used in a complex study. While Hart (1988/1989) only partially controlled for threats to both internal and external validity, analyses of data from the interviews with rural parents were appropriate, as were interpretation of the results. The investigators of the preceding studies demonstrated consistency between reporting the findings and presenting the conclusions.

Critical analysis of qualitative research. Analysis of the one qualitative physiologic study is found in Table 3.7. Zungu (1993) used strategies such as descriptive vividness, methodologic congruence, and heuristic relevance to ensure validity, but included little discussion about reliability. The author acknowledged that the interviews were a collaborative effort between informant and investigator, but did not explain how this was used as a strategy for reliability. The method of data analysis appeared appropriate in that categories were developed out of the data, listed in tables, and the author provided illustrative accounts of specific responses as examples. However, the author presented some inconsistencies in the findings. While discussing causes of visual impairment, the author focused on primary health care to prevent visual impairment. This is a good point, but inconsistent with the purpose of the study, that is, assessing life experiences of visually impaired adults.

Critical analyses of instrument development studies. Three physiologic mode studies focused on instrument development using elements of the RAM (Table 3.8). Joseph (1994) developed the Joseph Continence Assessment Tool (JCAT) to holistically assess postprostatectomy males before any bladder behavior interventions for urinary incontinence. The Prosthetic Problem Inventory Scale (Huber et al., 1988) was developed to identify problem areas in the use of prostheses by adults with lower leg amputations. O'Leary and colleagues, (1993) developed a 24-hour behavioral-log assessment, to be completed by family caregivers, that would provide a description of the adaptive and ineffective behaviors of people with AD.

Table 3.7 – Critical Analysis of Qualitative Physiologic Adaptive Mode Research (N=1)

Criteria	Evaluation		
	Yes	Partially	No
Design			
Strategies to ensure validity		18	
Strategies to ensure reliability			18
Data Analysis			
Appropriate method	18		
Interpretation of Results			
Consistency of findings with conclusions		18	

Key: 18=Zungu (1993)

Table 3.8 – Strategies Used in Instrument Development for Physiologic Adaptive Mode Research (*N*=3 studies)

Instrument Author(s)/Year	Reliability	Validity
6. Joseph Continence Assessment Tool (JCAT); Joseph, 1994	Winer's interclass correlation was .88 for both theoretical and practitioner experts. Content Kappa was used to determine the proportion of agreement among the expert raters.	Content validity was 77.5% for both theoretical and practitioner experts.
9. Prosthetic Problem Inventory Scale; Huber, Medhat, & Carter, 1988	Chronbach's Alpha coefficients were .83 for total scale and .97, .88, .95, and .90 for subscales of activities of daily living, social participation, sexual activity, & athletic participation, respectively.	Content validity – 46 items were generated from four dimensions of activities & reviewed by content experts. Construct validity was supported by linkage with theory & results of factor analysis with varimax rotation.
12. 24-Hour Behavioral Log assessment; O'Leary, Haley, & Paul, 1993	Stability assessed by comparing adaptive behaviors ($r=.80, p<.0001, n=32$) and ineffective behaviors ($r=.80, p<.0001, n=32$) on two consecutive 24-hour days.	Content validity was judged by expert family caregiver. Normal behaviors vs. problem behaviors were categorized according to RAM by two raters. Convergent & discriminant validity with MBPC was supported for adaptive behaviors ($r=-.75, p<.001$) and for ineffective behaviors ($r=.75, p<.001$) of the behavioral log assessment.

Joseph (1994) used 18 experts, nine theoretic and nine urologic practitioners, for content validity of the JCAT. Content validity for both groups was 77.5%. Reliability was assessed by Winer's interclass correlation (.88) and by Cohen's Kappa statistic. The concerns of the experts were theoretic, while practitioners focused on the feasibility and relevance of clinical applications.

The Prosthetic Problem Inventory Scale (Huber et al., 1988) measured four dimensions of activity performance. Reliability was supported by Cronbach alpha coefficients for the total scale and subscale scores. A linkage with theory and the results of a factor analysis provided support for construct validity.

The 24-Hour Behavioral Log Assessment (O'Leary et al., 1993) was developed to describe the behaviors of people with AD and was designed to be completed by family caregivers who lived with the patient. The measure was systematically developed in a number of stages, including analysis of available instruments to assess behavioral problems in AD patients, use of a preliminary version of the log (O'Leary, 1990/1991), and two experts to judge content validity. Reliability was supported with tests for stability, and tests for convergent and discriminate validity were completed with other appropriate measures.

Initial reliability and validity were established for all three physiologic mode instruments. In addition, all three instruments were theoretically related to the RAM. The JCAT (Joseph, 1994) was developed to reflect assessment of the four adaptive modes of the RAM. Huber and colleagues (1988) developed the Prosthetic Problem Inventory Scale to measure four dimensions of activities in people with prostheses. O'Leary and colleagues, (1993) distinguished normal versus problem behaviors in their 24-Hour Behavioral Log Assessment by using the terms adaptive and ineffective from the RAM.

Evaluation of Relationships to the Roy Adaptation Model

Thirteen physiologic adaptative mode studies were evaluated for relationships to the RAM. The studies meeting the criteria for both critical analysis and linkages with the model were then used to test propositions from the RAM.

Evaluation of Linkages to the RAM

An evaluation of the linkages between the 13 physiologic mode studies and the Roy Model is shown in Table 3.9. Linkages between the RAM and the research variables, empiric measures, and findings were evaluated for each of the studies. Most authors explicitly identified the model and linked the research variables with concepts of the RAM. Linkage of the research variables with empiric measures was explicitly identified in only seven

Table 3.9 – Evaluation of Linkages of Physiologic Adaptive Mode
Research with the Roy Adaptation Model (*N*=13)

| Linkages to RAM | Evaluation | | |
	Explicit	*Implicit*	*Absent*
Research variables	1,2,3,4,7, 10,13,14,17, 19,20,21	11	
Empirical measures	1,3,7,13, 14,19	2,4,11,17, 20,21	10
Findings	1,3,7,10, 13,14,17	2,20	4,11,19,21

Key: 1=Cheng & Williams (1989); 2=Harrison, Leeper, & Yoon (1990); 3=Norris, Campbell, & Brenkert (1981); 4=Shogan & Schumann (1993); 7=Gervasini (1994); 10=Medhat, Huber, & Medhat (1990); 11=O'Leary (1990/1991); 13=Cheng (1990/ 1991); 14=Calvillo (1991/1992); 17=Kelly (1993/1994); 19=Hunter (1991); 20=Pontious, Kennedy, Shelly, & Mittrucker (1994); 21=Hart (1988/1989)

studies. More than half of the researchers either explicitly or implicitly related the findings of the research study to the model, while this relationship was not evaluated in six studies.

The authors of the oxygenation studies were consistent in explicitly linking the research variables to the RAM. For example, the dependent variable in four of the studies using infants as subjects was arterial oxygen saturation levels. Because oxygenation is one of the basic needs identified by the model, common nursing activities related to diagnostic and treatment procedures were viewed as stimuli affecting oxygenation. Likewise, the findings of these studies could be used to support or refute specific propositions of the RAM.

While authors who investigated the need for activity and rest used various concepts for the dependent variable, the concepts were clearly related to the RAM. In two of these studies, the outcome measures were categorized as adaptive or ineffective according to the Roy typology of adaptive behaviors. Most of these authors related the findings to the model and indicated how stimuli affected adaptation.

Studies that examined sensory function focused on the phenomena of pain and visual impairment. In the two pain studies, the effect of specific contextual stimuli on sensation was clearly related to the model. Visual impairment in the elderly was the independent variable for both studies. A discussion of findings explicitly described outcomes consistent with the model. In the three studies focusing on neurologic function, the dependent variable was temperature. Again, common nursing activities and procedures were identified as stimuli relevant to the dependent variable. In these studies, the research variables were clearly linked to the RAM, and the empiric measures were implicitly linked to the research variables. However, in discussing the findings, only one author implied any relationship to the RAM.

An evaluation of the linkages between each of the 13 studies and the model supported the effectiveness of the RAM in guiding nursing research. The weakest area of linking the research to the model was in discussion of findings. When this linkage is made, according to standards for evaluation of conceptual models (Fawcett & Downs, 1992), significant credibility is added to the model.

Testing of Propositions from the RAM

Twelve of the physiologic mode studies met the criteria for testing propositions of the RAM. From the model propositions listed in Chapter 2, studies focusing on the physiologic adaptive mode tested five of the propositions (Table 3.10).

The model shows that the person or group has innate and acquired ways of adapting, and regulator and cognator processes affect adaptation in the individual. All of the studies examining oxygenation supported the proposition that innate, acquired ways of adapting were major influences of adaptation, given the same external stimuli. Further, the findings were consistent with the postulation of regulator and cognator processes being the active force of adapting. Neural and chemical channels were relevant to the individual variability of infants' return to baseline oxygenation levels. As a group, these studies provided support for a key proposition of the model.

A second proposition was related to the effect of external stimuli characteristics on adaptive responses. Findings from nine different studies supported this proposition. In the discussion of the theory of the adapting person, Roy (Roy and Roberts, 1981) concluded that internal and external stimuli have characteristics such as magnitude and clarity that influenced the functioning of the regulator and cognator. The related propositions indicated that in general (a) the magnitude of the stimuli influenced the magnitude of the regulator response and (b) that the optimum amount and clarity of internal and external stimuli influenced the adequacy of cognator processing. In four of the studies of oxygenation in low birth weight infants, the stimuli characteristics, diagnostic procedures and treatment procedures affected the levels of change in oxygenation. In some

Table 3.10 – Testing of Propositions from the RAM (N=12)

Propositions from the RAM	Ancillary and practice propositions	Supported by results	Not supported by results
1. At the individual level, regulator and cognator processes affect innate and acquired ways of adapting.	Changes in oxygenation were variable between subjects, given the same stimuli.	Cheng & Williams (1989); Harrison, Leeper, & Yoon (1990); Norris, Campbell, & Brenkert (1981); Shogan & Schumann (1993)	
3. The characteristics of the internal and external stimuli influence adaptive responses.	a. Some common diagnostic and treatment procedures place greater demands on the adaptive system.	Cheng & Williams (1989); Harrison, Leeper, & Yoon (1990); Norris, Campbell, & Brenkert (1981); Shogan & Schumann (1993)	
	b. Strong contextual stimuli can affect physiologic adaptation.	O'Leary (1990)/1991	O'Leary (1990/1991); Kelly (1993/1994)
	c. Strong contextual stimuli can affect social adaptation.	Kelly (1993/1994)	
	d. Pleasant stimuli can change adaptive behavior.	Cheng (1990/1991)	Cheng (1990/1991)
	e. Ethnicity and social class affected nurses' perceptions of patients' physiologic stimuli.	Calvillo (1991/1992)	
	f. Ethnicity and social class did not affect patients' perception of their own physiologic stimuli.	Calvillo (1991/1992)	
	g. Nurses' judgments are affected by contextual stimuli.	Pontious, Kennedy, Shelly, & Mittrucker (1994)	

(continued)

Table 3.10 (continued)

Propositions from the RAM	Ancillary and practice propositions	Supported by results	Not supported by results
7. The pooled effect of focal, contextual, and residual stimuli determines the adaptation level.	Stimuli can be identified that predict adaptive and ineffective responses in the physiological mode.	Gervasini (1994)	
9. The variable of time influences the process of adaptation.	Time is an important variable that affects measurement of responses in the physiological mode.	Hunter (1991)	
10. The variable of perception influences the process of adaptation.	a. Nurses' and patients' perceptions of the same events differ.	Calvillo (1991/1992)	
	b. Parents treat fever based on misperceptions	Hart (19881989)	

cases, the stimuli characteristic was clearly magnitude, for example, changes in the amount of illumination was most important. In other cases, the characteristic included other dimensions in addition to magnitude. For example, suctioning caused greater disturbance of oxygenation than heel stick caused. Although magnitude of the stimuli was one relevant characteristic, investigators noted that in this case, suctioning involved an interruption of the infant's airway by the catheter. The proposition is thus broadened to use the more general term characteristic rather than magnitude, which is only one dimension of the stimuli.

Contextual stimuli of unusual magnitude were a variable in four studies. The stimuli were all clinical conditions such as AD (O'Leary, 1990/1991) and visual impairment (Kelly, 1993/1994). When caregivers identified adaptive and ineffective behaviors of people with AD, the most ineffective activity was physical repetitive behaviors. Thus the ancillary proposition notes that strong contextual stimuli can affect social adaptation.

The general proposition was also not supported by the results of the studies using clinical conditions as the stimulus. O'Leary (1990/1991) found AD patients' sleep behaviors were mainly adaptive, as were the activities of leisure behaviors. In studying decreased vision in the elderly, Kelly (1993/1994) found minimal, if any, effects on daily life. In each of these cases, the individual innate and acquired ways of adapting, reflecting regulator and cognator processes, have more influence on adaptive responses than given external stimuli have. The relationship between the first two propositions needs to be clarified.

Cheng (1990/1991) investigated pleasant stimuli, such as social support, affecting measures of daytime sleep. The findings provide some support for the general proposition about external stimuli characteristics. However, the social support stimuli did not affect measures of sleep characteristics. The mixed results may reflect that individual variability, indicating differing regulator and cognator activity, may confound the effects of the characteristics of the external stimuli characteristics. The additional findings support explanation of why the studies related to clinical conditions had results that did not support the second proposition.

Two other studies lend support to the proposition that internal and external stimuli characteristics influence adaptive responses. Calvillo (1991/1992) found that ethnicity and social class affected nurses' perceptions of, but not patients' perceptions of pain. Pontious and colleagues, (1994) found that nurses' judgments were affected by contextual stimuli. The third proposition received moderate support from the physiologic adaptive mode research, but questions were raised about the relationship between the first and third propositions.

Roy (1976) defined adaptation as a function of the pooled effect of focal, contextual, and residual stimuli. Based on this assumption, a logically derived proposition was that stimuli can be identified to predict levels of adaptive and ineffective responses in the physiologic mode. The proposition was addressed in two studies. Gervasini (1994) generated a list of predictor variables that successfully classified 47.6% of septic patients and 81.5% of non-septic patients. The support for the proposition in the one study may be related to the degree of specificity used in the predictor stimuli, that is, Gervasini had specific outcome variables.

Results of one study provided support for the proposition that adaptation is a process that takes place over time (Roy & Andrews, 1991). In Hunter's (1991) study of axillary temperatures, time became an important variable affecting the measurement of adaptation. Therefore, the variable of time needs to be considered when conducting research focusing on the physiologic adaptive mode.

In summary, results of physiologic adaptive mode research that supported model propositions and those that did not provide support were discussed. The propositions evaluated here and those tested in the other content chapters are synthesized in Chapter 11, where the RAM's contributions to knowledge are examined through the testing of all propositions in the research reviewed.

Synthesis of Physiologic Mode Research: Contributions to Nursing Science

Contributions to nursing science were derived from the synthesis of 12 studies that met the criteria in testing of the model propositions. Studies are discussed in relation to contributions to clinical practice, research, and theory. Many of the findings relate to all three areas. Future directions for clinical practice, physiologic mode research, and model developed are addressed in relation to the RAM.

Applications to Nursing Practice

From knowledge developed through testing concepts and their relationships within the RAM, (Pollock, Frederickson, Carson, Massey, & Roy, 1994), clinical applications can be derived and implemented in the practice setting. Specifically, interventions can be proposed that promote or maintain physiologic adaptation in various populations and settings. The interventions are tested and refined before implementation in the practice setting. The twelve studies were examined for their applications to practice based upon previously developed categories (Table 3.11).

Four of the studies had potential for implementation in practice. Related to the physiologic need for protection, a clinical application from Gervasini's study (1994) was the ability to accurately predict which patients will develop a septic profile. Given the predictions, prevention principles may decrease the incidence of traumatic injury and the associated

Table 3.11 – Applications to Nursing Practice from Physiologic Adaptive Mode Research (*N*=12)

Category One: High potential for implementation
>   Gervasini (1994)
>   Hunter (1991)
>   Pontious, Kennedy, Shelly, & Mittrucker (1994)
>   Hart (1988/1989)

Category Two: Needs further clinical evaluation before implementation
>   Cheng & Williams (1989)
>   Harrison, Leeper, & Yoon (1990)
>   Norris, Campbell, & Brenkert (1981)
>   Shogan & Schumann (1993)

Category Three: Further research indicated before implementation
>   O'Leary (1990/1991)
>   Calvillo (1991/1992)
>   Cheng (1990/1991)
>   Kelly (1993/1994)

---

complications. Identified as predictors of a septic profile post trauma were two variables: patients who experienced a longer lag time and those who had higher injury severity scores. Trauma prevention programs need to focus on not only decreasing the incidence of trauma but also on identifying high risk behaviors and modifying behaviors to reflect a protective pattern. Both clinicians and the public need to be educated about delay in treatment of trauma.

Results from studies related to neurologic function of temperature can be confidently used in clinical practice due to the low risk for subjects. For example, findings indicated that three minutes is the clinically appropriate time for measuring axillary temperatures in healthy newborns because stabilization occurred within three minutes for 100% of the sample using two types of thermometers (Hunter, 1991). Similarly, results from Pontious and colleagues (1994) can be used with confidence in the clinical setting. They found TempaDOT the most clinically useful instrument, and the oral site accurate for measuring temperature of children in the acute care setting. They also made pertinent comments for temperature measurement when, axillary rather than oral temperatures were taken in younger children. Related to policies about the education of pediatric nurses was that the level of in-service education significantly affected all temperature readings obtained at any site and by any measurement instrument.

Based on the results of Hart's (1988/1989) study, nurses working with parents of school-aged children in rural areas, and possibly in other areas, can be more aware that these parents may have misperceptions about fever in their children. The parents may need instruction about the principles of management of fever, including accurate methods to measure temperature, correct medications to be used, and other appropriate methods to reduce fever.

Results from four studies need to be evaluated by clinical experts to determine if the interventions are appropriate for current use or if they need refinement or further evaluation in the clinical setting. Knowledge about the effects of various contextual stimuli on infants' arterial saturation levels (Cheng & Williams, 1989; Harrison et al., 1990; Norris et al., 1981; Shogan & Schumann, 1993) can be applied by nurses in efforts to prevent or minimize developmental problems in these children.

Likewise, results from these studies indicated factors to be considered regarding current nursing policies, such as those that affect parental touch for preterm infants (Harrison et al., 1990) and the amount of environmental lighting for preterm infants (Shogan & Schumann, 1993). Modifying types and the amount of touch based on the infant's behavioral and physiologic responses may be more appropriate. Parents could be taught to observe the infant's oxygen saturation monitors and alter their patterns of touching accordingly. Some procedures for infants may not need to be performed as frequently as current routine demands. For other procedures, making modifications that lessen the severity of the stress or alter the intensity of environmental stimuli without removing the therapeutic value may be possible (Norris et al., 1982; Shogan & Schumann, 1993).

Findings from four studies had potential for contributions to clinical practice but warranted further research. Clinical importance from O'Leary's (1990/1991) study was a better understanding of the sleep and activity behaviors of people with AD, because these behaviors were continuously recorded by caregivers for two consecutive days in behavior logs. Home visits made by the researcher in this study proved useful in obtaining additional information not only about effective and ineffective behaviors of the people with AD, but also about creative strategies caregivers used to prevent or decrease the ineffective activities. The home visits may also have been therapeutic for the caregivers based on the positive comments they made about enjoying visitors and needing to talk about their feelings with someone who understood.

Nurses need to be aware that their perceptions of patients' pain may be influenced by the ethnicity and social status of patients and that, according to Calvillo's (1991/1992) findings, nurses and patients have different perceptions of patients' pain. Implications for practice emphasized the need for nurses to be aware that their values influence how they evaluate pain in different cultural groups. Because the two ethnic groups investigated by Calvillo did not differ significantly on any measure of pain, nurses need to validate further how they are evaluating patients' pain in order to avoid inaccurate evaluation and control of pain.

Replication of the studies by Cheng (1990/1991) and Kelly (1993/1994) is warranted by their importance for nursing. While Cheng did not find any difference in the sleep patterns of adults with social support compared to patients without, further studies are needed to investigate the type and quality of the social support and whether the other confounding variables in the environment could be better controlled. Likewise, further study is needed to explain factors associated with adaptation in the elderly with visual problems.

Recommendations for Model-Based Research

Future directions for model-based research were identified from all studies that had applications to nursing practice, but were most obvious in category three where further testing was indicated. In addition, studies where findings were ambiguous or differed from previous research are priority areas for further clinical investigations.

Clinical investigations to assess individual variations in internal processes over time are warranted (Cheng & Williams, 1989; Harrison et al., 1990; Norris et al., 1982; Shogan & Schumann, 1993). Interventions aimed at keeping infants' oxygen saturation within normoxemic levels are indicated with larger samples in order to identify and quantify specific influences on oxygenation (Cheng & Williams, 1989). Other variables known to affect oxygenation of infants and of other populations need to be measured (Harrison et al., 1990; Norris et al., 1982; Shogan & Schumann, 1993).

The effect of environmental stimuli, such as age, stress, and nutrition, on the immune system need to be studied in relation to the process of protection (Gervasini, 1994). Using a behavior log to identify not only the frequency, but the types of effective and ineffective behaviors of adults with AD will be beneficial in future research endeavors (O'Leary, 1990/ 1991). Important implications for clinical research are the testing of interventions to reduce the frequency of ineffective behaviors and to increase the amount of adaptive behaviors. Creative nursing interventions are also indicated to help the caregiver cope with the realities of daily caring for people with AD.

Evaluation of nurses' perceptions of patients' pain, including the effects of ethnicity and social class, needs to be further investigated using the RAM. While Calvillo's (1991/1992) study focused on factors that influenced nurses' perceptions of patients' pain, it is possible that nurses evaluated patients' pain differently based on their own culture and sociodemographic characteristics. Several major avenues for adaptation research are the role of culture in the expression and assessment of pain, and the effect of the other three adaptive modes on the evaluation of patients' pain.

Further research on the neurologic function of temperature needs to include an assessment of temperature over time to determine the healthy newborn's ability for thermoregulation. Findings from Hunter's study (1991) indicate a basis for replication to study axillary temperature measurement in other infant groups, such as premature newborns and newborns who are small or large for gestational age. Also, the effects of the environment on the newborn's ability to adapt physiologically via thermoregulation needs to be considered in future studies. Findings from Pontious and colleagues (1994) emphasized that no procedure performed on patients is routine and that clinical research is warranted to determine the accuracy, reliability, validity, and cost effectiveness of all procedures and instruments used with patients. This study provided a model not only for guiding research about other procedures but also for using research to determine the best instrument or procedure to use in the clinical setting.

Hart's study (1988/1989) provided baseline data regarding the perceptions and management of fever by rural parents. Differences in rural versus urban parents' knowledge of fever could be studied under more controlled conditions. More important are experimental studies to determine the effectiveness of programs aimed at increasing parents' knowledge about fever and the management of it in their children.

To improve the efficacy of the RAM in guiding research,thereby, increasing contributions to nursing science, instruments that appropriately measure specific concepts of the model need to be identified. Initial progress and current limitations in this area are discussed in the chapter on measurement of the model. Instruments need to appropriately reflect the theoretic definitions and operational indicators of specific model variables under study. The primary contribution of the three instrument development studies focusing on specific aspects of physiologic adaptation, (Joseph, 1994; Huber et al., 1988; O'Leary et al., 1993) was operationalizing various concepts of the RAM. Many possibilities exist for instrument development for physiologic adaptive mode research using the RAM. Likewise, instruments are available that have been effectively used in physiologic adaptive mode research. Continued use and refinement of these instruments is indicated to develop clinical knowledge about adaptation to various health-related conditions. Reliable and valid instruments are needed to measure major concepts from the model in order to better guide physiologic nursing research.

Directions for Theory and RAM Development

Physiologic research based on the RAM contributed to identifying directions for further development of theory and the nursing model. Three clear directions were identified from the reported research. First, there was the need to examine the relationship between two model components, the innate and acquired ways of adapting, and the stimuli affecting levels of adaptation. Second, the mixed findings related to the characteristics of stimuli indicated further conceptual and theoretic development was needed in this area. Third, time as a potentially important concept needs to be included in theorizing about adaptation.

Among the key concepts of the RAM, the regulator and cognator were identified as the internal processes for innate and acquired ways of adapting. In addition, stimuli were identified as pooling with coping abilities to make up an adaptation level. The model has not addressed the interaction between the regulator and cognator and the stimuli. Examining this relationship could include linking the concepts either directly or indirectly through a third concept. In a given situation, theoretic concepts that determine the primacy of contribution of the regulator and cognator or of the stimuli to the behavioral outcome need to be identified. If the concepts can be related in a series of theoretic statements, hypotheses can be generated about their reciprocal influence in a given situation. Productive theory and model development can come from addressing such questions.

Based on the findings of reported research analyzed in this chapter, further conceptual clarity is offered to better understand the key concept of external stimuli. Whereas Roy (Roy & Roberts, 1991) identified magnitude and optimum amount of stimuli as important influences in the adequacy of regulator and cognator processing, the work reported here indicated that other characteristics of the stimuli were relevant. For example, the suction catheter may be a clear stimulus of relatively small magnitude, but its effect on oxygenation was great because of the characteristic that it could occlude the airway. Model development will take into account a broader range of characteristics of the stimuli. Further, in the studies that examined either strong or pleasant stimuli, the findings were mixed. Both sets of findings supported the need to clearly identify the stimuli characteristics and their effects in differing situations.

Finally, time was identified in one study as an important variable affecting measurement of adaptation. In related work on information processing, Roy (1988) identified time as a key variable for study. However, to date the concept of time has not been explored or integrated in the model or related theoretic work. Based on this analysis, the concept of time is potentially important for further RAM development.

Summary

Multidimensional theoretic frameworks that reflect a holistic approach, such as the RAM, are indicated for nursing studies because the discipline purports to focus on the whole person. Of the final 163 nursing studies included in this monograph, 21 focused primarily on physiologic adaptive mode and more than 55 included physiologic variables. This is twice the percent of physiologic studies recently identified by Pugh and DeKeyser (1995), who found that only 15% of recently reported nursing research focused on physiologic variables. Findings reported from the studies support the use of a holistic framework such as the RAM to increase the inclusion of physiologic variables in nursing investigations.

The numerous applications for nursing practice also support the value of using the RAM to guide physiologic adaptive mode research. Scholarly inquiry in the practice setting that is guided by a nursing model will not only inform proposed interventions, but allows for refining the theories and knowledge needed to direct clinical practice. Additionally, areas for further development of the physiologic adaptive mode will be made explicit from the empiric and clinical findings. Finally, using a nursing model to guide practice and research of physiologic phenomena will strengthen the relationships among theory, research, and practice. The contributions to nursing science from all RAM research, including the physiologic mode studies, are synthesized and addressed collectively in a later chapter.

References

Calvillo, E.R. (1991/1992). Pain response in Mexican-American and white non-Hispanic women. (Doctoral dissertation, University of California, Los Angeles, 1991). *Dissertation Abstracts International, 52*, 3524-B.

Calvillo, E.R., & Flaskerud, J.H. (1993). The adequacy and scope of Roy's adaptation model to guide cross-cultural pain research. *Nursing Science Quarterly, 6*, 118-129.

Cheng, L.C. (1991). Social support related to the sleep pattern in Southern Taiwanese hospitalized adults. (Master's thesis, University of Arizona, 1990). *Master's Abstracts International, 29*, 90.

Cheng, M. & Williams, P.D. (1989). Oxygenation during chest physiotherapy of very-low-birth-weight infants: Relations among fraction of inspired oxygen levels, number of hand ventilations, and transcutaneous oxygen pressure. *Journal of Pediatric Nursing, 4*(6), 411-418.

Fawcett, J., & Downs, F.S. (1992). *The relationship of theory and research.* (2nd ed.). Philadelphia: F.A.Davis.

Gervasini, A.A. (1994). Classification of trauma patients with a septic profile utilizing a predictor model. Unpublished doctoral dissertation, Boston College, Boston.

Gujol, M.C. (1994). A survey of pain assessment and management practices among critical care nurses. *American Journal of Critical Care, 3*(2), 123-128.

Harrison, L.L., Leeper, J. D., & Yoon, M. (1990). Effects of early parent touch on preterm infants' heart rates and arterial oxygen saturation levels. *Journal of Advanced Nursing, 15*, 877-885.

Hart, M.A. (1989). Rural parents' perception and management of fever in their school-age children. (Master's thesis, University of Florida, 1988). *Masters Abstracts International, 27*, 376.

Huber, P.M., Medhat, A., & Carter, M. C. (1988). Prosthetic Problem Inventory Scale. *Rehabilitation Nursing 13*(6), 326-329.

Hunter, L.P. (1991). Measurement of axillary temperatures in neonates. *Western Journal of Nursing Research 13*, 324-335.

Joseph, A.C. (1994). Content validity of the Joseph Continence Assessment Tool. Unpublished master's thesis, San Diego State University, San Diego.

Kelly, M. (1994). Visual impairment in the elderly and its impact on their daily lives. (Doctoral dissertation, Texas Women's University, 1993). *Dissertation Abstracts International, 54*, 5093-B.

Khanobdee, C., Sukratanachaiyakul, V., & Gay, J.T. (1993). Couvade syndrome in expectant Thai fathers. *International Journal of Nursing Studies, 30*, 125-131.

Medhat, A., Huber, P.M., & Medhat, M.A. (1990). Factors that influence the level of activities in persons with lower extremity amputation. *Rehabilitation Nursing 15*, 13-18.

Norris, S., Campbell, L.A., & Brenkert, S. (1981). Nursing procedures and alterations in transcutaneous oxygen tension in premature infants. *Nursing Research 31*, 330-336.

O'Leary, P. A. (1991). Family caregivers' log reports of sleep and activity behaviors of persons with Alzheimer's disease. (Doctoral dissertation, University of Alabama, 1990). *Dissertation Abstracts International,51*, 4780-B.

O'Leary, P.A., Haley, W.E., & Paul, P.B. (1993). Behavioral assessment in Alzheimer's disease: Use of a 24-hour log. *Psychology and Aging, 8*, 139-143.

Pontious, S., Kennedy, A.H., Shelly, S., & Mittrucker, C. (1994). Accuracy and reliability of temperature measurement by instrument and site. *Journal of Pediatric Nursing, 9*(2), 114-123.

Rustic, D.L. (1993). A study of somatic symptomatology: Occurrence and severity as reported by international graduate students at Michigan State University. (Master's thesis, Michigan State University, 1992). *Masters Abstracts International, 31*, 282.

Shogan, M.G., & Schumann, L.L. (1993). The effect of environmental lighting on oxygen saturation of preterm infants in the NICU. *Neonatal Network Journal of Neonatal Nursing, 12*, 7-13.

Zungu, B.M. (1993). Assessment of the life experiences of visually impaired adults in the Empangeni Region of Kwazulu. *Curationis: South African Journal of Nursing, 16*(4), 38-42.

Bibliography

Pollock, S.E., Frederickson, K., Carson, M.A., Massey, V.H., & Roy, C. (1994). Contributions to nursing science: Synthesis of findings from adaptation model research. *Scholarly Inquiry for Nursing Practice, 8*(4), 361-372.

Pugh, L.C. & DeKeyser, F.G. (1995). Use of physiologic variables in nursing research. *IMAGE: Journal of Nursing Scholarship, 27*, 273-276.

Roy, C. (1976). *Introduction to nursing: An adaptation model.* Englewood Cliffs, NJ: Prentice Hall.

Roy, C. (1988). Patient information processing and nursing research. In J. Fitzpatrick & R.L. Tauton (Eds.) *Annual review of nursing research, 6*, New York: Springer, 237-263.

Roy, C. & Andrews, H. (1991). *The Roy Adaptation Model: The definitive statement.* E. Norwalk, CT: Appleton & Lange.

Roy, C. & Roberts, S.L. (1981). *Theory construction in nursing: An adaptation model.* Englewood Cliffs, NJ: Prentice-Hall.

Chapter 4

Self-Concept Mode Research

In this chapter, research reported from 1970-1994 which focused primarily on the self-concept adaptive mode of the Roy Adaptation Model (RAM) is analyzed. Eighteen studies based on the RAM, including dissertations and theses, were categorized as self-concept mode research. Self-concept studies using either an experimental or quasi-experimental design are described in Chapter 9. Studies about adaptation in more than the self-concept mode and not focusing primarily on self-concept are included in Chapter 7.

Purposes

The purposes of this chapter are to (a) critically analyze research in the self-concept adaptive mode; (b) evaluate the relationship of self-concept mode research to the RAM; and (c) synthesize contributions of reported studies to nursing science. Contributions to nursing science include applications for nursing practice, recommendations for model-based self-concept research, and directions for further theory and RAM development of the self-concept mode. The criteria developed and the processes used by the research team for analysis and synthesis of the studies are explained in Chapter 2.

Background

The self-concept adaptive mode focuses specifically on person aspects. Self-concept examines the question "Who am I?" The basic need underlying the mode is psychic integrity, defined as the need to know who one is so that one can be or exist with a sense of unity (Roy & Andrews, 1991, 1999).

The self-concept mode consists of two subareas: the physical self and the personal self. The physical self includes body sensation and body image. Body sensation is the ability to feel and to experience self as a physical being, such as feeling sick or tired. Body image is one's views of one's body–as attractive or physically fit, for example. The personal self includes self-consistency, self-ideal, and moral-ethical-spiritual self. Self-consistency has to do with maintaining a consistent self-organization under such stress as a student's experience of anxiety before a test. Self-ideal is what one would like to be or what one is capable of doing, and is reflected, for example, in expressing a desire to be a lawyer. The moral-ethical-spiritual self includes the person's belief system and an evaluation of who one is, such as believing in the purposefulness of life (Roy & Andrews, 1991).

Self-esteem is inherent within each component of the self-concept mode. Self-esteem is one's perception of self-worth, and the level of self-esteem reflects self-concept. Behaviors related to self-esteem give insight into adaptation in the self-concept mode. Behaviors are evident through the person's appearance, actions, and comments (Roy & Andrews, 1991).

Critical Analysis of Self-Concept Mode Research

Critical analysis involves a description of each study, followed by the evaluation of studies according to the criteria described in Chapter 2.

Description of Reported Research

In the self-concept adaptive mode, 18 studies were categorized into three groups: (a) self-esteem and the self-concept ($n=10$), (b) self-concept and pregnancy ($n=2$), and (c) self-concept and chronic illness ($n=6$). Self-esteem, a person's perception of self-worth, is imbedded in each component of the self-concept mode (Roy & Andrews, 1991). Considerable research focused on the concept of self-esteem and its relationship to selected demographic and situational variables. Because achievement of maturation tasks affects a person's self-concept, other research examined the effect of pregnancy on self-concept. Acknowledging that the person's appraisal of the health-illness state is included in considerations of the physical self, other researchers studied the relationship between chronic illness and self-concept.

Self-esteem and the self-concept. In 10 of the 18 studies, the focus of the research was on self-esteem (Table 4.1). Holcombe (1985/1986) examined social support, perception of illness, and self-esteem in 50 women who had cervical, endometrial, or ovarian cancer. The women perceived receiving social support, primarily from their families. Self-esteem was related to perceptions of illness and perceptions of love, respect, and affirmation from the women's supportive others.

To determine the relationship among kindergarteners' self-esteem and maternal self-esteem, work status, and sociodemographic variables, Lavender (1988/1989) studied 130 mother-child dyads. Maternal employment, socioeconomic status, and birth order were not related to the child's self-esteem. However, child care arrangements (parental care), family structure (two-parent family), age (younger), and gender (male) were related to higher self-esteem in the kindergarten child.

McRae (1990/1991) studied 70 primiparous women age 30 years and older to determine the effect of self-esteem, ego development, and attitudes toward pregnancy and motherhood on adaptation to pregnancy and motherhood. Relationships existed among the symptoms reported during

Table 4.1 – Description of Studies About Self-Esteem and Self-Concept in the Self-Concept Adaptive Mode of the RAM (N=10)

Author(s) & Date	Purpose	Sample	Design	Findings
1. Holcombe (1985/1986)	To describe social support, perception of illness, and self-esteem of women with gynecologic cancer	Women with gynecologic cancer (N=50)	Correlational	Self-esteem was related to perceptions of illness and perceptions of love, respect, and affirmation from supportive others. Women with gynecologic cancer perceived that they received social support, primarily from family.
2. Lavender (1988/1989)	To determine the relationship between maternal self-esteem, work status, and socio-demographic characteristics and self-esteem of the kindergarten child	Mother-child dyads (N=130)	Correlational	There was no significant difference in self-esteem between kindergarten children of working mothers and those whose mothers did not work. There was a significant relationship between child care arrangements, family structure, age, gender, and self-esteem of kindergarten children.
3. McRae (1990/1991)	To determine the effect of self-esteem, ego development, and attitudes toward pregnancy and motherhood on adaptation to pregnancy and motherhood in primiparous women age 30 years and older	Primiparous women age 30 years and older (N=70)	Correlational	There was a relationship between self-esteem and symptoms reported during pregnancy, and between pregnancy symptoms and postpartum maternal-infant sensitivity. Age was correlated to ego development. *(continued)*

Table 4.1 (continued)

Author(s) & Date	Purpose	Sample	Design	Findings
4. Foster (1989/1990)	To determine the relationship between demographic variables and self-esteem of adolescent mothers, pregnant adolescents, and never pregnant adolescents	Adolescent mothers (n=107), pregnant adolescents (n=105), never-pregnant adolescents (n=300); N=512	Descriptive	There were no significant differences in self-esteem among the three groups. Self-esteem significantly increased with age in adolescent mothers and pregnant adolescents. Family structure was significantly related to self-esteem in never-pregnant adolescents.
5. Stein (1991/1992)	To explore relationships among the concepts of life events, self-esteem, and perceived powerlessness as experienced by adolescents	Adolescents 11-18 years of age (N=261)	Correlational	Perceived powerlessness and concepts of life events were predictive of adolescents' self-esteem. There was a significant difference among levels of self-esteem and powerlessness among adolescents of differing socioeconomic classes.
6. Robinson (1991)	To provide an understanding of the adolescent in relation to gender, sexual activity, pregnancy, and self esteem	High school students (n = 299); Pregnant adolescents (n = 16); (N=315)	Descriptive	There was no significant difference in self-esteem in relation to pregnancy, gender, and sexual activity. Males who had fathered a child had a lower level of self-esteem than males who had not fathered a child.

	Purpose	Sample	Method	Findings
7. Robinson & Frank (1994)	To examine the relationship between self-esteem, sexual activity, and pregnancy in a racially mixed sample of male and female teens	High school students (n = 299); Pregnant teens (n = 16); N=315	Descriptive	There were no differences in self-esteem in relation to gender, pregnancy, and sexual activity. Males who had fathered a child had lower self-esteem than non-fathers.
8. Edwards (1991/1992)	To determine if there were differences in self-esteem and sense of mastery between low income pregnant women who obtained adequate prenatal care and their counterparts who obtained inadequate prenatal care	Low income women in third trimester of pregnancy (N=102)	Descriptive	Women who obtained adequate prenatal care had higher self-esteem and sense of mastery, independent of the influence of education or level of poverty, than did women who did not obtain adequate prenatal care.
9. Christian (1993)	To determine the relationship between self-esteem and the number, frequency, and severity of symptoms of endometriosis	Women with endometriosis (N=23)	Correlational	There were no significant correlations between self-esteem and the number, frequency, and severity of symptoms. Symptoms of endometriosis interfered with activities of daily living.
10. Chen (1994)	To determine relationships among hearing handicap and loneliness and self-esteem	Elders age 65 and older with a hearing loss (N=88)	Correlational	Among women, the greater the hearing handicap, the greater the loneliness and the lower the self-esteem. Hearing handicap was not related to loneliness and low self-esteem in men.

pregnancy, self-esteem, and postpartum maternal-infant sensitivity. Ego development was related to age.

Four studies used adolescence as a contextual stimulus in self-esteem and adaptation. Foster (1989/1990) examined the relationships among age, race, grade, family structure, sexual activity, contraceptive use, and self-esteem of 107 adolescent mothers, 105 pregnant adolescents, and 300 never-pregnant adolescents. No differences were found in self-esteem among the three groups, but self-esteem significantly increased with age in the adolescent mothers and the pregnant adolescents. Never-pregnant adolescents had lower self-esteem if their mother and sibling had a child during adolescence or if only their sibling had a child during adolescence.

To examine the relationships among life events, perceived powerlessness, and self-esteem, Stein (1991/1992) studied 261 adolescents between the ages of 11 and 18. Feelings of powerlessness and an increased incidence of significant life events were predictive of low levels of self-esteem. Adolescents of lower socioeconomic status had lower levels of self-esteem and greater feelings of powerlessness than did their counterparts of higher socioeconomic status.

Robinson (1991) and Robinson and Frank (1994) studied 299 high school students and 16 pregnant adolescents to examine the relationships among self-esteem, sexual activity, gender, and pregnancy. No differences were found in self-esteem in regard to pregnancy, gender, and sexual activity. Males who had fathered a child had lower self-esteem than nonfathers had.

One hundred and two low income women in their third trimester of pregnancy were studied by Edwards (1991/1992) to determine differences in self-esteem and sense of mastery between those who obtained adequate prenatal care and those who obtained inadequate prenatal care. Both self-esteem and sense of mastery were higher among the women who obtained adequate prenatal care than in women who did not. Education and level of poverty influenced adequacy of prenatal care, but self-esteem and sense of mastery exerted an effect independent of education or poverty.

Christian (1993) studied 23 women to determine the relationship between self-esteem and the number, frequency, and severity of symptoms of endometriosis. The symptoms of endometriosis interfered with their activities of daily living, but no significant correlations appeared between self-esteem and the number, frequency, and severity of symptoms.

Chen (1994) studied 88 elders with a hearing loss to determine the relationships among hearing handicap, loneliness, and self-esteem. Hearing handicap was related to loneliness and low self-esteem in women but not in men. The greater the hearing handicap, the greater the loneliness and the lower the self-esteem.

Self-concept and pregnancy. Adaptation in the self-concept mode was examined in two studies in relation to pregnancy but self esteem was not specifically examined. (Table 4.2). Bergin (1985/1986) examined self-concept, depression, powerlessness, and feelings of loss of control in 15 marital dyads experiencing primary infertility. Infertility was associated with frustration, negative self-concept, powerlessness, and loss of control. Female partners were significantly more depressed than the males.

To determine differences in maternal identity between younger and older primiparae during the third trimester of pregnancy, Shaffer (1988/1989) studied 33 primiparous women. Age was not a significant factor in maternal identity, but the younger women perceived their somatic symptoms more negatively than did their older counterparts.

Self-concept and chronic illness. In 6 of the 18 self-concept studies, the research focused on adaptation to chronic illness (Table 4.3). To explore the process of sexual adaptation, Lamb (1991) interviewed 19 women who had undergone treatment for endometrial cancer. Sexual adaptation was a process that evolved over time and was enhanced by internal and external factors. The women experienced major changes in self-concept, self-esteem, body image, and sexual functioning.

Morris (1991/1992) studied 29 women newly diagnosed with breast cancer and undergoing adjuvant treatment to determine if a relationship between symptom distress and life quality existed. Symptom distress was negatively related to current life quality and to six-month predicted life quality. Chemotherapy was positively related to the number of symptoms experienced and negatively related to current life quality and six-month predicted life quality. Hormone therapy was negatively related to the number of symptoms experienced and positively related to current life quality and six-month predicted life quality.

Elders with and without cancer were studied by McGill (1991/1992) and McGill and Paul (1993) to determine the relationship between functional status and hope and to determine if differences existed between the two groups with respect to hope and functional status. Education, perceived financial status, and physical health were related to hope. However, no difference in hope was found between those under treatment for cancer and healthy age peers. Age and gender were not significantly related to hope.

A pilot study was conducted by Samaral and Fawcett (1992) of six women with breast cancer and their coaches who were participating in a cancer support group. Attendance ranged from 75% to 100% with illness being the primary reason for nonattendance. Participants learned skills and techniques and developed social supports that assisted them with adaptation.

Table 4.2 – Description of Studies About Self-Concept and Pregnancy in the Self-Concept Adaptive Mode of the RAM (N=2)

Author(s) & Date	Purpose	Sample	Design	Findings
11. Bergin (1985/1986)	To examine certain psychosocial and emotional reactions among married couples experiencing primary infertility	Married partners with primary infertility (N=30)	Descriptive	Female partners were significantly more depressed than were the male partners. Infertility was associated with stress, lowered self-concept, powerlessness, and loss of control.
12. Shaffer (1988/1989)	To determine if there was a difference in maternal identity between younger and older primiparae during the third trimester of pregnancy	Primiparae age 20-30 (n=20), age 35 and older (n=13); N = 33	Descriptive	There was no significant difference in maternal identity between younger and older primiparae during the third trimester of pregnancy. Younger primiparae perceived their somatic symptoms more negatively than did their older counterparts.

Table 4.3 – Description of Studies About Self-Concept and Chronic Illness in the Self-Concept Adaptive Mode of the RAM (N=6)

Author(s) & Date	Purpose	Sample	Design	Findings
13. Lamb (1991)	To explore the process of sexual adaptation in women treated for endometrial cancer	Women treated for endometrial cancer (N=19)	Grounded theory & Correlational	Sexual adaptation was a process that evolved over time in women who underwent treatment for endometrial cancer. Internal and external factors enhanced adaptation.

Study	Purpose	Sample	Design	Findings
14. Morris (1991/1992)	To determine if there was a relationship between symptom distress and life quality in women undergoing adjuvant treatment for breast cancer	Women newly diagnosed with breast cancer (N=29)	Correlational	Symptom distress was negatively related to current life quality and to 6 month predicted life quality. Chemotherapy was positively related to the number of symptoms experienced and negatively related to current life quality.
15. McGill (1991/1992)	To determine if there was a relationship between functional status and hope in elders with and without cancer and to determine if there were differences between these two groups with respect to hope and functional status	Elders under treatment in outpatient oncology clinic (n=86), healthy elders (n=88); (N=174)	Descriptive	Education, perceived financial status, and physical health were significantly related to hope. There was no significant difference in hope between elders with and without cancer. Time use and physical health were the only domains of functional status that predicted group membership. Age and gender were not significantly related to hope.
16. McGill & Paul (1993)	To determine if there was a relationship between functional status and hope in elderly people with and without cancer and to determine if there were differences between these groups with respect to hope and functional status	Adults ≥ 65 years, outpatients of an oncology clinic (n=86), healthy adults ≥ 65 (n=88)	Descriptive	Education, perceived financial status, and physical health were significantly related to hope. There was no significant difference in hope scores between the two groups. Time use and physical health were the only domains that allowed prediction of group membership. Age and gender were not significantly related to hope.

(continued)

Table 4.3 (continued)

Author(s) & Date	Purpose	Sample	Design	Findings
17. Samaral & Fawcett (1992)	To determine rates of attendance, reasons for attrition, training procedures, and content for cancer support groups	Women with breast cancer (n=6) and their coaches (n=6)	Descriptive	Attendance ranged from 75% to 100% with illness being the primary reason for nonattendance. Participants learned skills and developed social supports.
18. Bertch (1993/1994)	To describe the adaptation of persons with chronic obstructive pulmonary disease (COPD)	Oxygen dependent adults with COPD (N=56)	Correlational	Participants < 62 years of age had significantly lower life satisfaction than those > age 62. There were no differences in life satisfaction related to gender, race, marital status, education, length of time on oxygen, or amount of oxygen.

To describe the adaptation of persons with chronic obstructive pulmonary disease (COPD), Bertch (1993/1994) studied 56 adults who were oxygen dependent. Participants less than 62 years of age had lower life satisfaction than those age 62 and older. Race, gender, marital status, education, employment status, length of time on oxygen, and amount of oxygen were not related to life satisfaction.

Critical Analysis of Reported Research

Based on the description of the 18 studies reviewed in this chapter, research in the self-concept adaptive mode was critically analyzed and evaluated with respect to the quality of the research and the relationship to the RAM. From this analysis, contributions to nursing science were synthesized. As is typical in such investigations, reviews were limited to reports of studies as retrieved, with no additional information sought from the authors. Seventeen self-concept adaptive mode studies were quantitative, and one was qualitative. Critical analyses are presented separately for the quantitative and qualitative studies.

Critical analyses of quantitative research. Critical analyses of the 17 quantitative studies are presented in Table 4.4. In 10 of the 17 studies, measures to control for threats to internal validity were adequately addressed, while threats to external validity were adequately addressed in 11 of the studies.

In the quantitative studies, threats to validity were focused on several issues. History and maturation were potential threats to internal validity in the three studies in which data were collected during more than one time period. For example, Morris (1991/1992) analyzed data from 29 women whose ages ranged from 35 to 72 years old, who had received a variety of treatments for breast cancer and approximately half of whom worked at least part time. Data were collected at two times, 6 weeks apart. No measures were reported that addressed the potential threats to history and maturation. A pilot study briefly reported by Samaral and Fawcett (1992) did not include sufficient information to adequately address any of the threats to internal or external validity.

Instrumentation was a potential threat to internal validity in another quantitative study. Bergin (1985/1986) used research assistants but did not clearly report how the assistants were trained. Mortality was a potential threat to internal validity in the studies that collected data at more than one time. Three other studies also had a problem with loss of subjects. Bertch (1993/1994) had a 56% response rate and did not report any information on the 44% who failed to return the questionnaires. Similarly, Christian (1993) had a 47% response rate and did not report any information on the 53% who failed to return the questionnaires.

Sampling techniques affected both internal and external validity. Convenience samples were used in all the studies, but most researchers identi-

Table 4.4 – Critical Analysis of Quantitative Self-Concept Adaptive Mode Research (*N*=17)

Criteria	Evaluation		
	Yes	*Partially*	*No*
Design			
Threats to Internal Validity Controlled	1, 2, 4, 5, 8, 10, 12, 15, 16, 18	6, 9, 11	3, 7, 14, 17
Threats to External Validity Controlled	1, 2, 4, 5, 8, 10, 11, 12, 15, 16, 18		3, 6, 7, 9, 14, 17
Measurement			
Reliability of Instruments Addressed	1, 2, 3, 4, 5, 6, 7, 8, 10, 11, 12, 14, 15, 16, 18		9, 17
Validity of Instruments Addressed	1, 2, 3, 4, 5, 6, 7, 8, 10, 11, 12, 14, 15, 16, 18		9, 17
Data Analysis			
Appropriate	1, 2, 4, 5, 6, 7, 8, 9, 10, 11, 12, 14, 15, 16, 17, 18		3
Interpretation of Results			
Consistency of Findings with Conclusions	1, 2, 4, 5, 8, 9, 10, 11, 12, 15, 16, 18	17	3, 6, 7, 14

Key: 1=Holcombe, 1985/1986; 2= Lavender, 1988/1989; 3=McRae, 1990/1991; 4=Foster, 1989/1990; 5=Stein, 1991/1992; 6=Robinson, 1991; 7=Robinson & Frank, 1994; 8=Edwards, 1991/ 1992; 9=Christian, 1993; 10=Chen, 1994; 11=Bergin, 1985/1986; 12=Shaffer, 1988/1989; 14=Morris, 1991/1992; 15=McGill, 1991/1992; 16= McGill & Paul, 1993; 17=Samaral & Fawcett, 1992; 18=Bertch, 1993/1994 fied inclusion criteria and described the sample. However, McGill (1991/1992) and McGill and Paul (1993) eliminated subjects with cognitive impairment from part of the data analysis even though cognitive impairment was not identified as an exclusion factor before data were collected. Robinson (1991) and Robinson and Frank (1994) obtained students from university high schools, which may have introduced selection bias and affected generalizibility of the findings. The subjects who participated in Chen's (1994) and McRae's (1990/1991) studies were well educated. Couples studied by Bergin (1985/1986) were all Caucasian and the majority were Roman Catholic. Shaffer (1988/1989) and Morris (1991/1992) had small samples which were then divided into groups that may not have been representative of the population. Thus, representativeness of subjects was a threat to external validity in these studies.

Control of the environment was a threat to external validity in five quantitative studies. McRae (1990/1991) gave subjects the option to complete the instruments at home with specific instructions regarding time limitations. Out of 70 women, 68 elected to complete the questionnaires at home with no external control over the time or conditions under which the instruments were completed. Robinson (1991) and Robinson and Frank (1994) collected some data at a prenatal clinic and other data at high schools—very different environments. Morris (1991/1992) analyzed data that had been collected as part of another study and did not discuss the environment for data collection. The environment in which data were collected from the mothers of kindergarten children was not controlled by Lavender (1988/1989).

Consistency of treatment was adequately controlled in all of the studies. Control of extraneous variables was at least partially addressed by eight of the quantitative studies. However, Robinson (1991) and Robinson and Frank (1994) did not control for socioeconomic status or family environment. The other studies had a variety of extraneous variables that were not controlled.

Reliability and validity of the instruments were adequately addressed in all but two studies. Data analysis was not appropriate in one study; interpretation of the results was a problem in five studies. Samaral and Fawcett (1992) and Christian (1993) did not include any information about the reliability and validity of the instruments. McRae (1990/1991) planned to analyze data using stepwise multiple regression but reported the results as correlations. Also, higher scores on the symptom checklist represented less difficulty but were interpreted as more difficult, which made the interpretation of the data inconsistent with the findings. Robinson (1991) and Robinson and Frank (1994) did not specify an alpha level for statistical significance and accepted $p=<.088$ as statistically significant. In discussing conclusions, Morris (1991/1992) used two different scales for symptom distress without differentiating between the two.

The investigation of differences in self-esteem and sense of mastery between low-income pregnant women who obtain adequate prenatal care and their counterparts who obtain inadequate prenatal care (Edwards, 1991/1992) was one quantitative study in which most of the criteria for critical analyses were met. For example, pregnant women with concurrent illness or complications of pregnancy were not included. ANCOVA was used to control for level of poverty, age, education, race, marital status, parity, and number of preschoolers. All data were collected by the investigator in prenatal clinics associated with a state public health department. Consistent procedures were followed with each subject and were described clearly. The reliability and validity of the instruments was described, and the interpretation of the results was consistent with the data.

Critical analyses of qualitative research. Critical analyses of the one qualitative self-concept mode study is shown in Table 4.5. The one qualitative study demonstrated strategies to ensure validity, strategies to ensure reliability, appropriate methods for data analysis, and consistency between findings and conclusions.

Lamb (1991) demonstrated all of the criteria for validity: descriptive vividness, methodologic congruence, analytical preciseness, theoretic connectedness, and heuristic relevance. The experience of collecting the data; rigor in documentation, procedure, ethics, and auditability; identification of the decision-making processes to transform data; clarification of concepts and relationships among concepts; and recognition, relationship, and applicability of findings were all addressed. Lamb also demonstrated the criteria for reliability–researcher position, participant choice, social situation conditions, and methods of procedure. The method for data analysis, content analysis using the constant comparative method, was appropriate, and the interpretation of the results was consistent with the findings.

Evaluation of Relationships to the RAM

Based on critical analyses of the research, studies were included in the evaluation of relationships to the RAM if threats to internal or external validity were not a problem, if reliability and validity of instruments were addressed, if data analyses were appropriate, and if consistency was found between results and conclusions. Twelve of the 18 self-concept adaptive mode studies met the criteria for inclusion.

Evaluation of Linkages to the RAM

Evaluation of the linkages between the self-concept adaptive mode studies and the RAM is summarized in Table 4.6. The linkages between the research variables, empiric measures, findings, and the RAM were evaluated for each of the 12 studies.

Table 4.5 – Critical Analysis of Qualitative Self-Concept Adaptive Mode Research (*N*=1)

Criteria	Evaluation		
	Yes	*Partially*	*No*
Design			
Strategies to ensure validity used	13		
Strategies to ensure reliability used	13		
Data analysis			
Appropriate method	13		
Interpretation of results			
Consistency of findings with conclusions	13		

Key: 13=Lamb,1991

Most of the self-concept studies made explicit linkages of the research variables, empiric measures, and findings to the RAM. For example, Bertch (1994) identified COPD and its oxygen requirements as the focal stimulus, while gender, age, race, marital status, education, employment status, length of time on oxygen, and amount of oxygen were identified as contextual stimuli. The body's response to oxygenation was described as part of the physiologic mode and processed through the regulator. The Life Satisfaction Index was explicitly linked to the adaptive modes, and a person's level of life satisfaction was identified as an indicator of a response that could be adaptive or ineffective. The findings were discussed in relation to the RAM.

The study by Holcombe (1985/1986) is another example of a self-concept adaptive mode study that made explicit linkages of the research variables, empiric measures, and findings to the RAM. Cancer and its treatment were identified as stimuli. The person's perceptions of cancer and of social support operate through the cognator subsystem and affect that person's response to the stimuli. The person's level of adaptation was evidenced through the self-concept mode, specifically in the person's self-esteem. The empiric measures, Norbeck Social Support Questionnaire, Perception of Illness Questionnaire, and Coopersmith Self-Esteem Inventory were explicitly linked to the RAM. The findings were discussed in relation to the RAM.

Only one self-concept mode study did not link the findings to the RAM. Chen (1994) explicitly linked the research variables and empiric measures to the RAM but failed to link the findings to the RAM.

Testing of Propositions from the RAM

Criteria were developed to determine which quantitative and qualitative research studies would be included in the testing of RAM propositions. Studies were included if internal or external validity was not a problem, if consistency was found between results and conclusions, and if the variables were either explicitly or implicitly related to the RAM. Twelve of the 18 self-concept adaptive mode studies met the criteria for inclusion. From the Roy Model propositions listed in Chapter 2, studies in the self-concept adaptive mode were used to test six propositions (Table 4.7).

Six propositions from the RAM were supported or not supported by results of self-concept adaptive mode research. The proposition that, at the individual level, regulator and cognator processes affect innate and acquired ways of adapting, was supported by Edwards (1991/1992), who found that adequacy of prenatal care was related to self-esteem and sense of mastery. Participants with high self-esteem responded to pregnancy with the adaptive response of obtaining adequate prenatal care, while their counterparts with low self-esteem did not obtain adequate prenatal care, thereby demonstrating an ineffective response to pregnancy. Likewise subjects with a strong sense of mastery responded with the adaptive behavior of obtaining adequate prenatal care while those with a low sense of mastery responded with the ineffective behavior of failing to obtain adequate prenatal care.

The proposition that characteristics of the internal and external stimuli influence adaptive responses was supported by Lamb (1991) and Bertch (1993) but was not supported by McGill (1991/1992), McGill and Paul (1993), and Shaffer (1988/1989). Lamb found that internal and external factors enhanced adaptation. Internal factors included viewing self as strong, being a fighter, keeping busy, and feeling content with life. External factors included the strength derived from partner, family, friends, formal support groups, and religion.

As a contextual stimulus, age was related to life satisfaction (Bertch, 1993). Participants with COPD who were younger than 62 years of age had significantly lower life satisfaction scores than their counterparts who were 62 years of age or older. However, age was not significantly related to hope (McGill, 1991/1992; McGill & Paul, 1993) or to maternal identity (Shaffer, 1988/1989). In elders receiving outpatient treatment for cancer and among healthy elders, age was not significantly related to hope (McGill

Table 4.6 – Evaluation of Linkages to the RAM (*N*=12)

| | Evaluation | | |
	Explicit	*Implicit*	*Absent*
Research variables	1,2,4,5,8, 11,12,13,15, 16,18		
Empirical measures	1,2,4,5,8,10 11,12,13,15, 16,18		
Findings	1,2,4,5,8, 11,12,13, 15,16,18		10

Key: 1=Holcombe, 1985/1986; 2=Lavender, 1988/1989; 4=Foster, 1989/1990; 5=Stein, 1991/1992; 8=Edwards, 1991/1992; 10=Chen, 1994; 11=Bergin, 1985/1986; 12=Shaffer, 1988/1989; 13=Lamb, 1991; 15=McGill, 1991/1992; 16=McGill & Paul, 1993; 18=Bertch, 1993/1994

1991/1992; McGill & Paul, 1993). Shaffer 1988/1989 found no significant difference in maternal identity between younger and older primiparous women during the third trimester of pregnancy.

The proposition that adaptation in one mode is affected by adaptation in other modes through cognator and regulator connectives was supported by Chen (1994), McGill (1991/1992), McGill and Paul (1993), and Bergin (1985/1986). Even though these studies focused primarily on the self-concept mode, the effects on other modes was also a factor. Hearing handicap was related to loneliness and self-esteem (Chen). The greater the hearing handicap, the greater the loneliness and the lower the self-esteem. McGill and McGill and Paul found that physical health was related to hope. The intercorrelations of the domains of the Multilevel Assessment Instrument affirmed the interrelationships of the modes.

In a study of 15 marital partners with primary infertility, Bergin (1985/1986) found that infertility was associated with stress, lowered self-concept, feelings of powerlessness and frustration, and loss of control. The women had significantly higher depression scores than did the men, but the mean depression scores were within normal range.

The proposition that the combined effect of focal, contextual, and residual stimuli determines the adaptation level was supported by Lavender (1988/1989), Foster (1989/1990), Stein (1991/1992), McGill (1991/1992),

Table 4.7 – Testing of Propositions from the RAM (N=12)

Propositions from the RAM	Ancillary and practice propositions	Supported by results	Not supported by results
1. At the individual level, regulator and cognator processes affect innate and acquired ways of adapting.	Adequacy of prenatal care is related to self-esteem and sense of mastery.	Edwards (1991/1992)	
3. The characteristics of the internal and external stimuli influence adaptive responses.	a. Internal and external factors enhance adaptation.	Lamb (1991)	
	b. Life satisfaction is related to age.	Bertch (1993/1994)	
	c. Age is related to hope.		McGill (1991/1992) McGill & Paul (1993)
	d. Age is related to maternal identity.		Shaffer (1988/1989)
6. Adaptation in one mode is affected by adaptation in other modes through cognator and regulator connectives.	a. Hearing handicap is related to loneliness and self-esteem.	Chen (1994)	
	b. Physical health is related to hope.	McGill (1991/1992) McGill & Paul 1993)	
	c. Infertility is associated with stress, low self-concept, and powerlessness.	Bergin (1985/1986)	

7. The pooled effect of focal, contextual, and residual stimuli determines the adaptation level.	a. Child care arrangements, family structure, age, and gender are related to self-esteem of kindergarten children.	Lavender (1988/1989)
	b. Family structure is related to self-esteem in adolescents.	Foster (1989/1990)
	c. Powerlessness and life events are related to self-esteem in adolescents.	Stein (1991/1992)
	d. Education and perceived financial status are related to hope.	McGill (1992/1992) McGill & Paul (1993)
9. The variable of time influences the process of adaptation.	Sexual adaptation is a process that evolves over time.	Lamb (1991)
10. The variable of perception influences the process of adaptation.	a. Self-esteem is related to perceptions of illness, love, respect, and affirmation.	Holcombe (1985/1986)
	b. Perception of somatic symptoms varies with age.	Shaffer (1988/1989)

and McGill and Paul (1993). Lavender found that the contextual stimuli of child care arrangements, family structure, age, and sex were related to the self-esteem of kindergarten children. Being cared for by a parent, living in a two-parent family, being young, and being a male were related to higher self-esteem.

Foster (1989/1990) found that family structure was related to self-esteem in adolescents. If the female adolescent had never been pregnant but had a mother and sibling or a sibling who had a child during adolescence, her self-esteem was significantly lower than her counterpart whose mother or sibling had not had a child during adolescence.

Powerlessness and life events were related to self-esteem in adolescents (Stein, 1991/1992), with a significant difference between levels of self-esteem and powerlessness among adolescents of differing socioeconomic classes. An increased number of life events and feelings of powerlessness predicted lower levels of self-esteem among adolescents.

McGill (1991/1992) and McGill and Paul (1993) found that education and perceived financial status were related to hope. Inadequate income and education indicated that elders with lower socioeconomic status may be more susceptible to lower levels of hope.

The study conducted by Lamb (1991) supported the proposition that the variable of time influences the process of adaptation. The researcher found that sexual adaptation was a process that evolved over time. Consequently, sexual adaptation was viewed as the achievement of optimal sexual functioning and satisfaction and was seen as a process affected by both internal and external factors rather than a state.

The proposition that the variable of perception influences the process of adaptation was supported by Holcombe (1985/1986) and Shaffer (1988/1989). Holcombe found that self-esteem of women with gynecologic cancer was related to their perceptions of illness and their perceptions of love, respect, and affirmation from others. These women perceived that they received support primarily from family members or relatives. Shaffer found that perception of somatic symptoms varied with age. Younger primiparae perceived their physiologic functions more negatively than their older counterparts.

Synthesis of Self-Concept Mode Research: Contributions to Nursing Science

Contributions to nursing science were derived from critical analysis of self-concept research and from evaluation of relationships to the RAM. Studies are discussed in relation to their contributions to clinical practice, research, and theory. Contributions and recommendations for future work were identified in those studies that met the established guidelines. Twelve self-concept mode studies were included in the synthesis (Table 4.8).

Applications to Nursing Practice

Findings from the two studies which examined self-esteem in adolescents have high potential for implementation in nursing practice. High potential, or category one, is defined in Chapter 2, based on empiric support and clinical risk. Clinical implications from the study by Foster (1989/1990) would lead the nurse working with female adolescents to assess the self-concept mode to identify adaptive and ineffective behaviors and how the young woman values herself. If the adolescent had high self-esteem (adaptive behavior), nursing interventions could focus on maintaining that level of self-esteem. If the adolescent had low self-esteem (ineffective behavior), nursing interventions would emphasize improving the level of self-esteem. When working with adolescents whose sibling or whose mother and sibling had a child during adolescence, the nurse would assess self-esteem and plan interventions accordingly.

As a result of the study by Stein (1991/1992), nurses who work with adolescents need to assess for recent significant life events that have been perceived negatively or as uncontrollable. These adolescents may be at risk for feelings of powerlessness and low self-esteem. The nurse may be able to help identify choices and options which decrease the feelings of powerlessness and enhance self-esteem. When caring for ill adolescents, the nurse may find a risk for feeling powerless. Thus, providing opportunities to choose the timing and sequences of procedures may decrease feelings of powerlessness thereby increasing levels of self-esteem. Nurses

---

Table 4.8 – Potential for Implementation from Self-Concept Adaptive Mode Research (*N*=12)

Category One: High potential for implementation
    Foster (1989/1990)
    Stein (1991/1992)
    Edwards (1991/1992)
    McGill (1991/1992)
    McGill & Paul (1993)
    Chen (1994)
    Lavender (1988/1989)

Category Two: Needs further clinical evaluation before implementation
    Bertch (1993/1994)
    Holcombe (1985/1986)
    Lamb (1991)

Category Three: Further research indicated before implementation
    Bergin (1985/1986)
    Shaffer (1988/1989)

---

need to be aware that youth from lower socioeconomic strata are more likely to experience feelings of powerlessness and low self-esteem than those from higher strata. Consequently, interventions may be needed to encourage decision making and build self-esteem in these young people.

The findings from the study by Edwards (1991/1992) have application for nurses working with low-income women. Because high self-esteem and sense of mastery were associated with the adaptive response of obtaining prenatal care, assessment of self-esteem and sense of mastery is indicated. When assessment reveals problems in the self-concept adaptive mode, the nurse may intervene by managing stimuli to improve the woman's self-esteem and sense of mastery. This could result in the woman adapting more effectively to pregnancy by obtaining adequate prenatal care.

The findings from the study conducted by McGill (1991/1992) and McGill and Paul (1993) have high potential for implementation in nursing practice. When caring for elders, nurses need to promote physical health and consider the contextual stimulus of socioeconomic status in order to support hope and adaptation. If improving physical health and socioeconomic status is not possible, nurses need to assist clients in identifying other sources of hope and strategies to alleviate financial distress. For example, nurses may help clients to set and achieve short term goals to foster hope. Nurses may collaborate with family, friends, or social workers to help identify strategies that will alleviate financial distress.

Findings from the study by Chen (1994) have application to nurses working with the elderly who have a hearing handicap. Detection of hearing problems and early intervention promote independence, the ability to maintain contact with the environment, and self-esteem. Assisting the elderly to successfully adjust to hearing aids is a primary intervention. Nurses need to give special support to elderly women who have a hearing handicap as they may suffer more emotional difficulties than elderly men.

Assisting parents with understanding their child's development of self-esteem is an important responsibility for the practicing nurse. Many working mothers would benefit from the study conducted by Lavender (1988/1989) who found no significant difference in self-esteem scores between kindergarten children of working mothers and those whose mothers did not work. Nonworking mothers who choose not to supplement the family's income may be helped to learn that socioeconomic status was not related to self-esteem in the kindergarten child. When a kindergarten child has the contextual stimulus of living in a one-parent family structure, interventions may be needed to foster self-esteem.

Findings from three studies need further clinical evaluation before implementation (category two). Considering the focal stimulus of COPD with oxygen dependency and the contextual stimulus of age less than 62 years, clinical nurse experts need to assist with a long-term focus on adaptive processes when working with these clients. Collaboration with community resources in order to develop adaptive physiologic and psychosocial behaviors for persons with COPD is imperative if optimum life satisfaction is to be achieved (Bertch, 1993/1994).

Results from the studies by Holcombe (1985/1986) and Lamb (1991) also need further evaluation by clinical nurse experts before implementation. When confronted with the focal stimulus of gynecological cancer, nurses need to assess the need for social support and provide appropriate resources when indicated. Nurses can allow clients to express their concerns about the disease and then provide resources to meet their support needs. Continuity of care and nursing case management are imperative because sexual adaptation to endometrial cancer extends over a period of time.

Findings from two studies need further testing before implementation (category three). Results of the study by Bergin (1985/1986) need to be evaluated using a larger sample and examining the role of support groups with couples experiencing primary infertility. Bergin suggests that nurses refer these couples to support groups, but all of her subjects came from a support group and the effectiveness of this intervention was not examined. Whether support groups are appropriate for everyone experiencing infertility or whether they should be for women, for men, or for couples, is not known.

Findings from the study conducted by Shaffer (1988/1989) also need further testing before implementation. Although most threats to internal and exernal validity were controlled, the sample was small ($N=33$), especially in the group of older primiparae ($n=13$). The finding of no significant difference in maternal identity between younger and older primiparae during the third trimester of pregnancy may have been due to the small sample. Consequently, this finding needs additional study before being implemented in practice.

Recommendations for Model-Based Research

Future directions for model-based research were identified from all studies with applications to nursing practice but were most obvious in the studies where further testing was indicated. In addition, studies in which findings were equivocal or differed from previous research are priority areas for further research.

Methodologic studies to develop instruments based on RAM to measure self-concept and self-esteem in adolescents are needed (Foster, 1989/1990; Stein, 1991/1992). In addition, further analysis and instrument development of the powerlessness concept and life event scale for adolescents is warranted (Stein, 1991/1992). Improved measures for social support and hope in the elderly population are needed (McGill, 1991/1992; McGill & Paul, 1993).

Longitudinal studies are needed to examine changes in self-esteem and adaptation in adolescents (Foster, 1989/1990; Stein, 1991/1992); in children (Lavender (1988/1989); in women with gynecologic cancer (Holcombe, 1985/1986; Lamb, 1991); and throughout pregnancy and postpartum (Edwards, 1991/1992). Longitudinal studies are needed with elders to identify changes in functional status and hope over time (McGill, 1991/1992; McGill & Paul, 1993).

Intervention studies are needed to determine which techniques support hope and adaptation in elders (McGill, 1991/1992; McGill & Paul, 1993); to test interventions for increasing self-esteem and sense of mastery in low income women (Edwards, 1991/1992); and to explore strategies that foster social support and increase self-esteem in women with gynecologic cancer (Holcombe, 1985/1986; Lamb, 1991).

The variables affecting self-esteem of the kindergarten child, especially the father's influence and school environment, need further investigation (Lavender, 1988/1989). Delineation of internal and external factors influencing sexual adaptation of women with endometrial cancer requires additional study (Lamb, 1991). To identify variables that influence the amount and type of social support required by women with gynecologic cancer, further research is needed (Holcombe, 1985/1986).

The study conducted by Bergin (1985/1986) needs to be replicated using a larger sample that includes minority groups and persons from lower socioeconomic strata. In addition, the effect of infertility support groups needs investigation. Is a support group helpful to all infertile couples? Is it helpful for women, for men, or both? Does length of time experiencing infertility affect adaptation? What relationships exist among infertility and psychological, demographic, and coping variables?

The study conducted by Shaffer (1988/1989) needs to be replicated using a larger sample consisting of different age groups to determine whether the sample size influenced the findings. Women need to be studied over the entire child-bearing period to determine if maternal identity changes throughout pregnancy. To determine if age-specific differences exist in a primipara's perception of maternal identity, assessment tools need to be developed and tested. Consequently, numerous recommendations exist for model-based research from these self-concept adaptive mode studies.

Directions for Theory and RAM Development

Research in the self-concept adaptive mode contributed to identifying directions for further development of theory and the RAM. Three clear directions were identified from propositions tested by the reported research. First, the mixed findings related to the characteristics of the internal and external stimuli influencing adaptive responses indicated that further conceptual and theoretic development was needed in this area. Second, the manner in which regulator and cognator processes affect innate and acquired ways of adapting at the individual level needed further development. Third, the influence of time on the process of adaptation needed further clarification and development.

In four self-concept mode studies, the characteristic of age as a stimulus had mixed results. Roy (Roy & Andrews, 1991) clearly identified age as a contextual stimulus which is a factor in the developmental stage of the client and a common stimulus affecting adaptation. Age is to be assessed as part of the second level of assessment. The importance of age on urinary elimination was specific, but the effect of age on various psychosocial variables was less clear. Because age was a contextual stimulus in the reported research that both supported and did not support the proposition, future RAM development needs to consider clarifying the role of age as a contextual stimulus.

Only one self-concept adaptive mode study tested the proposition that regulator and cognator processes affect innate and acquired ways of adapting at the individual level. Stimuli activate the regulator and cognator coping mechanisms which result in behavioral responses. The first level of assessment involves gathering data about the person's behavior and level of adaptation (Roy & Andrews, 1991). Future RAM development needs to clarify strategies to assist with identifying regulator and cognator processes because this is a key proposition that requires assessment of behaviors that reflect adaptation.

The effects of the passage of time on the process of adaptation was examined in one self-concept study. In a review of research on human information processing, Roy (1988) identified this experience of time as a variable evident in the literature. Responses were varied according to the individual, and the need for adequate methods to study effects of time was apparent. However, the concept of time as a key variable has not been explored or integrated in the RAM. Based on this analysis, this concept of time is an important concept for future development of the RAM.

Summary

Theoretic frameworks that reflect a multidimensional holistic approach, such as the RAM, are important for nursing research because the discipline claims to focus on the whole person. Of the final 163 nursing studies included in this monograph, 18 focused primarily on the self-concept adaptive mode. The numerous applications for nursing practice also support the value of using the RAM to guide research in the self-concept adaptive mode. Scholarly inquiry in clinical practice that is guided by a nursing model not only will evaluate proposed interventions but will refine the theories and knowledge needed to direct nursing practice. In addition, areas for further development of the self-concept mode and the RAM will be made explicit from the empiric and clinical findings. Finally, using a nursing model to guide practice and research will strengthen the interrelationships among theory, research, and practice.

References

Bergin, M.A. (1986). Psychosocial responses of marital couples experiencing primary infertility (Doctoral dissertation, Temple University, 1985). *Dissertation Abstracts International, 46*, 2197-A.

Bertch, D.A. (1994). Life satisfaction of persons with chronic obstructive pulmonary disease (Master's thesis, Grand Valley State University, 1993). *Masters Abstracts International, 34*, 1165.

Chen, H-L. (1994). Hearing in the elderly: Relation of hearing loss, loneliness, and self-esteem. *Journal of Gerontological Nursing, 20*(6), 22-28.

Christian, A. (1993). The relationship between women's symptoms of endometriosis and self-esteem. *Journal of Obstetric, Gynecologic, & Neonatal Nursing, 22*, 370-376.

Edwards, M.R. (1992). Self-esteem, sense of mastery, and adequacy of prenatal care (Doctoral dissertation, University of Alabama at Birmingham, 1991). *Dissertation Abstracts International, 53*, 768-B.

Foster, P.L. (1990). The relationship between selected variables and the self-esteem in adolescent females (Doctoral dissertation, University of Alabama at Birmingham, 1989). *Dissertation Abstracts International, 50*, 3918-B.

Holcombe, J.K. (1986). Social support, perception of illness, and self-esteem of women with gynecologic cancer (Doctoral dissertation, The University of Alabama in Birmingham, 1985). *Dissertation Abstracts International, 47*, 1928-B.

Lamb, M.A. (1991). Sexual adaptation of women treated for endometrial cancer (Doctoral dissertation, Boston College, 1991). *Dissertation Abstracts International, 52*, 2994-B.

Lavender, M.G. (1989). The relationship between maternal self-esteem, work status, and sociodemographic characteristics and self-esteem of the kindergarten child (Doctoral dissertation, The University of Alabama in Birmingham, 1988). *Dissertation Abstracts International, 49*, 5229-B.

McGill, J.S. (1992). Functional status as it relates to hope in elders with and without cancer (Doctoral dissertation, The University of Alabama in Birmingham, 1991). *Dissertation Abstracts International, 53*, 771-B.

McGill, J.S., & Paul, P.B. (1993). Functional status and hope in elderly people with and without cancer. *Oncology Nursing Forum, 20*, 1207-1213.

McRae, M.G. (1991). Adaptation to pregnancy and motherhood: Personality characteristics of primiparas age 30 years and older (Doctoral dissertation, Boston University, 1990). *Dissertation Abstracts International,* 51, 3326-B.

Morris, B.C. (1992). Relationship between symptom distress and life quality in women with breast cancer undergoing adjuvant treatment (Master's thesis, The University of Arizona, 1991). *Masters Abstracts International,* 30, 300.

Robinson, R. B. (1991). The relation between self-esteem and pregnancy in adolescent males and females. Unpublished master's thesis, Florida State University, Tallahassee.

Robinson, R.B., & Frank, D. I. (1994). The relation between self-esteem, sexual activity, and pregnancy. *Adolescence,* 29(113), 27-35.

Roy, C., & Andrews, H. (1991). *The Roy Adaptation Model: The definitive statement.* Norwalk, CT: Appleton & Lange.

Roy, C., & Andrews, H. (1999). The Roy Adaptation Model (2nd ed.). Stamford, CT: Appleton & Lange.

Samaral, N., & Fawcett, J. (1992). Enhancing adaptation to breast cancer: The addition of coaching to support groups. *Oncology Nursing Forum,* 19, 591-596.

Shaffer, F.H. (1989). A comparison of maternal identity in younger and older primiparae during the third trimester of pregnancy (Doctoral dissertation, University of Alabama at Birmingham, 1988). *Dissertation Abstracts International,* 49, 4236-B.

Stein, P.R. (1992). Life events, self-esteem, and powerlessness among adolescents (Doctoral dissertation, Texas Woman's University, 1991). *Dissertation Abstracts International,* 52, 5195-B.

Bibliography

Roy, C. (1988). Human information processing. In J.J. Fitzpatrick, R.L. Taunton, & J.Q. Benoliel (Eds.), *Annual review of nursing research* (Vol. 6, pp. 237-262). New York: Springer.

Chapter 5

Role Function Mode Research

In this chapter we analyze research reported from 1970 through 1994 which was focused primarily on the role function adaptive mode of the Roy Adaptation Model (RAM). Twenty-one studies based on the RAM, including dissertations and theses, were categorized as role function mode research. Role function mode studies in which either an experimental or quasi-experimental design were used are in Chapter 9, except for one (Fawcett, Pollio, et al., 1993) which was part of a program of research and is included in this chapter. Studies that investigated adaptation in more modes than the role function mode and were not focused primarily on the role function mode are included in Chapter 7.

Purposes

The purposes in this chapter are to (a) critically analyze research in the role function adaptive mode, (b) evaluate the relationship of role function mode research to the RAM, and (c) synthesize contributions of reported studies to nursing science. Contributions to nursing science include applications for nursing practice, recommendations for model-based role function mode research, and directions for further theory and RAM development of the role function mode.

Background

The role function adaptive mode focuses specifically on the roles a person occupies in society. The basic need underlying the mode is social integrity, defined as the need to know who one is in relation to others, so that one can act appropriately (Roy & Andrews, 1991). Roles are classified as primary, secondary, and tertiary. The primary role determines the majority of behaviors and is influenced by age, developmental stage, and sex as with a 28-year-old, young adult woman. Secondary roles such as wife, mother, and nurse are assumed in order to complete the tasks associated with a primary role. Tertiary roles represent ways in which persons meet their obligations associated with secondary roles, such as the nurse being chair of a patient education committee (Roy & Andrews, 1991;1999).

Instrumental and expressive behaviors are associated with each role and provide an indication of social adaptation relative to role function. The goal of instrumental or goal-oriented behavior is role mastery, the demonstration of behavior that meets societal expectations. Instrumental behaviors are usually physical actions. The goal of expressive behavior is direct feedback from others. Expressive behaviors involve feelings and attitudes and result from interactions (Roy & Andrews, 1991).

Critical Analysis of Role Function Mode Research

Critical analysis of role function mode research has descriptive and analytic steps. First, the studies are briefly described, then they are analyzed according to the evaluative criteria developed by the BBARNS' team and described in Chapter 2.

Description of Reported Research

In the role function adaptive mode, 21 studies were categorized into four groups: (a) functional status instrument development ($n=5$), (b) adaptation to maternal role ($n=6$), (c) adaptation to cesarean birth ($n=7$), and (d) interactive roles ($n=3$). Functional status, defined as primary, secondary, and tertiary role behaviors, was derived from the role function mode of the RAM, and instruments were developed to assess functional status during selected life stages. The maternal role has three phases: childbearing, childbirth, and child rearing (Roy & Andrews, 1991). Considerable research was focused on the phases of adaptation to the maternal role with several researchers concentrating specifically on adaptation to cesarean birth. Emphasizing that roles exist in relationship to another person (Roy & Andrews, 1991), other researchers examined interactive roles.

Functional status instrument development. In 5 of the 21 studies, the focus of the research was to develop instruments to measure functional status (Table 5.1). These instruments were developed to measure functional status after childbirth (Fawcett, Tulman, & Myers, 1988), functional status during pregnancy (Tulman, Higgins, et al., 1991), paternal functional status during pregnancy and postpartum (Tulman, Fawcett, & Weiss, 1993), functional status in women who have cancer (Tulman, Fawcett, & McEvoy, 1991), and functional status in the elderly (Paier, 1994).

Each Inventory of Functional Status contained subscales which encompassed the dimensions of the roles of that life stage. The number of subscales varied from four to seven, and each subscale was classified as primary, secondary, or tertiary role behaviors. Primary role behaviors were represented by personal care activities. Secondary role behaviors were addressed by household, childcare, infant care, occupational, and educational activities. Tertiary role behaviors were represented by social and community activities. In all of the functional status instruments, higher scores indicated greater functional status. The section on critical analysis of instrument development studies and Table 5.7 contain information about reliability and validity of the instruments.

Table 5.1 – Description of Studies About Functional Status Instrument Development in the Role Function Mode of the RAM (N=5)

Author(s) & Date	Purpose	Sample	Design	Findings
1. Fawcett, Tulman, & Myers (1988)	To develop an instrument to assess functional status after childbirth	Women in 6th-10th week postpartum (N=76)	Instrument development	Development of Inventory of Functional Status after Childbirth. Reliability supported by Cronbach's alpha, item to subscale score, subscale to total score, and test-retest coefficients. Content validity supported by Popham's average congruency score. Construct validity supported by the subscale structure.
2. Tulman, Higgins, Fawcett, Nunno, Vansickel, Haas, & Speca (1991)	To develop an instrument to measure functional status during pregnancy	Pregnant women, most in third rimester (N=192)	Instrument development	Development of Inventory of Functional Status Antepartum Period. Reliability supported by item to subscale score, subscale to total score, and test-retest coefficients. Content validity supported by Popham's average congruency score. Construct validity partially supported by subscale structure and contrasted groups.

(continued)

Table 5.1 (continued)

Author(s) & Date	Purpose	Sample	Design	Findings
3. Tulman, Fawcett, & Weiss (1993)	To develop an instrument to measure paternal functional status during pregnancy and postpartum	Expectant fathers (*n*=125), new Fathers (*n*=57); *N*=182	Instrument development	Development of Inventory of Functional Status Fathers. Reliability supported by item to subscale score and subscale to total score coefficients. Content validity supported by Popham's average congruency score. Construct validity partially supported by subscale structure.
4. Tulman, Fawcett, & McEvoy (1991)	To develop an instrument to measure functional status in women who have cancer	Women under treatment in an ambulatory oncology clinic (*N*=100)	Instrument development	Development of Inventory of Functional Status Cancer. Reliability supported by item to subscale score, subscale to total score, and test-retest coefficients. Content validity supported by Popham's average congruency score. Construct validity was partially supported by subscale structure and contrasted groups.
5. Paier (1994)	To develop and determine psychometric properties of an instrument that measures functional status in usual role activities of well elderly	Independent residents of life care community (*n*=130) and community dwelling (*n*=24); *N*=154	Instrument development	Development of Inventory of Functional Status in the Elderly. Reliability supported by item to subscale score and subscale to total score. Test-retest reliability not supported. Content validity supported by content experts. Construct validity was supported by examining subscale correlations and by contrasted groups.

The Inventory of Functional Status After Childbirth (IFSAC) contained 36 items arranged in five subscales encompassing the dimensions of infant care, self-care, household activities, social and community activities, and occupational activities (Fawcett et al., 1988). Three versions of the instrument were developed sequentially. The earlier versions were semi-structured questionnaires and led to refinement of the IFSAC. Items were rated on a 4-point scale. Items rated not applicable were excluded from score calculations.

The Inventory of Functional Status—Antepartum Period (IFSAP) had 44 items arranged in six subscales encompassing the dimensions of childcare, personal care, household activities, social and community activities, educational activities, and occupational activities (Tulman, Higgins, et al., 1991). The IFSAP was developed as the antepartum counterpart of the IFSAC. Items were rated on a 3-point scale; items marked not applicable were excluded from the score.

The Inventory of Functional Status—Fathers (IFS-F) contained 51 items arranged in seven subscales encompassing the dimensions of childcare, infant care, personal care, household activities, social and community activities, educational activities, and occupational activities (Tulman et al., 1993). The IFS-F was developed as the paternal counterpart of the IFSAP and the IFSAC. Items were rated on a 4-point scale; items marked not applicable were excluded from the score.

A scale focused on cancer patients, the Inventory of Functional Status—Cancer (IFS-CA) had 39 items arranged in four subscales encompassing the dimensions of personal care, household and family activities, social and community activities, and occupational activities (Tulman, Fawcett, et al., 1991). The IFS-CA was developed to assess self-reported performance of primary, secondary, and tertiary role behaviors in women with cancer. Items were rated on a 4-point scale with a not applicable option.

The 48 items of the Inventory of Functional Status in the Elderly (IFSITE) were arranged in six subscales encompassing the dimensions of personal care, household activities, social and community activities, volunteer/work activities, care of another, and leisure activities (Paier, 1994). The IFSITE was developed to measure functional status in the usual role activities of the well elderly. Items for the scale were generated from content analysis of 14 interviews conducted with community-dwelling elderly. Items were rated on a 4-point scale with a not applicable code for items never engaged in by the respondent.

Adaptation to maternal role. In 6 of the 21 studies, the focus of the research was adaptation to the role of mother (Table 5.2). Tulman, Fawcett, Groblewski, and Silverman (1990) used the IFSAC in a longitudinal study to explore changes in role performance during the first 6 months following childbirth. Data were collected at 3 and 6 weeks and at 3 and 6 months postpartum. While significant changes in functional status were found over the 6 months, many women had not resumed their usual level of activities by the end of the project. Less than 30% of the women had resumed their usual levels of household, social, self-care, or occupational activities at the end of the traditional 6-week postpartum recovery period.

Tulman and Fawcett (1990) further analyzed the data to explore differences between employed and nonemployed mothers. Mothers who were employed at 6 months postpartum were more likely to have regained their usual level of energy and have infants that slept through the night than those mothers not employed. Overall, however, employed and nonemployed mothers were more alike than different in the various areas of functional status during the first 6 months after childbirth.

In a qualitative descriptive study, Nyqvist and Sjoden (1993) operationalized the RAM in a neonatal intensive care unit (NICU). Mothers' advice on how to facilitate breast-feeding in the NICU was divided into themes and categories and then classified according to the adaptive modes of the RAM. Three nurses classified the answers, which were then compared in five different ways. The researchers concluded that the overall percentage of agreement indicated that the RAM was easy to understand and apply even after a brief introduction. However, considerable overlap of the modes and lack of distinction among modes existed.

In two studies, investigators examined birth as the focal stimulus with primiparous mothers. Razmus (1993/1994) compared maternal adaptation at 3 months postpartum between mothers who delivered term infants and those who delivered preterm infants. When the timing of the birth, the contextual stimulus, was preterm the mothers scored significantly lower on the total positive affects scale and on the joy, contentment, and vigor subscales.

Legault (1990/1991) interviewed 10 first-time mothers to examine what stimuli influenced adaptation during the transition to motherhood. Mothers without postpartum depression had realistic expectations of motherhood, effective coping behaviors, and an adequate support network, while those with postpartum depression did not exhibit these characteristics.

Teenage pregnancy was used as an independent variable to study adaptation to maternal roles, tasks, and behaviors (Nwoga, 1990/1991). The twenty-nine 18- and 19-year-old women were found to perceive themselves as able to adapt to maternal roles. Family experiences with teen pregnancies was significantly related to adaptation.

Adaptation to cesarean birth. In 7 of the 21 role function adaptation mode studies, the focus of the research was cesarean delivery (Table 5.3). All of the studies represented a program of research initiated with a qualitative descriptive study to determine the needs of cesarean birth parents

Table 5.2 – Description of Studies About Adaptation to Maternal Role in the Role Function Mode of the RAM (*N*=6)

Author(s) & Date	Purpose	Sample	Design	Findings
6. Tulman, Fawcett, Groblewski, & Silverman (1990)	To explore changes in and variables associated with role performance in the form of functional status during the first six months following childbirth	Women who delivered healthy, full-term infants (*N*=97)	Correlational	There were significant changes in functional status between 3 and 6 weeks and between 6 weeks and 3 months, but not between 3 and 6 months.
7. Tulman & Fawcett (1990)	To describe differences because of employment status in selected variables and functional status during the first 6 months following childbirth	Women who delivered healthy, full-term infants (*N*=92)	Correlational	Employed and nonemployed mothers were more alike than different in relation to functional status during the 6 months postpartum. Mothers employed at six months were more likely to have fully regained their physical energy, have infants that slept through the night, and have better relationships with husbands than mothers not employed.
8. Nyqvist & Sjoden (1993)	To determine the interrater agreement in classification of mothers' comments and advice, and to analyze this information according to the RAM	Mothers of full-term infants admitted to NICU (*N*=178)	Qualitative-descriptive	Comments divided into themes and categories. Interrater reliability established for classification of themes according to RAM. The degree of agreement ranged between 74% and 92%. Considerable overlap of the adaptive modes was reported.

(continued)

Table 5.2 (continued)

Authors(s) & Date	Purpose	Sample	Design	Findings
9. Razmus (1993/1994)	To compare adjustment at three months post birth between mothers of term and preterm infants	Primiparous mothers; term birth (*n*=46) preterm birth (*n*=55); N=101	Descriptive	Mothers who delivered preterm infants had significantly lower joy, contentment, vigor, and total positive affect scores than mothers who delivered term infants.
10. Legault (1990/1991)	To access key factors influencing maternal role transition	First time mothers with depression (*n*=5) and no depression (*n*=5)	Qualitative-descriptive	When compared with women who had no postpartum blues or depression, women with postpartum depression had unrealistic expectations of motherhood, ineffective coping behaviors, and a limited support system resulting in delayed adaptation and negative self-concept.
11. Nwoga (1990/1991)	To investigate how pregnant teenage girls perceive they adapt to maternal roles, tasks, and behaviors	Pregnant 18-19 year olds (N=29)	Correlational	Pregnant teenagers perceive themselves as able to adapt to maternal roles, tasks, and behaviors.

(Fawcett, 1981). Content analysis was used to analyze data obtained from open-ended questionnaires completed separately by 24 husbands and wives who had experienced cesarean birth within the preceding seven years. Responses and needs were identified in each adaptive mode.

Based on Fawcett's (1981) initial findings, an antenatal education program of cesarean birth information was developed and tested by Fawcett and Burritt (1985). The program consisted of an educational pamphlet about cesarean birth and a follow-up home visit or telephone call. Fifteen couples who experienced an unplanned cesarean birth after attending Lamaze classes completed open-ended questionnaires about their reactions to the program. Data were categorized according to adaptive modes and classified as adaptive or ineffective. The educational pamphlet was found to be informative and reassuring and the follow-up visit or telephone call provided an opportunity for clarification of pamphlet information. Parents exhibited adaptive and ineffective responses in all four modes. In general, the responses were more positive than usually reported, which may be attributed to the effects of the educational program.

Using data from the 39 women who participated in the preceding two studies and 173 women from another study, Reichert, Baron, and Fawcett (1993) compared responses to planned and unplanned cesarean birth. Content analyses of data from open-ended questionnaires found that women who had planned cesarean deliveries had more adaptive and fewer ineffective responses than women who had unplanned cesarean deliveries.

The antenatal cesarean birth education program developed by Fawcett and Burritt (1985) was further tested by Fawcett and Henklein (1987) to compare responses of vaginally delivered and cesarean delivered parents. Content analyses of the data from the open-ended questionnaires revealed that most of the parents' information needs were met, regardless of the method of delivery.

In the next step of testing the education program, Fawcett, Pollio, and colleagues (1993) conducted a quasi-experimental study. The experimental group attended childbirth preparation classes in which a pamphlet developed by Fawcett and Burritt (1985) about cesarean birth was included. The comparison group attended classes based on the standard curriculum for childbirth preparation. All adaptive modes were examined. No differences between the groups were found in perception of the birth experience, physical distress, self-esteem, functional status, feelings about the baby, or quality of the marital relationship. The authors questioned whether it was realistic to expect the effects of an intervention made several weeks before birth to remain effective until several weeks postpartum.

Two different contextual stimuli, the effects of culture and past experience, were examined for their effects on adaptation to cesarean birth.

Table 5.3 – Description of Studies About Adaptation to Cesarean Birth in the Role Function Mode of the RAM (N=7)

Author(s) & Date	Purpose	Sample	Design	Findings
12. Fawcett (1981)	To determine reactions, needs, and suggestions of mothers and fathers to cesarean birth	Married couples who had cesarean births (N=24)	Qualitative-descriptive	Fathers and mothers had many unmet needs throughout the cesarean birth experience. Parents needed information about cesarean birth, support and guidance, and needed ability to fulfill anticipated roles.
13. Fawcett & Burritt (1985)	To develop and test an antenatal education program of cesarean birth information	Couples who experienced cesarean birth after attending Lamaze classes (N=15)	Qualitative-descriptive	The educational program was beneficial in that it met most of the information needs of the parents. Wives and husbands had responses in all four modes.
14. Reichert, Baron, & Fawcett (1987)	To compare the findings of three studies of women's responses concerning planned and unplanned cesarean birth	Women who had cesarean births Study 1 (n=24); Study 2 (n=15); tudy 3 (n=173); N=212	Qualitative-descriptive	Dominant responses were happiness and excitement accompanied by disappointment about need for cesarean delivery. Women who had planned cesarean deliveries had more adaptive and fewer ineffective responses than women who had unplanned cesarean deliveries.
15. Fawcett & Henklein (1987)	To compare responses of vaginally delivered and cesarean delivered parents to an antenatal educational program	Women (n=44) and their male partners who attended Lamaze classes (N=86)	Qualitative-descriptive	Educational program was effective and met most of parents' information needs, regardless of method of delivery.

16. Fawcett, Pollio, Tully, Baron, Henklein, & Jones (1993)	To compare effectiveness of two types of antenatal childbirth preparation classes on maternal reactions to unplanned cesarean delivery	Women who had unplanned cesarean birth (N=122) experimental group (n=74); control group (n=48)	Quasi-experimental	No differences between groups in perception of birth experience, physical distress, self-esteem, functional status, feelings about the baby, or quality of the marital relationship.
17. Fawcett & Weiss (1993)	To extend knowledge of cultural influences on adaptation to cesarean birth	Cesarean-delivered women (N=45); Caucasian (n=15), Asian (n=15), Hispanic (n=15)	Descriptive & Qualitative-descriptive	No substantial differences in adaptation to cesarean birth for the three cultural groups.
18. Fawcett, Tulman, & Spedden (1994)	To compare women's reactions to their experiences of vaginal birth after cesarean with reactions to their previous cesarean birth	Women who experienced vaginal birth after an earlier cesarean (N=32)	Descriptive	Significantly greater proportion of adaptive responses to the vaginal birth after an earlier cesarean birth than to the previous cesarean birth.

Fawcett and Weiss (1993) found no differences in adaptation to cesarean birth among Asian, Caucasian, and Hispanic women. Using content analysis of an open-ended questionnaire, no differences in the proportions of adaptive and ineffective responses for the three cultural groups were identified. An equal number of adaptive and ineffective responses across the adaptive modes were found.

Using previous birth experiences as a contextual stimulus, Fawcett, Tulman, and Spedden (1994) examined women's responses to vaginal birth after a previous cesarean section. They found a greater proportion of adaptive responses to the vaginal birth after a cesarean than to the previous cesarean delivery. However, the mean score on the Perception of Birth Scale was lower than the means previously reported for vaginally delivered women. Each woman was asked to comment on her reactions to the vaginal birth experience and to the previous cesarean birth experience. A significant association was found between the type of delivery and the adaptive and ineffective responses.

Interactive roles. For studies in this category, researchers examined roles related to people in reciprocal roles. Three of the role function mode adaptation studies were focused on such interactive roles (Table 5.4). Friedemann and Andrews (1990) used the RAM to explore facilitating factors in the process of stress transmission from parent to child. In single-parent families, neither assistance with child rearing nor support of extended family made a difference in the occurrence of children's behavior problems. No differences in total behavior problems were found between single-parent and two-parent families, but more school suspensions were found in single-parent families.

Weiss (1990/1991) examined 102 primiparous couples to describe marital interdependence and adaptation to parenthood. A relationship existed between the husband's and wife's adaptation to parenthood. Expectations for interdependence within the postpartum marital relationship were predictive of the realities of interdependence actually experienced.

The effect of attending a group role-play program on role adequacy of pediatric outpatients undergoing surgery and their mothers' state anxiety was studied by Kiker (1983). No differences were found in children's role adequacy based on attendance at the role-play program when age, gender, and mothers' state anxiety were controlled. Also, there was no difference in mothers' state anxiety when trait anxiety was controlled. The researcher concluded that the RAM was not supported in that the role-play program did not enhance role adequacy.

Critical Analysis of Reported Research

Based on the description of the 21 studies reviewed, research in the role function mode was critically analyzed and evaluated with respect to

Table 5.4 – Description of Studies About Interactive Roles in the Role Function Mode of the RAM (N=3)

Author(s) & Date	Purpose	Sample	Design	Findings
19. Friedemann & Andrews (1990)	To explore the role of facilitating factors in the process of stress transmission from parent to child	Single-parent families (n=103); two-parent families (n=271); (N=374)	Descriptive	In single-parent families, neither assistance with child rearing nor support of extended family made a significant difference in occurrence of children's behavior problems. However, there was no difference in total behavior problems between single-parent and two-parent families, but there were more school suspensions in single-parent families.
20. Weiss (1990/1991)	To describe changes in marital interdependence and adaptation to parenthood as expectations become realities of parenthood	Primiparous couples (N=102)	Correlational	Expectations for interdependence were predictive of realities of postpartum interdependence. The greatest interdependence was in the affective dimension. Scores indicated effective adaptation to parenthood.
21. Kiker (1983)	To compare role adequacy between pediatric outpatients who attend a group role-play program and those who do not attend the program and to compare state anxiety between mothers who attend a group role play with their children and mothers who do not attend	Children ages 3-9 years undergoing eye, ear, nose, or throat outpatient surgery (n=50) and their mothers (n=50)	Descriptive	No differences between the groups in children's role adequacy when controlling for preoperative role adequacy, mothers' state anxiety, and age and gender of the child. No differences between groups in mothers' state anxiety when effects of trait anxiety and age and gender of child controlled.

the quality of the research and the relationship to the RAM. Reviewers, however, were limited to reports of studies as retrieved with no additional information sought from the researchers. In some cases, the analyses might not reflect the author's original intent. Ten role function mode adaptation studies were quantitative, six were qualitative, and five focused on instrument development. Critical analyses are presented separately for the quantitative, qualitative, and methodologic studies.

Critical analyses of quantitative research. Critical analyses of the 10 quantitative studies are presented in Table 5.5.

In 4 of the 10 studies, measures to control for threats to internal validity were adequately addressed, but threats to external validity were a problem in all of the studies. History and maturation were potential threats to internal validity in four of the five studies in which data were collected more than one time. Kiker (1983) controlled maturation by using age as a covariate and controlled history by using a comparison group taken from the same population as the treatment group. Mortality was an issue in the study by Weiss (1990/1991). Although 78% of the sample completed the study, no description was included of how the subjects who dropped out compared to those who completed the study. Consistency of measurement or instrumentation was not a threat to internal validity in any of the quantitative studies.

Sampling techniques affected both internal and external validity. Convenience samples were used in all the studies, but most researchers identified inclusion criteria and described the sample. However, Friedemann and Andrews (1990) used data from a larger sample and did not describe the subjects used for their analysis. Fawcett, Pollio, and colleagues (1993) recruited additional subjects for their control group from a postpartum unit and did not report how these subjects compared with the subjects recruited from the childbirth education classes. Fawcett and colleagues (1994) had a small sample that was diverse in experiences related to vaginal births after cesareans and relied on the women's being able to accurately recall previous cesarean birth experiences. Many of the samples were predominately white, upper-middle class, well-educated adults which limited generalizability of findings. Thus, representativeness of the sample or equivalence of groups was a threat, or partial threat, to external validity in all the studies.

The environment and extraneous variables were at least partially controlled in half the studies. Control of measurement was a threat for Friedemann and Andrews (1990) as they analyzed data previously collected as part of a larger study. Consistency of treatment was not a problem in the three studies which had comparison groups (Fawcett, Pollio, et al., 1993; Kiker, 1983; Razmus, 1993/1994).

Table 5.5 – Critical Analysis of Quantitative Role Function Mode Research (*N*=10)

Criteria	Evaluation		
	Yes	*Partially*	*No*
Design			
Threats to internal validity controlled	19, 16, 17, 21	6, 7, 11, 18	19, 20
Threats to external validity controlled		9, 17, 21	6, 7, 11, 16, 18, 19, 20
Measurement			
Reliability of instruments addressed	6, 7, 9, 16, 17, 18, 20, 21		11, 19
Validity of instruments addressed	6, 7, 16, 17, 18, 20, 21	9, 11	19
Data Analysis			
Appropriate	6, 7, 9, 16, 17, 18, 20, 21		11, 19
Interpretation of Results			
Consistency of findings with conclusions	6, 7, 9, 16, 17, 18, 20, 21	11, 19	

Key: 6=Tulman et al.,1990; 7=Tulman & Fawcett,1990; 9=Razmus,1993/1994; 11=Nwoga,1990/1991; 16=Fawcett, Pollio, et al.,1993; 17=Fawcett & Weiss,1993; 18=Fawcett et al.,1994; 19=Friedemann & Andrews,1990; 20=Weiss,1990/1991; 21=Kiker,1983

Reliability and validity of the instruments were not adequately addressed in three studies. Data analysis and consistency of interpretation of results were not adequately addressed in three of the studies. Friedemann and Andrews (1990) did not address instrument reliability or validity and used *t*-tests to analyze nominal and ordinal level data. Nwoga (1990/1991) partially addressed instrument validity but not reliability. In addition, measurements of dichotomous and interval data were combined for analysis and the number of subjects varied without explanation. These two studies had only partial consistency between the data and the findings and conclusions.

The comparison of maternal adjustment at 3 months postpartum between mothers of term and preterm infants (Razmus, 1993/1994) was one quantitative study in which most of the criteria for critical analyses were adequately addressed. For example, sample inclusion criteria clearly identified infant gestational age, size, primiparous birth, lack of severe congenital anomalies, and time in hospital, as well as whether the mother was living with the father of the infant.

The investigation of cultural influences on adaptation to cesarean birth (Fawcett & Weiss, 1993) was another quantitative study where most of the criteria for critical analyses were met. For example, all subjects were recruited from the same hospital, detailed demographic characteristics for each cultural group were reported, and statistically different characteristics were included. The testing environment was controlled, and there was consistency of measurement. Cronbach's alpha for the study was reported for the Perception of Birth Scale, and content validity was addressed.

Critical analyses of qualitative research. Critical analyses of the six qualitative studies are presented in Table 5.6. In all studies, strategies to ensure validity and appropriate methods for data analysis were followed. In one study, no strategies to ensure reliability were found, and in one study only partial consistency between findings and conclusions was found.

Regarding strategies to ensure validity, three of the six studies had evidence of descriptive vividness, methodologic congruence, analytical preciseness, theoretic connectedness, and heuristic relevance. Fawcett (1981) did not demonstrate descriptive vividness while Nyqvist and Sjoden (1993) only partially demonstrated methodologic congruence. Theoretic connectedness was only partially met in another study (Fawcett & Henklein, 1987). In five studies strategies such as describing contextual conditions, participant selection, and procedural stages for data collection were used to ensure reliability. In addition, Nyqvist and Sjoden (1993) obtained feedback from participants. Legault (1990/1991) acknowledged the researcher position by developing a semi-standardized interview, and clearly identifying the researcher's role in the setting, to further enhance reliability. However, Fawcett (1981) did not address researcher position or report the pro-

Table 5.6 – Critical Analysis of Qualitative Role Function Mode Research
(_N_=6)

Criteria	Evaluation		
	Yes	_Partially_	_No_
Design			
Strategies to ensure validity used	8, 10, 12, 13, 14, 15		
Strategies to ensure reliability used	8, 10, 13, 14, 15		12
Data Analysis			
Appropriate method	8, 10, 12 13, 14, 15,		
Interpretation of Results			
Consistency of findings with conclusions	10, 12, 13, 14, 15	8	

Key: 8=Nyqvist & Sjoden, 1993; 10=Legault, 1990/1991; 12=Fawcett, 1981;
13=Fawcett & Burritt, 1985; 14=Reichart et al., 1993; 15=Fawcett & Henklein, 1987

cedural stages for data collection and analysis. Thus, sufficient information to ascertain reliability was not ensured.

In all six studies appropriate methods of data analysis such as content analysis were used. However, themes formulated under each category were not discussed in the report of one study (Nyqvist and Sjoden 1993). These investigators had only partial consistency between the findings and conclusions.

Critical analyses of instrument-development studies. Five role function mode studies were focused on development of instruments to measure functional status at different developmental stages (Table 5.7). Steps taken to establish reliability and validity were similar for all five instruments.

Procedures used to establish content validity of the IFSAC (Fawcett et al., 1988) were described. Seven professionally educated women who had experienced childbirth within the preceding year served as content experts. The average congruency score was 84.4% after the first round and 96.7% after the second round. The sample used to determine reliability

Author(s) Year	Reliability	Validity
1. Inventory of Functional Status after Childbirth (IFSAC) Fawcett et al., 1988	Cronbach's alpha coefficients were .76 for total scale and ranged from .56 to .98 for subscales. Item to subscale coefficients ranged from .51 to .78. Subscale to total coefficients ranged from .23 to .89. Test-retest was .86 for total scale with subscales ranging from .48 to .93.	Content - Popham's average congruency score of 96.7% after two rounds. Construct - subscale correlations ranged from .01 to .53. No significant difference between contrasted groups.
2. Inventory of Functional Status Antepartum Period (IFSAP) Tulman, Higgins et al., 1991	Item to subscale coefficients ranged from .57 to .87. Subscale to total coefficients ranged from .53 to .90. Test-retest reliability was .90 for total scale with subscales ranging from .27 to .93.	Content - Popham's average congruency score of 92.6% after two rounds. Construct - subscale correlations ranged from -.11 to .97. Significant differences between contrasted groups. (t=-3.28, p<.001; F=18.99, p<.0005).
3. Inventory of Functional Status Fathers (IFS-F) Tulman et al., 1993	Item to subscale coefficients ranged from .54 to .75. Subscale to total coefficients ranged from .31 to .61.	Content - Popham's average congruency score of 86% after two rounds. Construct - subscale correlations ranged from -.02 to .69.
4. Inventory of Functional Status Cancer (IFS-CA) Tulman, Fawcett, et al., 1991	Item to subscale coefficients ranged from .56 to .82. Subscale to total coefficients ranged from .73 to .92. Test-retest reliability was .91 for total scale with subscales ranging from .43 to .96.	Content - Popham's average congruency score of 98.5% after three rounds. Construct - subscale correlations ranged from .33 to .62. Significant difference between contrasted groups (t=-4.24, p<.001).

(continued)

Table 5.7 *(continued)*

Author(s) Year	Reliability	Validity
5. Inventory of Functional Status in the Elderly (IFSITE) Paier, 1994	Item to subscale coefficients ranged from .42 to .68. Subscale to total coefficients ranged from .41 to .77. Test-retest reliability was .21 for total scale with subscales ranging from .00 to .34.	Content - Panel of experts (n=10). Construct - subscale correlations ranged from .10 to .47. Significant difference between contrasted groups (F=359.9, p<.0005).

and construct validity consisted of 76 women who were 6 to 10 weeks postpartum. Reliability coefficients were somewhat variable, but acceptable for a newly developed instrument. The instrument was tested on a fairly small sample (n=76). Because some subscales were not applicable to all subjects, the number of responses was small. For example, the occupational activities subscale had only 15 subjects for internal consistency and 3 for test-retest. Vaginally and cesarean delivered women were used as contrasted groups. The lack of significant differences may be due to a blurring of variances by 6 to 10 weeks postpartum rather than a failure of the IFSAC to detect differences. Correlations among the subscales indicated the five subscales did not measure exactly the same thing although some overlap did occur.

Content validity of the IFSAP was established (Tulman, Higgins, et al., 1991) with 21 pregnant women who had no major complications and served as content experts. The average congruency score was 88.3% after the first round and 92.6% after the second round. The sample used to determine reliability and construct validity consisted of 192 pregnant women recruited from childbirth preparation classes and from private obstetric practices. Reliability coefficients were acceptable for a newly developed instrument. Test-retest coefficients were adequate except for the Personal Care Activities subscale (r=.27). In three comparisons of contrasted groups, no differences were found between homemakers and women employed outside the home. However, women who had children had a significantly higher functional status than women who had no children (t=-3.28, p<.001). Also, women categorized into one of four groups based on restrictions during pregnancy were found to have significantly different functional status scores (F=18.99, p < .0005). Correlations among the subscales indicated that the six subscales did have considerable overlap. For example, the dimension of household activities overlapped with social and community, childcare, occupational, and educational activities.

However, the dimension of personal care activities was relatively independent.

Eleven expectant fathers and 13 new fathers, all of whose partners were participating in a study of maternal functional status, served as content experts for the IFS-F (Tulman et al., 1993). For the first round, antepartum and postpartum versions of the IFS-F were used. The average congruency scores were 82% and 86%, respectively. Based on the results, a single version of the IFS-F was developed. The congruency score was 86% after the second round. The sample used to determine reliability and construct validity consisted of 125 expectant fathers and 57 new fathers. Reliability coefficients were somewhat variable, but acceptable for a newly developed instrument. No test-retest reliability was reported. Correlations of the subscales revealed the six subscales were relatively independent with the exception of household and childcare activities. No contrasted groups construct validity was reported.

Appropriate procedures to establish content validity of the IFS-CA (Tulman, Fawcett, et al., 1991) were described. Sixteen women receiving outpatient chemotherapy for breast cancer served as content validity judges. The average congruency score was 93.7% after the first round, 97.6% after the second round, and 98.5% after the third round. The sample used to determine reliability and construct validity consisted of 100 women from an ambulatory oncology clinic at an urban medical center. Reliability coefficients were somewhat variable, but acceptable for a newly developed instrument. The method used for the test-retest reliability could have affected the results. For example, subjects were given two copies of the IFS-CA and told to complete one that day and the other IFS-CA at home in 4 to 7 days and return both in a stamped envelope. The subjects might have completed both copies at the same time or used the first copy to guide answers for the second copy. Correlations indicated that the four subscales were not independent. For example, the household and family activities subscale overlapped with social and community, personal care, and occupational activities subscales. Women who were in active treatment for cancer were contrasted with those who had completed treatment. Total functional status was significantly higher for those who had completed treatment (t=-4.24, p<.001).

Procedures to establish content validity of the IFSITE (Paier, 1994) were described, but the researcher did not always follow the criteria that had been established. Five community-dwelling elders and five long-term health-care providers served as content experts; however, the community-dwelling elders seemed to have difficulty understanding the process and frequently had differing opinions about endorsement of an item. Consequently, eight items not receiving the 80% average congruency score were included in the IFSITE. The number of rounds and the final average congruency score were not reported. The sample used to determine reliability and construct validity consisted of 154 well elders. Reliability coefficients were somewhat variable, but most were acceptable for a newly developed instrument. Test-retest reliability was not acceptable. The researcher thought this might have been attributable to the four-week test-retest interval, which was viewed as being too long. Correlations indicated that the six subscales were mostly independent, although some moderate overlap did occur. Community-dwelling elderly and nursing home residents were used as contrasted groups. As expected, functional status was significantly higher for the community-dwelling elderly $(F=359.9, p < .0005)$.

Evaluation of Relationships to the RAM

Criteria were developed to determine which quantitative and qualitative studies to include in the evaluation of relationships to the RAM. Methodologic studies were excluded because their focus was on instrument development. Studies were included if internal or external validity was not a problem, if reliability and validity of instruments were addressed, if data analysis was appropriate, and if consistency between results and conclusions was present. Eight of the 21 role function mode studies met the criteria for inclusion.

Evaluation of Linkages to the RAM

Evaluation of the linkages between the role function mode studies and the RAM is summarized in Table 5.8. The linkages among the research variables, empiric measures, and findings and the RAM were evaluated for each of eight studies.

Most of the role function mode investigators made explicit linkages of the research variables, empiric measures, and findings to the RAM. In four of the role function studies a linkage between the empiric measures and the RAM, was implied, while in one study the linkage was absent. In only one study was the research variables link to the RAM not explicit; the linkage was implied in that study.

Nyqvist and Sjoden (1993) did not completely link empiric measures to the RAM. Data were collected through telephone interviews asking mothers two questions related to advice about breast-feeding of infants in the NICU. Answers were classified and divided according to themes and categories. The authors did not describe the processes used to accomplish this classification; however, these themes and categories were then classified according to the adaptive modes of the RAM. These classifications were compared in five ways to test interrater reliability.

Razmus (1993/1994) used the Affects Balance Scale (ABS) to measure the mother's adjustment to the preterm and term birth experience in the self-concept mode. The ABS was used to measure eight affect states, four positive and four negative. Linkages between the ABS and the RAM were implicit rather than explicit.

Reichert and colleagues (1993) implied a linkage between the empiric measure and the RAM. The investigators used an open-ended questionnaire to collect data about what emotional and physical responses were to cesarean birth, what needs existed during cesarean birth, and what could have been done by whom to improve the experience. An explicit link between the questionnaire and the RAM was not found.

In a related study, Fawcett and Burritt (1985) made the link explicit by including the questionnaire and details about an educational pamphlet that represented the four adaptive modes of the RAM. However, in an extension of the preceding study, the only link to the RAM was through the educational pamphlet. Thus, the link with the research variables was implied, but no links with the empiric measures or the finding existed (Fawcett & Henklein, 1987). Kiker (1983) used the Prehospital Behavior Questionnaire to measure the child's role adequacy before outpatient surgery. An identical questionnaire identified as the Posthospital Behavior Questionnaire, was used a week after the child's surgery to measure role adequacy following outpatient surgery. A linkage between the behavior questionnaire and role adequacy was implied.

Testing of Propositions from the RAM

According to the criteria discussed in Chapter 2, studies were included in testing of RAM propositions if they were analytically sound and had adequate links to the Roy Model. Seven of the 21 role function mode studies met the criteria for inclusion. From the RAM propositions listed in Chapter 2, findings from studies in the role function mode were used to test five of the propositions (Table 5.9).

Table 5.8 – Evaluation of Linkages to the RAM (N=8)

	Evaluation		
	Explicit	*Implict*	*Absent*
Research variables	8,9,10,13,14 17,21	15	
Empirical measures	10,13,17 21	8,9,14,	15
Findings	8,9,10,13, 14,17,21		15

Key: 8=Nyqvist & Sjoden, 1993; 9=Razmus, 1993/1994; 10=Legault, 1990/1991; 13=Fawcett & Burritt, 1985; 14=Reichert et al., 1993; 15=Fawcett & Henklein, 1987; 17=Fawcett & Weiss, 1993; 21=Kiker, 1983.

Five propositions from the RAM were supported or not supported by role function adaptive mode research. The proposition that characteristics of the internal and external stimuli influence adaptive responses was supported by Razmus (1993/1994). When examining the adaptation of primiparous mothers, Razmus found that the contextual stimulus of preterm birth resulted in less adaptive responses in new mothers. The mothers who delivered at term had higher scores on the total positive affects scale and on the joy, contentment, and vigor subscales than did the mothers who delivered preterm infants.

The study conducted by Legault (1990/1991) supported the proposition that the characteristics of the internal and external stimuli influence the adequacy of cognitive and emotional processes. The researcher found that the new mother "was influenced by internal and external stimuli which triggered her regulator and cognator coping mechanisms" (p. 103). The mothers with symptoms of postpartum depression exhibited ineffective behaviors, had ineffective role transition, and struggled to balance secondary roles. The mothers without symptoms of postpartum depression exhibited adaptive behaviors, were able to assume the new role of mother, and had more tertiary roles.

The proposition that adaptation in one mode is affected by adaptation in other modes through cognator and regulator connectives was supported by Legault (1990/1991) and Nyquist and Sjoden (1993). Legault found many overlapping factors affecting both the self-concept and role function modes. Nyqvist and Sjoden found considerable overlap of the four adaptive modes when data were classified by three nurses. The main problem encountered during the data classification process was a lack of clarity in the distinction among modes. This was especially true for the psychosocial modes of self-concept, role function, and interdependence. The authors concluded that this overlap confirmed the complexity of nursing situations that often have several overlapping patient needs. Roy (Roy & Andrews, 1991) refers to the overlap among modes as reflecting holism and uses the image of a kaleidoscope to represent new patterns developing as perspective is changed.

The proposition that the pooled effect of focal, contextual, and residual stimuli determines the adaptation level was supported by Reichert and colleagues (1993) and was both supported and not supported by Fawcett and Weiss (1993). Reichert and colleagues (1993) found that women who received regional anesthesia for the cesarean delivery had more adaptive responses than those women who had general anesthesia. The women who had planned cesarean births had more adaptive responses than those who had unplanned cesarean deliveries. The presence of the partner for the cesarean delivery appeared to influence the mother's adaptation but could not be statistically analyzed because almost all partners were present for the birth.

Table 5.9 – Testing of Propositions from the RAM (N=7)

Propositions from the RAM	Ancillary and practice propositions	Supported by results	Not Supported by results
3. The characteristics of the internal and external stimuli influence adaptive responses.	Preterm birth is related to less effective adaptive responses in new mothers.	Razmus (1993/1994)	
4. The characteristics of the internal and external stimuli influence the adequacy of cognitive and emotional processes.	Postpartum depression is related to ineffective role behaviors.	Legault (1990/1991)	
6. Adaptation in one mode is affected by adaptation in other modes through cognator and regulator connectives.	a. Overlapping factors affect self-concept and role function.	Legault (1990/1991)	
	b. Patients' needs represent three psychosocial modes.	Nyqvist & Sjoden (1993)	
7. The pooled effect of local, contextual, and residual stimuli determines the adaptation level.	a. Type of anesthesia for cesarean birth influences adaptation.	Reichert, Baron & Fawcett (1993)	
	b. Preparation for cesarean delivery influences adaptation.	Fawcett & Weiss (1993)	
	c. Culture affects adaptation to cesarean birth.		Fawcett & Weiss (1993)
12. Nursing assessment and interventions relate to identifying and managing input to adaptive systems.	a. Education about cesarean birth meets information needs of cesarean birth parents.	Fawcett & Burritt (1985)	
	b. Group role play programs enhance role adequacy.		Kiker (1983)

On the other hand, Fawcett and Weiss (1993) did not find that the contextual stimuli of culture affected adaptation to cesarean birth. They found no differences in the proportions of adaptive and ineffective responses among Caucasian, Hispanic, and Asian women. However, global adaptation was higher for women who felt prepared for a cesarean birth than for those who did not feel prepared.

The proposition that nursing assessment and interventions relate to identifying and managing input to adaptive systems was supported by Fawcett and Burritt (1985), but was not supported by Kiker (1983). Fawcett and Burritt found that reading of a cesarean-delivery educational pamphlet based on the four adaptive modes and posteducation follow-up resulted in meeting most of the information needs of the cesarean-birth parents. Kiker did not find that a group role play program enhanced role adequacy in children having outpatient surgery. However, the author stated that the routine preoperative teaching given to all children may have provided sufficient input regardless of participation in the role-play program. Kiker also stated that better instruments to measure role behaviors should be used.

Synthesis of Role Function Mode Research: Contributions to Nursing Science

Contributions to nursing science were derived from critical analysis of role function mode research and from evaluation of relationships to the RAM. Studies are discussed in relation to their contributions to clinical practice, research, and theory. The contributions and recommendations for future work are identified in studies that met the established guidelines for critical analysis. Thus, studies were not included if threats to internal or external validity were found, if the interpretation of results and conclusions were inconsistent, or if the variables or empiric measures were not explicitly or implicitly linked to the RAM.

Consequently, 14 studies were eliminated from the synthesis of role function mode research. Faulty methodology—numerous threats to internal and external validity—was present in eight studies. Content was an issue in three studies where inconsistencies between the interpretation of results and the conclusions were present. Methodologic studies were excluded. Therefore, seven role function mode studies are included in the synthesis.

Applications to Nursing Practice

The findings from the study conducted by Legault (1990/1991) have high potential for use in nursing practice (Table 5.10). These are referred to as category one, as defined in Chapter 2, considering empiric evidence and risk to patients. Nurses are in positions to help primiparous women develop realistic expectations of motherhood, effective coping behaviors, and support systems. When teaching prenatal education classes or delivering prenatal care, nurses can assist women to identify and use resources to ease the role transition required with motherhood. Women and their significant others can be taught about postpartum depression so it can be detected and treated as soon as possible. Early diagnosis and support would facilitate the new mother's adaptation and enhance her relationship with her child. These interventions have high benefit with low associated risks.

Nurses are routinely involved in prenatal education classes, and content about cesarean delivery is an essential component of the classes. The cesarean delivery educational pamphlet developed by Fawcett and Burritt (1985) has a high potential for meeting the information needs of parents. Follow-up phone calls or home visits are important in that they help to reinforce the content and emphasize the need to prepare for the possibility of a cesarean birth.

Related to the attitudes of women toward cesarean birth, clinical applications from the study by Reichert and colleagues (1993) are specific to nursing interventions during the cesarean delivery. Nurses in the delivery room need to provide information about the birth process while being supportive. Because women need their partners with them throughout labor and delivery, nurses can advocate for policies that allow family members to be present whenever possible. In addition, nurses are able to facilitate contact between the mother and the newborn without compromising the physiologic needs of the newborn.

Similarly, contributions from Fawcett and Weiss (1993) reinforced the need for nurses to provide support and information about cesarean birth and to facilitate both the presence of partners and contact with the newborn. Nursing care during cesarean birth needs to include conveying a feeling of care and concern, not just technical expertise. Health care professionals need to be sensitive to cultural differences without invoking preconceived expectations.

The findings from the study by Nyqvist and Sjoden (1993) have high potential for use in nursing practice. Nurses can encourage persistence and confidence in a new mother's ability to breastfeed, can promote early extensive physical contact with the newborn, and can supply structured information on breastfeeding. Facilitation of private, undisturbed parent/ infant contact and active parent participation in the infant's care and feeding were found to be important.

Findings from one research study need further clinical evaluation before use (category two). Considering the contextual stimulus of preterm birth, clinical nurse experts need to assess further the adaptation process of mothers who delivered preterm infants and to provide anticipatory guidance before discharge of the infant from the NICU. In addition, clinical nurse experts may be able to facilitate interaction between parents and community resources that could promote adaptation and positively influence adequate emotional processes (Razmus, 1993/1994).

Findings from one research study need further testing before implementation (category three). Results of the study conducted by Kiker (1983) did not support the use of a group role-play program to enhance role adequacy in children undergoing outpatient surgery. Consequently, the implementation of such programs needs further development and testing to determine their effectiveness in various ages, types of surgery, and cultures. Variables influencing role adequacy in children should be identified.

Recommendations for Model-Based Research

Future directions for model-based research were identified from all studies that had applications to nursing practice but were most obvious in the studies for which further evaluation and testing were indicated. In addition, studies where findings were equivocal or different from previous research are priority areas for further research.

Studies in which researchers examine the incidence, influencing factors, and effects of postpartum depression are indicated. Variables such as the father's role throughout pregnancy and postpartum, the ways women develop realistic expectations of motherhood, a woman's relationship with her mother, and the effect of other secondary and tertiary roles on adaptation should be examined in future research. Nursing interventions that can be implemented prenatally to promote realistic expectations of motherhood need to be developed and tested (Legault, 1990/1991).

Table 5.10 – Potentials for Implementation from Role Function Mode Adaptation Research (*N*=7)

Category One: High potential for implementation
  Legault (1990/1991)
  Fawcett & Burritt (1985)
  Reichert, Baron, & Fawcett (1993)
  Fawcett & Weiss (1993)
  Nyqvist & Sjoden (1993)

Category Two: Needs further clinical evaluation before implementation
  Razmus (1993/1994)

Category Three: Further research indicated before implementation
  Kiker (1983)

Identifying the evolving needs of cesarean birth parents and designing nursing interventions to meet those needs are both warranted (Fawcett & Burritt, 1985; Fawcett & Weiss, 1993; Reichert et al., 1993). The effects of cesarean birth education content and teaching strategies employed in childbirth preparation classes require further testing (Fawcett & Burritt, 1985).

Studies are recommended in which investigators explore environmental and physical variables such as complications during pregnancy and postpartum, extent of prenatal care, and support systems associated with maternal adaptation following preterm birth. The role of the father's involvement in the care of the preterm infant and the effect of that care on maternal adaptation should be examined. Nursing interventions aimed at enhancing maternal adaptation following a preterm birth need to be developed and tested (Razmus, 1993/1994).

While the nursing intervention of conducting a group role-play program to enhance role adequacy in children undergoing outpatient surgery was not supported, other variables such as the age of the child, the recency of the role-play program, and the effects of routine preoperative teaching should be investigated. Better instruments to measure role adequacy in children need to be developed and tested (Kiker, 1983).

Initial psychometric testing of the various inventories of functional status (Fawcett et al., 1988; Tulman et al., 1993; Tulman, Fawcett, et al., 1991; Tulman, Higgins, et al., 1991; Paier, 1994) indicated that further testing was warranted. Refining the instruments with additional testing of reliability and validity is recommended. The value of these instruments in facilitating research based on the RAM is yet to be fully realized. These instruments can be a useful resource for future model-based research.

Directions for Theory and RAM Development

Role function mode research based on the RAM contributed to identifying directions for further developing theory and the nursing model. Two clear directions were identified from propositions tested by the reported research. First, examining the pooled effect of stimuli on adaptation level is indicated. Second, the mixed findings related to the nursing interventions enhancing adaptation by managing input to adaptive systems indicated that further conceptual and theoretic development is needed in this area.

One of the key relationships proposed by the RAM is that the stress placed by focal, contextual, and residual stimuli on the person's coping abilities results in behavior which indicates whether one is coping effectively. The second level of assessment involves identifying the internal and external stimuli influencing behavior. Roy clearly identifies culture as a contextual stimulus (Roy & Andrews, 1991). However, during acculturation, if or when the birth culture ceases to have an effect is not clear. Because culture was the only contextual stimulus in the reported research that did not support the proposition, future RAM development needs to consider clarifying the role of culture as a contextual stimulus in a variety of situations.

Because of the conflicting findings related to the role of nursing interventions enhancing adaptation by managing input, further conceptual and theoretic clarification is warranted. All stimuli that exert a positive influence should be supported (Roy & Andrews, 1991). Education is one of the most frequently identified contextual stimuli. If intellectual stimulation does not appeal to the person, other stimuli would be identified. Thus, when considering the holistic nature of the adaptive system, the total effect of a selected contextual stimulus may be difficult to distinguish. In the studies in which support for the proposition was lacking, additional educational contextual stimuli were present but were not measured. Consequently, future theory and RAM development should emphasize the total effect of contextual stimuli.

In addition, two propositions were supported by only one study each. These two propositions—the characteristics of the internal and external stimuli influence adaptive responses, and the characteristics of the internal and external stimuli influence the adequacy of cognitive and emotional processes—need further testing.

Summary

Theoretic frameworks that reflect a multidimensional holistic approach, such as the RAM, are important for nursing research because the profession claims to focus on the whole person. Of the 163 nursing studies included in this monograph, 21 focused primarily on the role function adaptive mode. Findings reported from RAM-based studies supported the use of a holistic framework, such as the RAM, to enhance understanding of role function mode variables in clinical situations.

The many applications for nursing practice also support the value of using the RAM to guide role function mode research. In clinical practice, scholarly inquiry guided by a nursing model not only will validate proposed interventions but will refine the theories and knowledge needed to direct nursing practice. In addition, areas for further development of the role function mode and the RAM will be made explicit from the empiric and clinical findings. Finally, using a nursing model to guide practice and research will strengthen the interrelationships among theory, research, and practice.

References

Fawcett, J. (1981). Needs of cesarean birth parents. *Journal of Obstetric, Gynecologic, & Neonatal Nursing, 10,* 372-376.

Fawcett, J., & Burritt, J. (1985). An exploratory study of antenatal preparation for cesarean birth. *Journal of Obstetric, Gynecologic, & Neonatal Nursing, 14,* 224-230.

Fawcett, J., & Henklein, J.C. (1987). Antenatal education for cesarean birth: Extension of a field test. *Journal of Obstetric, Gynecologic, & Neonatal Nursing, 16,* 61-65.

Fawcett, J., Pollio, N., Tully, A., Baron, M., Henklein, J.C., & Jones, R.C. (1993). Effects of information on adaptation to cesarean birth. *Nursing Research, 42,* 49-53.

Fawcett, J., Tulman, L., & Myers, S.T. (1988). Development of the Inventory of Functional Status after Childbirth. *Journal of Nurse Midwifery, 33,* 252-260.

Fawcett, J., Tulman, L., & Spedden, J.P. (1994). Responses to vaginal birth after cesarean section. *Journal of Obstetric, Gynecologic, & Neonatal Nursing, 23,* 253-259.

Fawcett, J., & Weiss, M.E. (1993). Cross-cultural adaptation to cesarean birth. *Western Journal of Nursing Research, 15,* 282-297.

Friedemann, M-L., & Andrews, M. (1990). Family support and child adjustment in single parent families. *Issues in Comprehensive Pediatric Nursing, 13,* 289-301.

Kiker, P.M. (1983). Role adequacy of pediatric outpatients undergoing surgery (Doctoral dissertation, Texas Women's University, 1983). *Dissertation Abstracts International, 44,* 1782 -B.

Legault, F.M. (1991). Adaptation within the role function and self-concept modes among women during the postpartum period (Master's thesis, D'Youville College, 1990). *Masters Abstracts International, 29,* 439.

Nwoga, I. A. A. (1991). Adaptation to maternal roles, tasks, and behaviors by pregnant teenage girls (Master's thesis, D'Youville College, 1990). *Masters Abstracts International, 29,* 97.

Nyqvist, K.H., & Sjoden, P-O. (1993). Advice concerning breast-feeding from mothers of infants admitted to a neonatal intensive care unit: The Roy Adaptation Model as a conceptual structure. *Journal of Advanced Nursing, 18,* 54-63.

Paier, G.S. (1994). Development and testing of an instrument to assess functional status in the elderly (Doctoral dissertation, University of Pennsylvania, 1994). *Dissertation Abstracts International, 55,* 1806-B.

Razmus, I.S. (1994). Maternal adjustment to premature birth: Utilizing the Roy Adaptation Model as a theoretical framework (Master's thesis, Grand Valley State University, 1993). *Masters Abstracts International, 32,* 1375.

Reichert, J.A., Baron, M., & Fawcett, J. (1993). Changes in attitudes toward cesarean birth. *Journal of Obstetric, Gynecologic, and Neonatal Nursing, 22,* 159-167.

Roy, C., & Andrews, H. (1999). *The Roy Adaptation Model.* Stamford, CT: Appleton & Lange.

Tulman, L., & Fawcett, J. (1990). Maternal employment following childbirth. *Research in Nursing & Health, 13,* 181-188.

Tulman, L., Fawcett, J., Groblewski, L., & Silverman, L. (1990). Changes in functional status after childbirth. *Nursing Research, 39,* 70-75.

Tulman, L., Fawcett, J., McEvoy, M.D. (1991). Development of the Inventory of Functional Status—Cancer. *Cancer Nursing, 14,* 254-260.

Tulman, L., Fawcett, J., & Weiss, M. (1993). The Inventory of Functional Status—Fathers: Development and psychometric testing. *Journal of Nurse Midwifery, 38,* 276-282.

Tulman, L., Higgins, K., Fawcett, J., Nunno, C., Vansickel, C., Haas, M.B., & Speca, M.M. (1991). The Inventory of Functional Status—Antepartum Period: Development and testing. *Journal of Nurse Midwifery, 36,* 117-123.

Weiss, M.E. (1991). The relationship between marital independence and adaptation to parenthood in primiparous couples (Doctoral dissertation, University of San Diego, 1990). *Dissertation Abstracts International, 51,* 3783-B.

Bibliography

Roy, C. (1988). Human information processing. In J. J. Fitzpatrick, R. L. Taunton, & J.Q. Benoliel (Eds.), *Annual review of nursing research 4,* pp. 237-263). New York: Springer.

Roy, C., & Andrews, H. (1991). *The Roy Adaptation Model: The definitive statement.* Norwalk, CT: Appleton & Lange.

Chapter 6

Interdependence Mode Research

This chapter includes a review of research reported between 1970 and 1994 which focused primarily on the interdependence adaptive mode of the Roy Adaptation Model (RAM). Twenty studies based on the RAM, including nine articles, seven dissertations, and four theses focused mainly on the interdependence mode. In all studies, the interactions of people with others to meet their social needs were investigated.

Purposes

The purposes of this chapter are to (a) critically analyze interdependence adaptative mode research, (b) evaluate the relationship of interdependence mode research to the RAM, and (c) synthesize contributions of the reported studies to nursing science. Contributions to nursing science include applications for nursing practice, recommendations for model-based interdependence mode research, and directions for further theory and RAM development of the interdependence mode.

Background

The interdependence mode involves interaction with others. Through this mode, individuals meet their affectional needs (Roy & Andrews, 1991). In the interdependence mode, the person is striving to achieve affectional adequacy through interaction, communication, and mutual nurturing. Affectional adequacy is described in this mode as the giving and receiving of love, value, and respect.

An adaptive response is observed in the establishing of mutually satisfying relationships or a freely chosen state of aloneness; whereas an ineffective response may include loneliness, separation, or alienation. In this mode, the specific relationships of significant others and support systems are examined. A significant other is the individual to whom the most meaning or importance is given, while support systems are persons, groups, or animals that contribute to meeting a person's interdependence needs.

In the theoretic development of the interdependence mode, propositions are derived that relate the regulator and cognator subsystems to interdependence mode adaptation. Adaptation in the interdependence mode, therefore, refers to adaptive and ineffective subsystem activity related to significant others and support systems.

Critical Analysis of Interdependence Mode Research

Each study in this chapter will be critically analyzed; that is, a brief description of the reported research will be followed by analysis according to established guidelines related to validity, reliability, data analysis, and findings.

Description of Reported Research

Studies of the interdependence adaptative mode were focused on significant others, support systems, or the ineffective responses of loneliness and abuse. For clarity of presentation, or the 20 studies were categorized as investigations of interdependence functioning of (a) significant others (n = 8), (b) significant others as caregivers (n = 5), (c) support systems (n = 3), and (d) loneliness and abuse (n = 4).

Significant others. In five of the eight studies categorized as investigating the interdependence needs of patients and/or their significant others (Table 6.1), researchers focused on the spouses of post-operative surgical patients. The female spouses of coronary artery bypass surgery (CABG) patients were the subjects of three studies conducted by Artinian (1988/1989, 1991, 1992). Using a longitudinal design, the author examined the sources of stress identified as hardships and demands associated with cardiac surgery. The mediators of stress were identified as social support, coping responses, and perception of illness severity. The manifestations of stress were identified as the spouses' stress responses (Artinian, 1988/1989). As derived by the author from the RAM, the model indicated relationships among the variables. The focal stimulus was the patient's recovery from CABG surgery—with social support, hardship, and demands being viewed as contextual stimuli. Internal processing was represented by the spouse's perception of the partner's illness severity and active and avoidance coping, while behavioral output was identified as physical and mental stress, role strain, and marital quality. Data were collected at two points. Time one (T1) data collection was conducted in the hospital with questionnaires and self-report scales; time two (T2) data were collected 6 weeks later at home using mailed questionnaires. The data presented four major findings: (a) social support was positively related to active coping and dyadic adjustment, (b) hardships and demands were negatively related to stress responses, (c) perception of illness severity was negatively related to stress responses, and (d) avoidance coping was positively related to stress responses. Using regression analysis, findings indicated that (a) social support accounted for 21% of the variance, (b) perception of illness severity added 12% to the explained variance, and (c) hardships and demands accounted for an additional 6% of variance. Data to determine which nursing interventions were viewed as supportive or nonsupportive by spouses were also collected. Results indicated that unfamiliarity of hospi-

Table 6.1 – Description of Studies About Relationships of Significant Others and/or Patients in the Interdependence Mode of the RAM (N = 8)

Author(s) & Date	Purpose	Sample	Design	Findings
1. Artinian (1988/1989)	To explore the stress process of the patient's spouse over time and to test relationships predicted by use of the model	Female spouses of coronary artery bypass (CABG) patients (N=86)	Correlational	Social support was significantly related to active coping and dyadic adjustment. Avoidance coping was significantly related to stress. Hardships and demands and perceptions of illness severity were significantly negatively related to stress. Regression indicated that social support explained 21% of the variance, perception of illness severity added 12%, while hardships and demands added 6%. Unfamiliarity of hospital environment and lack of information made hospitalization more difficult for spouses.
2. Artinian (1991)	To describe stress-process variables in spouses of CABG patients during hospitalization (T1) and 6 weeks after discharge (T2)	Females spouses of CABG patients (n=86)	Descriptive	Women reported an average number of family life changes and high levels of social support at T1 and T2. Physical and mental symptoms of stress were high at T1 but significantly less at T2. Marital quality was average at T1 but significantly less at T2. Husband's self-care activities, uncertainty, and husband's physical and mental symptoms were concerns at T2.

(continued)

Table 6.1 *(continued)*

Author(s) & Date	Purpose	Sample	Design	Findings
3. Artinian (1992)	To describe the stress process variables in spouses of CABG patients 1 year (T3) after CABG surgery	Female spouses of CABG patients (N=49)	Descriptive	Social support was moderate and significantly less at T3. Women still perceived their husbands as having some illness severity at T3, but significantly less than at T1 and T2. Symptoms of stress continued and role strain was significantly greater at T3 than at T1 or T2, while marital quality remained constant with T2. Spouses reported making several life-style changes.
4. Gardner (1994)	To describe the adaptation of spouses after their partner's open heart surgery (OHS) using the theory of person as an adaptive system	Spouses of OHS patients (N=45)	Correlational	The state of marital relationship explained 28% of the variation in spousal adaptation, while no other predictor variables accounted for a significant portion of the variance. No differences existed between gender in psychosocial adaptation. Highest percentage of ineffective adaptation occurred in the self-concept and interdependence modes while the greatest problems identified occurred in the interdependence and role function modes.

5. Silva (1987)	To identify and categorize the needs of spouses of surgical patients within the RAM	Spouses of surgical patients with a benign condition (N=75)	Descriptive	The most important needs included reassurance about quality of care, availability of staff, and clarity of information provided. Factor analysis indicated that needs were present in all four modes of the RAM, but in a different pattern than indicated by the model.
6. Bradley & Williams (1990)	To describe and compare the pre-operative concerns of open heart surgery (OHS) patients with concerns of their significant others (SOs).	Pairs of OHS patients and their SOs (N=21)	Correlational	Similar concerns were the effectiveness of the surgery in improving the patient's condition, surviving the surgery, and the development of post-operative complica-tions. Differences included high levels of concern by patients regarding resumption of activity, lifestyle modifica-tions, and understanding the surgical procedure, while SOs were most concerned about understanding the ICU environment, providing emotional support, and paying bills.

(continued)

Table 6.1 (continued)

Author(s) & Date	Purpose	Sample	Design	Findings
7. Grinspun (1991)	To describe the influence of the head injury patient's condition on spouse's adaptation and to describe factors that spouses identified as influencing adaptation	Spouses of head injury patients (N=40)	Correlational	The higher the communication and behavioral deficits the lower the level of spousal adaptation. There was no evidence of link between categories of time since injury, physical deficits, and spousal adaptation. Obtaining information and emotional support influenced spousal adaptation.
8. Baker (1993)	To determine the effects of the presence of a spouse on stroke patients' adaptation	Charts of stroke patients who received rehabilitation (N=67)	Descriptive	Married stroke patients who completed rehabilitation achieved a significantly higher level of adaptation than comparable patients without a spouse.

tal environment and lack of information about the patient's surgery and progress made hospitalization more difficult for spouses.

Using the same methods as those of the previous study, Artinian (1991) published results that focused on the life changes made by spouses. Results indicated that the women who participated in the study reported an average number of family life changes and high levels of social support at T1 and T2. They perceived their husband's illness severity at the extreme end of the continuum at both T1 and T2. Physical and mental symptoms of stress were high at T1 but significantly less at T2. Marital quality was average at T1 but significantly less at T2. Hospital environment, lack of information, and behaviors of family members were frequently reported to make hospitalization more difficult. Husband's self-care activities, uncertainty, physical and mental symptoms were concerns that spouses frequently reported at T2.

Artinian (1992) then conducted a 1-year (T3) follow-up study of the same subjects. The purpose was to describe spouses' life stressors, supports, perceptions of illness severity, role strain, physical and mental symptoms of stress, and marital quality 1 year after their husbands' CABG surgeries. Of the original 86 study participants, 49 women participated in the follow-up study. Results indicated that social support was moderate and significantly less at T3 than at T1 and T2. Women still perceived their husbands to have some illness severity 1 year after surgery, although this variable decreased significantly at T3. They continued to have physical and mental symptoms of stress and had significantly greater role strain than during T1 and T2. Spouses reported making several life-style changes in diet and activity to promote their husbands' recoveries from T2 to T3. Marital quality remained constant.

Gardner (1994) replicated a portion of Artinian's studies by examining the various concepts of spousal adaptation that explained marital quality. The primary focus of the study was interdependence, although other psychosocial concepts were measured. The focal stimulus remained the partner's open heart surgery, but contextual stimuli for this study were partner's health status before surgery, length of time since diagnosis of heart disease, number of years married, and the general state of the marital relationship. This study included both male and female spouses to identify gender differences in adaptation. Findings indicated that the state of marital relationship explained 28% of the variation in spousal psychosocial adaptation. The highest percentage of ineffective adaptive responses occurred in the domains of social environment and psychological distress—specifically behaviors in the self-concept and interdependence modes, respectively. The greatest problems identified by the spouses occurred in the interdependence and role function modes.

Two additional studies examined the interdependence needs of spouses of surgical patients (Silva, 1987; Bradley & Williams, 1990). The focal stimulus for Silva's study was the needs of spouses that trigger regulator and/or cognator coping mechanisms leading to adaptation in the four modes. The most important needs identified by spouses were related to reassurance about quality of patient care, availability of hospital staff, and understandability of information provided about the patients' hospitalizations and surgeries. While the results of factor analysis identified the interdependence needs of spouses, the other four modes were also reflected.

Bradley and Williams (1990) compared the preoperative concerns of open-heart surgery patients with the concerns of their significant others. The focal stimulus was identified as the surgery and contextual stimuli included educational level, age, marital status, prior surgeries, and prior myocardial infarctions. The concerns of both patients and significant others were categorized according to the four modes of the RAM and compared. Multiple concerns were reported with some similarities and some differences between patients and their significant others. Similarities included concerns about the effectiveness of the surgery in improving the patient's condition, surviving the surgery, and the development of post-operative complications. Differences included high levels of concerns by patients regarding resumption of activity, life-style modifications, and understanding the surgical procedure, while significant others were most concerned about understanding the intensive care environment, providing emotional support, and paying bills.

Grinspun (1991) studied the influence of the condition of head injured patients on their spouses' adaptation. The patient's condition, including physical condition and communication and behavioral deficits, was the focal stimulus with spousal adaptation viewed as the response to the stimulus. Findings indicated that (a) the more the communication and behavioral deficits, the lower the level of spousal adaptation, (b) time since injury and physical condition were not related to spousal adaptation, and (c) obtaining information and emotional support influenced spousal adaptation.

Baker (1993) conducted a chart review to identify the effect of a spouse on the adaptation of stroke patients who had completed rehabilitation. The presence of a spouse was a contextual stimulus which could influence patient adaptation after a stroke. The study's findings supported the hypothesis that patients who had a stroke and completed a rehabilitation program would achieve a higher level of adaptation if they had a spouse than would comparable patients without a spouse.

Family caregiving research. Research related to the interdependence mode and family caregiving was reported in five studies. Four of these studies were focused on providing care for the elderly or for adult patients with specific needs, while one study was focused on the empowerment process of mothers with chronically ill children (Table 6.2).

The burden of providing care for the elderly was examined by Smith (1989/1990) who sampled 36 caregiver daughters at the onset of the study and 6 weeks later. No significant relationships between change in caregiver burden and change in the four adaptive modes could be found during the time frame for this study. Findings indicated that caregiving had been an ongoing process which had begun informally before participation in the study. Caregiver burden scores indicated a high moderate perception of burden that remained stable throughout the study.

Perkins (1987/1988) studied relationships among interdependence, caregiver burden, and adaptation in 72 family caregivers and 72 frail elderly. Caregivers for the elderly included spouses, children, or other relatives who had lived with the person at least 6 months before the study. Caregiver burden was operationalized as subjective and objective burden. Subjective burden included the stressful feelings, attitudes, and emotions expressed by family caregivers. Objective burden involved the stressful events, happenings, and activities experienced by family caregivers. Major findings included the subjective burden of caregiving increasing when the elderly person's mental health was poor and decreasing as affection for the elderly increased. The elderly people's affection for the caregivers was significantly greater than the caregivers' affection for the elderly. Conversely, the caregiver's obligation to care for the elderly was greater than the elderly person's feeling that caregivers had the responsibility to provide care. Additional findings included that caregiving was less of a burden when assumed over time, than when assumed in a crisis situation.

Smith, Mayer, Parkhurst, Perkins, and Pingleton (1991) examined how caregivers adapt to having ventilator-dependent adults at home. The focal stimulus was a family member requiring home care which affected caregiver adaptation in the four modes of the RAM. The authors found that caregivers perceived their functioning as satisfactory and identified themselves as coping effectively. Interview data reflected both positive and negative responses to caregiving with the majority of responses being concerned with role mastery, self-concept, and interdependence functioning. Positive themes reflected confidence in ventilator care, satisfaction with the decision to provide home care, and improved quality of life. Negative caregiver themes reflected the burden of caregiving, patient dependence, resentment, and hopelessness. Of the small number of caregiver responses categorized as physiologic, few indicated that the role of caregiver affected physical health.

Physical health being unaffected by the caregiving role was also indicated in the study by the Smith, Moushey, Ross, and Geiffer (1993) study, in which 85% of the subjects stated that their health was good and had not changed within the last 3 months. However, 30% reported increased fatigue. In this qualitative study, investigators examined the responsibili-

Table 6.2 – Description of Studies About Relationships of Significant Others as Caregivers in the Interdependence Adaptive Mode of the RAM (N=5)

Author(s) & Date	Purpose	Sample	Design	Findings
9. Smith (1989/1990)	To examine the adaptation of middle-aged daughters to caregiving for a dependent, elderly parent	Primary caregiver daughters (N=36)	Correlational	There were no significant relationships between caregiver burden and change in the four adaptive modes.
10. Perkins (1987/1988)	To identify the relationships among interdependence, caregiver burden, and adaptation in the homebound, frail elderly	Elderly (n=72) and caregivers (n=72)	Correlational	Caregiver subjective burden increased when the elderly's mental health was poor, and decreased when affection for the elderly was high. Caregivers experienced less burden when adjustment to the caregiving role was developed over time. The elderly person's affection for the caregiver was significantly greater than the caregiver's affection for the elderly. The caregiver's obligation to care for the elderly was greater than the elderly's feelings that the caregiver should be responsible for their care.
11. Smith, Mayer, Parkhurst, Perkins, & Pringleton (1991)	To determine how caregivers adapt to having ventilator dependent adults at home	Related caregivers of adult ventilator patients (N=20)	Descriptive	Caregivers perceived their functioning as satisfactory and identified themselves as coping effectively. Interview data reflected both positive and negative responses to caregiving. Physical health was not affected by caregiving.

12. Smith, Moushey, Ross, & Geiffer (1993)	To examine the responsibilities and reactions of family caregivers who have a relative dependent on total parenteral nutrition (TPN)	Relatives of TPN dependent patients and 1 self caregiver (*N*=20)	Qualitative Case Study	Physical health was not affected by caregiving. Family responsibilities had changed since the initiation of home TPN. Caregivers mastered TPN technology and felt capable and successful in their caregiving role.
13. Gibson (1993/1994)	To describe the process of empowerment in mothers of chronically ill children	Mothers of neurologically impaired children (*N*=12)	Qualitative descriptive	The outcome of the empowerment process was participatory competence. Mothers developed the necessary knowledge, competence, and confidence for participation in their children's health care decisions.

ties and reactions of family members who provided home care to a relative dependent on total parenteral nutrition (TPN). Interview data reflected that responsibilities within the family changed since the initiation of home TPN, that caregivers mastered TPN technology, and that caregivers felt capable and successful in their caregiving role.

The process of empowerment in the mothers of hospitalized chronically ill neurologically impaired children was explored in a qualitative study by Gibson (1993/1994). The author identified interdependence as embedded in the empowerment process. Empowerment existed in a relationship with others when the mother felt understood, when requests and suggestions were considered, and when cooperative relationships with others were developed. The outcome of the empowerment process was participatory competence where the mothers developed and employed the necessary knowledge, competence, and confidence for participation in their children's health care decisions.

Support systems. In three studies, researchers explored the relationships of support systems to the interdependence mode of the RAM (Table 6.3). Short (1994) developed the Interdependence Questionnaire to assess interdependence adaptation of newly delivered mothers. The questionnaire included the following categories of interdependence functioning as described in the model: significant other, support systems (extended family), support systems (friendships), and feeling alone or lonely. The items addressed both giving and receiving behaviors in the areas of love, support, value, and security in the four identified categories. The questionnaire was a 45-item, five-point Likert-type scale with scores ranging from 1 (*strongly disagree*) to 5 (*strongly agree*). Results of the pilot test indicated that support systems (friendships) had the highest mean score, followed by significant other, support systems (extended family), and feeling alone or lonely, respectively.

Two studies were focused upon the relationship of support systems to interdependence adaptation. In the first study, the grief responses of widows ($N = 65$) during their second year of bereavement were studied (Robinson, 1991/1992). The focal stimulus was the loss of a spouse; contextual stimuli were social support, social network, education, income, and religious or spiritual beliefs. Coping responses were viewed as cognator functioning and grief responses represented adaption outcomes. Findings indicated that widows with more social support had higher coping scores and lower grief responses.

Eves (1992/1993) found that parents who were members of a support group for parents of developmentally disabled children possessed more adaptive coping mechanisms and fewer child care concerns than parents who were not members of such a group. In addition, fathers were as likely as mothers to access a large number of social support systems. The focal

Table 6. 3 – Description of Studies About Relationships of Support Systems in the Interdependence Adaptive Mode of the RAM (N = 3)

Author(s) & Date	Purpose	Sample	Design	Findings
14. Short (1994)	To evaluate the interdependence functioning of mothers after childbirth	Newly delivered mothers (N=10)	Instrument Development	Support systems (friendships) had the highest mean score followed by significant other, support systems (extended family), and feeling alone or lonely.
15. Robinson (1991/1992)	To examine the grief responses of widows during their second year of bereavement and to identify variables which influence the grief process	Widows in their second year of bereavement (N=65)	Correlational	Widows with more social support had higher coping scores and lower scores for grief response.
16. Eves (1992/1993)	To identify the concerns, support systems, and coping strategies of parents of developmentally disabled children	Parents of developmentally disabled children (N=48)	Correlational	Parents who are members of a parent support group possessed more adaptive coping mechanisms and had fewer concerns about resources for child care than parents who were not members of a support group. Fathers were as likely as mothers to access support systems.

stimulus for this study was caring for a developmentally disabled child which initiated coping behaviors leading to adaptation.

Abuse and loneliness research. In four studies, abusive relationships and loneliness were examined. In the two studies that explored abuse, Brown (1989/1990) focused on elder abuse, while Limandri (1985) focused on abused women (Table 6.4). Through examination of case files (Brown, 1989/1990) the characteristics of the abused and abuser, types of abuse, reporting sources of abuse, and causal factors were identified. The RAM theoretic framework was used to describe the health professional's role when working with the abused and abuser, but data were not collected about providing care for either group. Results indicated that the most common form of abuse was physical violence perpetrated on white elderly females by males living in the same household. Abuse was most often reported by hospitals or clinics.

Limandri (1985) examined the relationship of the independent variables of abuse, self-esteem, perceived role conflict, and social support, with the dependent variable of help-seeking behaviors, among 40 abused women. The focal stimuli were the women's perceptions of the severity of abuse, the escalation or extension of violence, and the identification of women as recipients of abuse. Contextual stimuli included the woman's general mental health, her experience with crises, her role socialization, and her social support. Results indicated that none of the independent variables were significantly related to the dependent variable.

Research related to the ineffective response of loneliness was the subject of two studies. Calvert (1989) examined the extent to which interaction with an animal reduced loneliness in 65 nursing home residents. The focal stimulus was feelings of alienation which resulted in loneliness. Contextual stimuli included poor health, lack of social contact, and institutionalization. Pet interaction was viewed as a contextual stimulus that would reduce loneliness. Findings indicated that residents who had higher levels of interaction with a pet program experienced significantly less loneliness than those who had lower levels of such interaction.

In the second study, Pruden (1991/1992) examined the relationships among adaptation, social support, and loneliness in 35 dyads with one partner having been diagnosed with chronic obstructive pulmonary disease (COPD). Focal stimuli included the increasing disability and escalating nature of COPD, which would compromise independence and dyadic adaptation. Results indicated that a negative significant correlation existed between dyadic adaptation and loneliness and between social support and loneliness, that is, couples with high levels of social support experienced higher levels of adaptation and less loneliness.

In this section, interdependence mode adaptation as an outcome has been defined in differing ways in a variety of samples. Investigators have found it an important variable to study and have derived implications

Table 6.4 – Description of Studies About Relationships of Abuse and Loneliness in the Interdependence Adaptive Mode of the RAM (N = 4)

Author(s) & Date	Purpose	Sample	Design	Findings
17. Brown (1989/1990)	To examine the characteristics of the abused elderly and abuser, types of abuse, sources, and causal factors	Case management files selected at random (N=57)	Descriptive	Physical violence perpetrated on white elderly females by males living in the same household was the most common form of abuse reported. Abuse was most often reported by employees of hospitals or clinics.
18. Limandri (1985)	To examine the relationship of abuse to self-esteem, perceived role conflict, social support, and help-seeking behaviors	Abused adult women (N=40)	Correlational	Level of self-esteem, perceived role conflict, and functional social support were not significantly related to help-seeking behaviors.
19. Calvert (1989)	To examine the extent to which interaction with an animal reduces loneliness in nursing home residents	Nursing home residents (N=65)	Descriptive	Nursing home residents who had greater levels of interaction with a pet program experienced less loneliness than those who had lower levels of interaction with a pet program.
20. Pruden (1991/ 1992)	To test the theory of interdependence derived from the RAM by examining the relationships of social support, loneliness, and adaptation in dyads where one partner had chronic obstructive pulmonary disease (COPD)	COPD patients and their spouses (N=35)	Correlational	Couples with high levels of social support had higher levels of adaption and less loneliness than did couples with lower levels of social support.

from their findings that will be discussed in the synthesis section of this chapter.

Critical Analysis of Reported Research

Based on the description of the 20 studies reviewed for the interdependence mode, each study was critically analyzed with respect to the quality of the research. Of the 20 interdependence studies, 17 were quantitative, either descriptive or correlational, two were qualitative, and one focused on instrument development. Critical analyses are presented separately for the quantitative, qualitative, and instrument-development studies.

Critical analysis of quantitative research. Critical analyses of the 17 quantitative studies are presented in Table 6.5. In most of the studies, measures were taken to at least partially control for the threats to internal and external validity. Instrument reliability was addressed in 85% of the studies, and validity in 90%. In all studies, the data were appropriately analyzed. Two studies lacked a consistency of findings with conclusions.

Of the 17 quantitative studies, 16 included attempts to control for threats to internal validity. History and mortality were issues in the longitudinal studies (Artinian, 1988/1989, 1991; Smith, 1989/1990). Artinian attempted to control for history by including life events in the 12 months before the study as an independent variable, while Smith made no efforts to control for history. An alternative hypothesis to the Smith study, which was acknowledged by the author, was that the absence of change in the dependent variable of caregiver adaptation, was caused by assumption of the caregiving role before the time of the first data collection for the study.

Likewise, mortality was an issue in both studies. Smith (1989/1990) recruited 72 volunteers as subjects, but identified 36 subjects as the sample. The author did not identify if subjects dropped out of the study before or during data collection and provided no explanation why subjects withdrew from the study or how subjects remaining in the study differed from subjects who withdrew from the study. In comparison, Artinian (1988/ 1989) accounted for all actual and potential subjects. She identified the number of potential subjects who met eligibility requirements, the number who consented to participate, and the number who did not complete and return the questionnaires. In the follow-up study (Artinian, 1992) the 43% mortality rate was accounted for and reasons were given for the loss of subjects. Subjects who remained in the study were not compared to subjects who withdrew.

Maturation was a threat to only one of the longitudinal studies. Artinian's (1992) follow-up study was conducted 1 year after the original study; therefore, there was ample opportunity for changes to occur within the subjects between the first study and the follow-up study. In the other longitudinal studies (Artinian, 1988/1989, 1991; Smith, 1989/1990), data

Table 6.5 – Critical Analysis of Quantitative Interdependence Adaptive Mode Research (*N*=17)

Criteria	Evaluation		
	Yes	*Partially*	*No*
Design			
Efforts to control for threats to internal validity	1,2,3,4,5,6,10, 11,15,16,18,19,20	7,8,9	17
Efforts to control for threats to external validity	1,2,4,6,10,11, 15,20	3,5,7,8,9, 16,19	17,18
Measurement			
Reliability of instruments addressed	1,2,3,4,5,9, 10,11,15,16, 18,19,20	7	6,8,17
Validity of instruments addressed	1,2,3,4,5,6,7,9, 10,11,15,16, 18,19,20		8,17
Data Analysis			
Appropriate	1,2,3,4,5,6,7,8,9, 10,11,15,16, 17,18,19,20		
Interpretation of Results			
Consistency of findings with conclusions	1,2,3,4,5,6,7,9,10, 11,15,16,18,19,20		8,17

Key: 1=Artinian, 1988/1989; 2=Artinian, 1991; 3=Artinian, 1992; 4=Gardner, 1994; 5=Silva, 1987; 6=Bradley & Williams, 1990; 7=Grinspun, 1991; 8=Baker, 1993; 9=Smith, 1989/1990; 10=Perkins, 1987/1988; 11=Smith, Mayer, Parkhurst, Perkins, & Pringleton, 1991; 15=Robinson,1991/1992; 16=Eves, 1992/1993; 17=Brown, 1989/ 1990; 18=Limandri, 1985; 19=Calvert, 1989; 20=Pruden, 1991/1992.

collection times were 6 weeks apart. The 6-week time frame was probably not sufficient to have produced significant differences in the dependent variables.

Smith and colleagues (1991) were better able to control for threats to internal validity than were Baker (1993) and Brown (1989/1990). Smith and colleagues trained two research assistants to use a structured interview guide to collect data, while in both the Baker and Brown studies multiple individuals contributed to the data sets. Neither investigator addressed interrater reliability nor addressed the training of data collectors.

Baker examined the charts of stroke patients who received rehabilitation. The Barthel Index was used to evaluate patients' level of adaptation before and after rehabilitation. Many people rated the patients' adaptation level. The author did not indicate their level of training. Likewise, Brown examined case management files from an adult protective services agency. The files contained information from differing sources, resulting in conflicting and missing data. The researcher did not completely describe the procedures used to collect data or address the resolution of the problems with missing data. In both the Brown and Baker studies, a rival hypothesis may have been that the change in the dependent variables was a result of different individuals contributing to the data sets.

Most investigators had well-defined procedures and selection criteria for inclusion of subjects. For example, in the eight studies in which spouses were subjects, some of the selection criteria were no common law marriages (Baker, 1993), spouses living together without the immediate threat of divorce or separation (Gardner, 1994), spouses of patients undergoing major surgery and expecting a benign outcome (Silva, 1987), and the exclusion of spouses of patients who had a cardiac arrest (Gardner, 1994) or other active cardiovascular or pulmonary disease (Pruden,1991/1992).

In the studies of significant others as subjects, a variety of relationships were identified. Smith's (1989/1990) sample included primary caregiver daughters, while the remaining authors included children, friends, and extended family members. Bradley and Williams (1990) used the selection criteria of the patient selecting a significant other from the categories of spouse, other immediate family member, relative, or friend. In studies that addressed caregiver adaptation, Perkins (1987/1988) included only caregivers who had lived with the frail elderly for a minimum of 6 months, while Smith, Mayer, and colleagues (1991) included any relatives who provided daily care of patients requiring mechanical ventilation.

Both Robinson (1991/1992) and Calvert (1989) had well-developed subject selection criteria. Robinson limited participation to widows 45 years or older who were in their second year of bereavement. Calvert (1989) administered an assessment tool to nursing home residents to test orientation, memory, and ability to perform serial mental operations. Only residents who were able to answer the questions correctly without assistance were included in the study. Eves (1992/1993) and Limandri (1985) had less well-developed selection criteria. Eves included parents of children with developmental disabilities without regard to severity, while Limandri used a self-selected sample of abused women with no inclusion criteria regarding type, severity, recency, or duration of abuse.

In all but two of the quantitative studies, researchers included attempts to control for threats to external validity. Authors attempted to control the environment, extraneous variables, consistency of procedures, and generalizability of findings to other populations. In only one study (Calvert,

1989), consistency of treatment was partially addressed by grouping levels of pet interaction.

Several authors attempted to control the environment by limiting data collection locations. The majority of authors collected data in hospitals, in homes, and by mail. Robinson (1991/1992) collected data in both the homes of subjects and in a hospice. The author did not specify the reason for data collection in the hospice, but does state that several subjects were contacted through a local hospice program. Limandri (1985) collected instrument data from 37 subjects at the time of personal contact, while 3 subjects later returned questionnaires by mail. In two studies (Baker, 1993; Brown, 1989/1990), data were collected by non-reactive means through the use of hospital charts and case files. In three studies, data were elicited from both patients and significant others. Bradley and Williams (1990) collected data independently from patients and significant others, while in the other two studies (Perkins, 1987/1988; Pruden, 1992), subjects may or may not have been together during data collection. Both authors allowed subjects to remain together if they desired.

All authors attempted to control for some extraneous variables through the collection of demographic and descriptive information about their subjects. Demographic information commonly included age, marital status, ethnic background, religious preference, employment status, family income, living arrangements, and, in some studies, health information. In most instances, this information was thoroughly analyzed and provided important sample characteristics. In addition to using demographic information, Artinian (1988/1989, 1991,1992) controlled for the extraneous variable of life changes within the year previous to the spouses' CABG surgeries by including the changes as an independent variable. Conversely, Limandri (1985) did not control for the severity or type of abuse and did not include either of these factors as independent variables.

Consistency during data collection was an issue in five studies. Authors (Perkins, 1987/1988; Robinson, 1991/1992; Calvert, 1989; Pruden, 1991/1992) reported reading instruments to some subjects, but not to others, which may have affected subjects' responses. Subjects may have responded to tones or inflections in an investigator's voice, thereby influencing independent and dependent variables. But given the age and illnesses of the subjects being sampled, the reading of instruments seems to be appropriate to ensure that the subjects understood what information the researcher was requesting. For some subjects, reading instruments may be the only method of data collection which ensures accuracy.

Convenience sampling was used in 14 studies, limiting the generalizability of findings from these samples to other populations. Perkins (1987/1988) selected subjects randomly from an active caseload at a community health nursing agency, while Brown (1989/1990) used a systematic sampling technique by including every third abuse case file. Purposive sampling which included 20 out of 23 families with a member requiring mechanical ventilation at home in a Midwestern metropolitan area was used by Smith and colleagues (1991). Three authors attempted to increase the generalizability of their studies by data comparison. Smith (1989/1990) compared her sample to a national survey of caregivers, while Silva (1987) compared data with the normal curve. Limandri (1985) compared the demographic data from her sample to the characteristics of abused women from three previous studies conducted by other authors.

Regarding measurement issues, the majority of authors sufficiently addressed instrument validity and reliability to allow the reader to determine the appropriateness of the instruments. Bradley and Williams (1990) omitted reliability data for their author-generated instruments about the concerns of open-heart surgery patients and their significant others. Grinspun (1991) used a scale in one instrument with a low reliability coefficient. Several authors reported reliability for the study sample, and one author (Grinspun, 1991) computed the reliability of an author-generated instrument on a pilot sample. Allowing for issues of retrospective data from charts and file review, the authors did not specifically address validity or reliability (Baker, 1993; Brown 1989/1990). In both of these studies, instrumentation consisted of tabulating data from the chart or case file.

All authors appropriately analyzed data. In most of the studies consistency between findings and conclusions was found. In two studies (Baker, 1993; Brown, 1989/1990), the authors drew conclusions that were not consistent with the findings. Baker discussed specific mechanisms by which spouses facilitated adaptation, such as buffering stress, assisting with independent living, and responding to a changing environment. Survey data collected by the author consisted of information about adaptation and the presence or absence of a spouse, not about how the spouse facilitated adaptation. Brown drew conclusions about the internal and external stressors affecting the abuser, while the data collected did not identify any stressors affecting the abuser.

Critical analysis of qualitative research. Evaluation of the two interdependence mode qualitative studies is presented in Table 6.6. Smith, Moushey, and colleagues (1993) used a case study approach to examine caregiver adaptation in relatives of patients receiving TPN. A semistructured interview guide was developed by the investigators and reviewed by experts familiar with home care and qualitative methods of data gathering. The same interview guide had been used to gather data for a previous study of family caregivers of patients on home mechanical ventilators (Smith et al., 1991). The authors used approaches such as descriptive vividness, analytical preciseness, and theoretic connectedness to ensure validity. Data were gathered by either telephone or home visits, thereby limiting methodological congruence. Strategies to ensure reliability included the use of two research assistants to collect data with an interrater reliability of 95%. Participants in the study included 19 relatives of patients receiving TPN and one patient who lived alone and provided all of his own care. The inclusion of the self-caregiver affects the generalizability of the findings. The structured interview guide asked questions such as "How have the responsibilities of family members changed since (patient's name) has been receiving TPN at home?" and "Family members have many emotional reactions to the changes in the person they are caring for. What have been your experiences with these responses?" Answers to these questions might be different for patients providing their own care.

Gibson (1993/1994) described the empowerment process in mothers of neurologically impaired children and used strategies such as descriptive vividness, methodological congruence, and analytical preciseness to ensure validity. The author provided vivid accounts of specific examples of the empowerment process. Consistency was achieved by coding each transcript three separate times and by having a second person randomly validate that coding. The author implemented multiple strategies to ensure reliability such as providing extensive descriptions so that others may reach a conclusion about whether transferability is possible by triangulating data from multiple sources and by addressing personal competence and bias. For both studies, the method of data analysis was appropriate and there was consistency of findings with conclusions.

Critical analysis of an instrument-development study. Short (1994) developed a tool to evaluate the interdependence needs of new mothers (Table 6.7). The Interdependence Questionnaire identified four categories

---

Table 6.6 – Critical Analysis of Qualitative Interdependence Mode Research (*N*=2)

Criteria	Evaluation		
	Yes	*Partially*	*No*
Strategies for validity	13	12	
Strategies for reliability	13	12	
Data Analysis appropriate	12,13		
Consistency of findings with conclusions	12,13		

Key: 12=Smith, Moushey, Ross, & Geiffer, 1993; 13= Gibson, 1993/1994

---

of interdependence needs according to the RAM: (a) significant other, (b) support systems (extended family), (c) support systems (friendships), and (d) feelings of loneliness. Items included in the questionnaire addressed both giving and receiving behaviors in the areas of love, support, value, and security in the four identified categories.

A review of the questionnaire for content validity was completed by a maternal-child clinician and a researcher familiar with the RAM. The author stated that revisions to the instrument were made after the review, but did not specify what revisions were made or how many items were revised. The content validity is limited. Measured by the Spearman-Brown prophecy formula, the instrument reliability was 0.88. The instrument appears to have beginning support for reliability, but has been used only with a small sample ($N = 10$ new mothers).

Evaluation of Relationships to the RAM

After the critical analysis of each of the interdependence adaptative mode studies, those that met the criteria were evaluated for relationships to the RAM. Evaluation consisted of examining the research variables, empiric measures, and findings for each study, and identifying the strength of their relationship to the model. The findings of the studies with analytic strength and adequate links to the model are used to test propositions derived from the model.

Evaluation of Linkages to the RAM

Evaluation of the linkages between the 15 interdependence adaptive mode studies and the RAM is summarized in Table 6.8. Most authors explicitly identified the model and linked research variables, empiric measures, and findings to the model. Several authors examined their variables by extending the model concepts. Gibson (1993/1994) conceptualized the process of empowerment, while Artinian (1988/1989, 1991, 1992) conceptualized multiple parts of the model to explain stress process variables over time.

Table 6.7 – Strategies Used in Instrument Development for Interdependence Adaptation Research ($N=1$)

Author/Year	Reliability	Validity
14. Short (1994)	Spearman-Brown split-half 0.88	Content validity judged by a maternal-child clinician and a researcher familiar with RAM.

In 15 of the studies, model linkages between research variables and empiric measures were explicitly identified. The weakest area of relating research to the model was in the discussion of the findings, where three authors implied the model linkages. Evaluation of the linkages supported the effectiveness of the RAM in guiding nursing research.

Table 6.8 – Evaluation of Linkages of Interdependence Adaptive Mode Research with the Roy Adaptation Model (N=15)

Linkages to RAM	Evaluation		
	Explicit	*Implict*	*Absent*
Research variables	1,2,3,4,5,7,9,10,11, 12,13,15,16,19,20		
Empirical measures	1,2,3,4,5,7,9,10,11, 12,13,15,16,19,20		
Findings	1,2,4,5,7,10,11,13, 15,16,19,20	3,9,12,	

Key: 1=Artinian, 1988/1989; 2=Artinian, 1991; 3=Artinian, 1992; 4=Gardner, 1994; 5=Silva, 1987; 7=Grinspun, 1991; 9=Smith, 1989/1990; 10=Perkins, 1987/1988; 11=Smith, Mayer, Parkhurst, Perkins, & Pringleton, 1991; 12=Smith, Moushey, Ross, & Geiffer, 1993; 13=Gibson, 1993/1994; 15=Robinson,1991/1992; 16=Eves, 1992/1993; 19=Calvert, 1989; 20=Pruden, 1991/1992

Testing of the RAM Propositions

Criteria were developed to determine if the results of research using the RAM supported the propositions of the model. In studies which were focused on the interdependence adaptive mode, 15 were examined for the relationships of study findings to major model propositions.

Data from studies of the interdependence mode were used to test six of the propositions from the RAM, as noted in Table 6.9. Three of these propositions had several ancillary propositions. The ancillary propositions are specific statements that relate to the interdependence mode. The propositions were based on existence and relational statements with model concepts, definitions, and assumptions in the published works of Roy (Roy & Roberts, 1981; Roy & Andrews, 1991).

The model shows that at the individual level regulator and cognator processes affect innate and acquired ways of adapting. In six studies, researchers supported the proposition that changes in interdependence

Table 6.9 – Testing of Propositions from the RAM (N=15)

Propositions from the RAM	Ancillary and practice propositions	Supported by results	Not supported by results
1. At the individual level, regulator and cognator processes affect innate and acquired ways of adapting.	a. Changes in interdependence adaptation are affected by innate and acquired ways of coping.	Artinian (1988/1989); Artinian (1991); Artinian (1992); Eves (1993); Smith, Mayer, Parkhurst, Perkins, & Pringleton (1991); Robinson (1991/1992)	
	b. Changes in interdependence adaptation are affected by perception.	Artinian (1988/1989); Artinian (1991); Artinian (1992); Silva (1987)	
3. The characteristics of the internal and external stimulus influence adaptive responses.	a. A focal stimuli affecting a significant other can affect interdependence adaptation.	Artinian (1988/1989); Artinian (1991); Artinian (1992); Gardner (1994); Grinspun (1991); Eves (1992/1993); Perkins (1987/1988); Smith, Mayer, Parkhurst, Perkins, & Pringleton (1991); Smith, Moushey, Ross, & Geiffer (1993); Gibson (1993/1994); Pruden (1991/1992); Robinson (1991/1992)	

	Proposition	Citations
	b. Social support can affect interdependence adaptation.	Artinian (1988/1989); Artinian (1991); Artinian (1992); Eves (1992/1993); Pruden (1991/1992); Robinson (1991/1992)
	c. Marital quality can affect interdependence adaptation.	Artinian (1988/1989); Artinian (1991); Artinian (1992); Gardner (1994)
	d. Gender affects interdependence adaptation.	Gardner (1994); Eves (1992/1993)
	e. Loneliness can affect interdependence adaptation.	Calvert (1989) Pruden (1991/1992)
	f. Caregiving places greater demands on the interdependence adaptive system.	Smith, Mayer, Parkhurst, Perkins, & Pringleton (1991) Smith, Moushey, Ross, & Geiffer (1993); Gibson (1993/1994); Perkins (1987/1988)
3.	The characteristics of the internal and external stimuli influence adaptive responses.	Smith (1989/1990)
4.	The characteristics of the internal and external stimuli influence the adequacy of cognitive and emotional processes	
	Social support affects cognitive and emotional processes.	Eves (1992/1993) Robinson (1991/1992)

(continued)

Table 6.9 (continued)

Propositions from the RAM	Ancillary and practice propositions	Supported by results	Not supported by results
6. Adaptation in one mode is affected by adaptation in other modes through cognator and regulator connectives.	Interdependence adaptation influences physiological adaptation.	Smith, Mayer, Parkhurst, Perkins, & Pringleton (1991); Smith, Moushey, Ross, & Geiffer (1993)	
9. The variable of time influences the process of adaptation.	a. Spouses adapt to their partner's condition over time.	Artinian (1988/1989); Artinian (1991); Artinian (1992)	
	b. Adaptation to caregiving occurs over time.	Perkins (1987/1988) Grinspun (1991)	Smith (1989/1990)

adaptation are affected by innate and acquired coping mechanisms. Further, these findings were consistent with postulating cognator processes being active forces of adaptation. Perceptual information processing, learning, judgment, and emotion were relevant to the cognator subsystem responses identified in these studies. Artinian (1988/1989, 1991, 1992) examined perception of illness severity as a cognator variable, and results indicated that perception was consistently related to adaptation. Likewise, understanding information, a cognator processing activity, was consistently rated important by the spouses of surgical patients (Silva, 1987). In all the studies in which the effects of cognator processes on adaptation were examined, researchers supported the proposition.

A second proposition was related to the effects of internal and external stimuli on adaptive responses. Findings from 13 studies supported this general proposition by supporting one or more of the five ancillary propositions. Roy and Roberts (1981) identified that stimuli have characteristics such as magnitude and clarity that influence cognator and regulator functioning. In the related propositions it was noted that, in general, the magnitude of the focal or contextual stimuli influenced cognator processing and adaptive output.

In several studies, the proposition that a focal stimulus affecting a significant other influences adaptation was supported. In each of these studies, the focal stimuli were illness, disability, or death of a significant other which affected adaptation in the interdependence mode. The focal stimuli were of sufficient magnitude to activate cognator and regulator subsystems and produce adaptive responses.

The two contextual stimuli of social support and marital quality were both found to affect adaptation in the interdependence mode. In all six of the studies in which social support was examined, the higher the level of social support the higher the level of adaptation. Likewise, in all four studies in which marital quality was examined, investigators found that the higher the marital quality, the higher the level of adaptation. In addition to the finding that significant others affect adaptation, the findings provide support for the model tenet that the focus of the interdependence mode is the relationships of significant others and support systems, and that these relationships meet the person's need for affectional adequacy.

In the two studies in which the effects of gender on adaptation were examined, researchers found that gender was not a factor. Gardner (1994) found no significant differences between genders in scores for psychosocial adaptation in response to their partners' open-heart surgery. Spouses, whether male or female, adapted similarly to the same focal stimuli. Eves (1992/1993) found that both mothers and fathers of developmentally disabled children equally accessed social support, and had similar adaptive coping mechanisms.

The ancillary proposition that loneliness affects interdependence mode adaptation was supported by two studies. In the first study, Calvert (1989) found that nursing home residents with higher levels of interaction with a pet experienced less loneliness. In the second study, Pruden (1991/1992) found that the greater the feelings of loneliness the lower the level of adaptation, and that the higher the level of social support the lower the feelings of loneliness. These findings supported the proposition that ineffective responses such as loneliness occur when the individual's needs for affectional adequacy are unmet, and that the external stimuli of social support contributes to the meeting of these needs. Therefore, in these studies social support or interaction with a pet decreased feelings of loneliness, and contributed to adaptation in the interdependence mode.

In four studies, the ancillary proposition that caregiving places demands on the interdependence adaptive system was supported, while investigators in one study failed to support this proposition. In each study, caregiver adaptation was the dependent variable, while the focal stimulus was the person needing care. Results of these studies indicated that caregivers adapt to the focal stimulus over time and that important contextual stimuli affecting adaptation include development of knowledge and skills necessary to provide care. Smith (1989/1990) failed to support this ancillary proposition in the study in which caregiver burden was measured twice, first when caregiving responsibilities were assumed or increased and again in 6 weeks. The respondents indicated that caregiving had been an ongoing process which had begun informally before participation in the study. Caregiver burden remained stable throughout the 6 weeks of the study; as a result, a change in caregiver burden and a change in adaptation could not be assessed. These results indicated, however, that even though length of time in that role may be an important variable in assessing caregiver adaptation, it has not been adequately studied.

The proposition that the characteristics of internal and external stimuli influence adequacy of the cognitive and emotional processes was supported by two studies (Eves, 1992/1993; Robinson, 1991/1992). The external stimuli of social support was related to more adaptive coping mechanisms and was a reflection of the adequacy of the cognitive and emotive processes. Robinson found that widows with more social support had higher coping scores and lower grief responses. Eves found that parents who had more adaptive coping mechanisms had more social support and fewer concerns about resources for child care. These findings support the model tenet that cognator activities involve cognitive and emotional processes. These processes include arousal, attention, perception, concept formation, and memory. Social support influences the processes leading to adaptation; in turn, the processes also influenced social support.

In two studies (Smith et al., 1991; 1993) the proposition that adaptation in one mode is affected by adaptation in other modes was supported.

In these studies, adaptation in the interdependence mode influenced adaptation in the physiologic mode. Family caregivers in both studies reported feeling successful in their caregiving roles and identified themselves as coping successfully in all four adaptive modes. Physical health was not affected by caregiving. These findings support the model proposition that each adaptive mode is linked to other adaptive modes by means of major cognator and regulator connectives. When individuals perceive themselves as coping effectively, an overall sense of well being may enhance adaptation in each of the four modes.

Results of six studies provided mixed support for the proposition that the variable of time influenced the process of adaptation. In the studies conducted by Artinian (1988/1989, 1991, 1992), spousal adaptation to their partner's open-heart surgery changed over the length of the studies, while in the Grinspun (1991) study, findings indicated no evidence of a link between time since injury and spousal adaptation. Likewise, in both caregiver studies in which time was examined, the results were mixed. In the Perkins' study (1987/1988), caregiver burden was less when adjustment to the caregiver role developed over time. Smith (1989/1990) found no change in caregiver adaptation during the 6 weeks of her study. The mixed results from these studies indicate that the variable of time warrants further study to more adequately identify the relationship.

In summary, results of the interdependence mode adaptation research were used to test five propositions of the RAM. Results that did or did not support the propositions were discussed. Research results that did not support the propositions were identified, and directions for further work were proposed. The propositions evaluated here, and those tested in the other content chapters, are synthesized in Chapter 11 which views contributions to knowledge from the perspective of testing all the model propositions.

Synthesis of Interdependence Mode Research: Contributions to Nursing Science

Of the 20 interdependence adaptative mode studies in this chapter, 15 were synthesized to derive contributions to nursing science. These 15 studies met given research criteria and demonstrated links to the model. Future directions for clinical practice, research, and model development are addressed in relation to the RAM.

Applications to Nursing Practice

Nursing knowledge can be developed through testing model concepts and proposing nursing interventions which can be implemented in the practice setting (Pollock, Frederickson, Carson, Massey & Roy, 1994). Specifically, interventions can be posed that promote or maintain adaptation

Table 6.10 – Potential For Implementation From Interdependence Adaptive Mode Research (*N*=15)

Category One: *High potential for implementation*
Artinian (1988/1989)
Artinian (1991)
Artinian (1992)
Gardner (1994)
Silva (1987)
Perkins (1987/1988)
Grinspun (1991)
Smith, Mayer, Parkhurst, Perkins, & Pringleton (1991)
Gibson (1993/1994)
Robinson (1991/1992)
Eves (1992/1993)
Calvert (1989)
Pruden (1991/1992)

Category Two: *Needs further clinical evaluation before implementation*
Smith, Moushey, Ross, & Geiffer (1993)

Category Three: *Further research indicated before implementation*
Smith (1989/1990)

---

in the interdependence mode in various populations and settings. Interventions need to be tested and refined before implementation in the practice setting.

Studies reviewed in this chapter were examined for applications to practice within three categories: (a) high potential for implementation, (b) needs further evaluation before implementation, and (c) further testing warranted before implementation (Table 6.10). Thirteen studies were deemed to meet criteria for inclusion in Category 1. All of these studies contained support for empiric relationships from which to derive effective interventions that did not pose harmful risks to subjects. One study met the criteria for Category 2 but further evaluation was needed before implementation. In Category 3, investigators for one study indicated that while no current application for practice could be found, potential existed for relevancy after additional testing.

Results from six studies inferred that nurses should actively assess important contextual stimuli that influence the needs of significant others and use that assessment to identify significant others who may exhibit ineffective adaptive responses. In addition to assessing the needs of significant others, nurses need to devote more nursing time and attention to meeting these needs. Because of the effects on marriage of increased hardships and demands, nurses should assess the general state of the marital relationship (Gardner, 1994) and identify spouses who are experiencing these difficulties (Artinian, 1988/1989). Silva (1987) and Artinian (1991) point out that the nursing role includes acting as change agent to remove personal and institutional barriers which significant others perceive as impediments to meeting their needs. The need for increased nursing assessment of significant others applies to caregivers (Perkins, 1987/1988) and the spouses of head-injured patients (Grinspun, 1991). In particular, investigators found that poor mental health or impaired cognitive status of the patient decreased caregiver adaptation. The need for nurses to continue assessing for the effects of stress 1 year after open-heart surgery or bereavement was identified by Artinian in three studies (1988/1989, 1991,1992) and by Robinson (1991/1992) in one study. The time for adaptation after severe focal stimuli may indeed be longer than is recognized by most nurses. Consequently, nurses can be taught to assess the needs of significant others on a long-term basis.

The necessity of planning to meet the needs of significant others was identified by two authors (Artinian, 1988/1989, 1991, 1992; Grinspun, 1991). Planned attempts need to be made by nurses to offer emotional support to meet the needs of significant others and to incorporate these needs into the total plan of care. A planned approach would lessen the possibility that the needs of significant others would not be identified or would be inadequately assessed.

Significant others, caregivers, and parents all identified the need for increased information about the condition of the patient and current care. Therefore, the need for information was a recurring theme of investigators in the results of eight studies (Artinian, 1988/1989, 1991, 1992; Grinspun, 1991; Robinson, 1991/1992; Silva, 1987; Smith et al., 1991; 1993). In addition to providing significant others with this information, nurses should share expectations for future care and condition with significant others. Nurses can educate significant others so that they can distinguish between normal and abnormal developments (Artinian, 1991; Robinson, 1991/1992). Knowing what to expect and being able to recognize what is common or what is deviant would provide significant others with a better sense of control over the situation. In addition to educating significant others about patient care and concerns, nurses need to help significant others become aware of the effects of the focal stimulus on their own adaptation. Significant others need to know that their experiences are shared by others and that they can improve their adaptation through education in stress management techniques (Artinian, 1992).

Importance of support groups and emotional support was identified by six authors (Artinian, 1992; Gardner 1994; Gibson, 1993/1994;

Grinspun, 1991; Smith et al., 1991; 1993). Significant others need support groups to share their feelings, learn new coping skills, and identify positive contextual stimuli in their lives, which could enhance adaptation. Nurses can be instrumental in the development of support groups and in the provision of support group information to significant others. Providing emotional support, a traditional nursing activity, should be expanded. Gibson (1993/1994) specifically recommended that nurses offer emotional support by listening, understanding the need for hyper-vigilance, providing guidance, and acting as a patient and family advocate. In addition, Gibson also advocated assignment of a nurse who can visit on a long-term basis for affirmation, encouragement, information, and guidance to each family with a chronically ill child.

The need for patient and family advocacy was also addressed by Perkins (1987/1988) and Smith and colleagues (1991). Perkins recommended nurses prevent early or inappropriate admission of the elderly to long-term care facilities by encouraging supportive family relationships and by encouraging caregivers to maintain their own quality of life, in addition to providing care for the client. Likewise, Smith, Mayer, and colleagues recommended that nurses support families in their caregiving roles and help caregivers recognize their own psychosocial and physical needs.

Calvert (1989) identified specific nursing actions to help alleviate loneliness in nursing home residents. Nurses can organize pet programs in settings where loneliness may occur such as personal care homes and adult day care centers. Calvert also recommended that nurses employed in institutions with pet programs, encourage pet rounds so pet interaction is distributed among all resident. Pet programs provide a simple effective contextual stimulus that reduces loneliness and increases adaptation.

Findings from one research study need further evaluation before implementation. Smith and colleagues suggested that nurses assist family caregivers in identifying time periods when adaptation can be maintained by assistance from home health nurses. Assessment criteria arc needed for home health nurses to identify times when caregiver adaptation could be improved by external assistance. These assessment criteria will have to be identified before the finding can be implemented.

Findings from one research study need further testing before implementation. Results of the study by Smith (1989/1990) did not support a change in caregiver burden during the 6 weeks of the study, and the relationship between change in caregiver burden and the change in the four modes of the RAM could not be assessed. Subjects reported caregiving as being gradually assumed over time. Consequently, the development of caregiving, change in caregiver burden, and adaptation in the four modes of the RAM needs further development and testing to determine how caregiving is assumed in families over time.

Recommendations for Model-Based Research

Future directions for model-based research were identified from all researchers with studies that had applications to nursing practice. Studies in which findings were ambiguous or differed from previous research are priority areas for further clinical investigations.

Researchers of studies in which innate and acquired ways of coping were tested found that coping affected adaptation. According to the RAM, the cognator subsystem of the coping mechanism involves the knowledge, perception, and skill possessed by the person to assist in coping with environmental stimuli; therefore, perceptions can also affect coping. Two major avenues for future adaptation research would be to identify factors that influence perceptions and to explore the relationship between perceptions and innate and acquired ways of coping. Positive perceptions may be related to active coping, while negative perceptions may be related to avoidance coping. This relationship remains unexplored.

Findings from the studies in which investigators evaluated the characteristics of internal and external stimuli and the effects of these stimuli on interdependence mode adaptation supported predictions based on the model regarding relationships among the variables of significant other, social support, loneliness, and interdependence adaptation. Although this support seems sufficient, model development would benefit from future research assessing the influence of common stimuli on interdependence mode adaptation. According to the RAM, common stimuli include culture, belief systems, family dynamics, developmental stage, integrity of adaptive modes, cognator effectiveness, and the environment (Roy & Andrews, 1991).

None of the studies included in this section had children as subjects. The interdependence mode is one of the two modes present at birth (Roy & Andrews, 1991); therefore, an important addition to research on the model would be studies in which the development of this mode in children were examined. Other potential areas of research include: (a) testing prospectively derived specific interventions to reduce the frequency of ineffective behaviors and to increase the frequency of interdependence adaptive behaviors, (b) identifying contextual stimuli that differentiate between effective and ineffective responses to similar stimuli, (c) categorizing the intensity and magnitude of focal and contextual stimuli so adaptation can be predicted in the interdependence mode, and (d) identifying the effect of passing time on interdependence mode adaptation.

The effects of sociodemographic variables such as gender, and situational variables such as marital quality, on the adaptive process need further exploration. Findings from the studies in which the effect of marital quality was tested indicated that a positive relationship existed between marital quality and adaptation (Artinian 1988/1989, 1991, 1992; Gardner, 1994).

Studies should be replicated in both healthy and ill populations. The possibility exists that marital quality is involved in role adaptation, which would provide support for the model proposition that adaptation in one mode affects adaptation in other modes. Investigators of two studies (Gardner, 1994; Pruden, 1991/1992) identified that gender does not affect interdependence mode adaptation. Studies examining the influence of gender on adaptation in other populations is indicated.

Findings from the two studies that examined loneliness indicated that loneliness decreases dyadic adaptation (Pruden, 1991/1992) and can be modified by contextual stimuli (Calvert, 1989). The use of a contextual stimulus such as pet interaction to increase adaptation provides specific interventions that can be implemented in nursing practice. Results from Calvert's study serve as a model for guiding interdependence mode adaptation research for the development and testing of other interventions that can be used in the clinical setting. According to concepts of the RAM, the clinical art and science of nursing is the knowing of human processes in health and illness and planning nursing care with individuals and groups to enhance their adaptation (Roy & Andrews, 1991). Future research should be conducted to design and evaluate the effectiveness of interventions that could enhance interdependence mode adaptation. Further research is needed to examine the effects of caregiving on adaptation. Gibson (1993/1994) found that mothers who developed empowerment experienced adaptive changes by developing the knowledge, competence, and confidence to participate in their children's health care decisions. An important area of model-based research would be to identify individuals who are adapting successfully to severe stimuli, and to examine the effect of multiple contextual stimuli on adaptation. Contextual stimuli include other variables such as empowerment, culture, and spirituality.

Additional research is indicated to identify the effects of social support on cognitive and emotional processes. In two studies findings indicated that social support affects coping mechanisms (Eves, 1992/1993; Robinson, 1991/1992). However neither study indicated social support characteristics that were beneficial. Viable areas for future model-based research include which characteristics of social support influence coping, and whether certain characteristics are associated with active or avoidance coping. In addition, researchers should examine the effects of social support on adaptation of significant others.

Evaluation of the effects of interdependence mode adaptation on physical adaptation in the caregiver role deserves further study. In two studies, researchers found that physical health was not affected by the caregiving role (Smith et al., 1991; 1993). These findings need additional support from future longitudinal studies to examine if caregiver health remains stable over years, instead of months. In addition, the role of other contextual and residual stimuli such as age, physical condition, and baseline health should be examined for potential effects on the physical health of caregivers.

The effects of time on the process of adaptation is another productive area for future research. Findings are mixed from the six studies that included time as a variable. Artinian (1988/1989; 1991) and Smith (1989/1990) examined significant other adaptation 6 weeks after the occurrence of the focal stimulus. Artinian (1988/1989; 1991) found a change in the four adaptive modes over 6 weeks, while Smith did not. Likewise, Perkins (1987/1988) found that caregiver burden was less when adjustment to the caregiving role occurred over time, and Smith (1989/1990) found the assumption of the caregiving role occurred gradually. These seemingly inconsistent results may be explained by the magnitude of the focal stimulus and the effect of differing contextual stimuli over time. The focal stimulus of a spouse's CABG surgery may have greater magnitude than the assumption of gradual caregiving responsibilities for the elderly. Grinspun (1991) found no evidence that time since head injury affected spousal adaptation. Again, interaction of the magnitude of the focal stimulus and the contextual stimuli over time may account for this finding. The mixed results from these studies indicate that further research needs to be conducted to clarify the effects of time on adaptation in the interdependence mode. Studies should be designed to identify how the process of adaptation developed over time as the caregiving role is assumed or maintained.

To improve the effectiveness of the RAM in guiding research, instruments that measure specific concepts of the model need to be developed and tested. Reliable and valid measures of each adaptative mode are needed to ensure a holistic view of the adaptive person. The instrument developed by Short (1994) appropriately measured the concepts of the interdependence mode. This instrument put into operation the model concepts of significant other, support systems (friendships), support systems (extended family), and loneliness. Possibilities exist for an entire program of research related to developing measures for interdependence mode functioning. In addition, many effective instruments are available for use in interdependence mode adaptation research. These instruments, including initial progress and current limitations, are discussed in Chapter 10 on measurement of the model.

Directions for Theory and RAM Development

Interdependence mode research based on the RAM contributed to identifying directions for further theory and model development. Two clear directions were identified: first, a need to examine the relationship between the characteristics of stimuli and the effects of these characteristics on adaptation, and second, a need to examine further theoretic development of the effects of the variable of time and the characteristics of the stimuli.

A major model proposition is that the characteristics of the internal and external stimuli influence adaptive response. Roy has identified (Roy & Roberts, 1981) magnitude and optimum amount of stimuli as characteristics that influence the adequacy of regulator and cognator processing, thereby affecting adaptation. The investigators included in this mode have identified other characteristics besides magnitude that influence adaptation. For example, both Grinspun (1991) and Perkins (1987/1988) indicated that mental health and behavior affected adaptation in significant others more than physical health does, although the need exists to identify characteristics of mental health and behavior that would determine magnitude. Future model development requires consideration of a broader range of stimuli characteristics and their effects on adaptive responses in different situations.

Based on the findings of reported research analyzed in this chapter, further conceptual clarity is needed concerning the variable of time. Roy (1988) has identified time as a key variable for study, but to date, this concept has not been explored or integrated in the model or related theoretic work. Therefore, the concept of time is potentially important for further RAM development.

Summary

Research that focused primarily on the interdependence mode of the RAM was presented in this chapter. Of the 163 nursing studies included in this monograph, 20 were identified for inclusion in research that focused on the interdependence adaptive mode. Studies were critically analyzed, the relationships of the studies to the RAM were evaluated, and the contributions of the studies to nursing science were shown. Findings from these studies support the use of the RAM in guiding nursing practice and research of interdependence mode phenomena and strengthen the interrelationships among theory, research, and practice.

References

Artinian, N.T. (1989). The stress process within the Roy adaptation framework: Sources, mediators and manifestations of stress in spouses of coronary artery bypass patients during hospitalization and six weeks post discharge (Doctoral dissertation, Wayne State University, (1988). *Dissertation Abstracts International, 49*, 5225-B.

Artinian, N.T. (1991). Stress experience of spouses of patients having coronary artery bypass during hospitalization and 6 weeks after discharge. *Heart & Lung, 20*, 52-59.

Artinian, N.T. (1992). Spouse adaptation to mate's CABG surgery: 1-year follow-up. *American Journal of Critical Care, 1*(2), 36-42.

Baker, A.C. (1993). The spouse's positive effect on the stroke patient's recovery. *Rehabilitation Nursing, 18,* 30-33

Bradley, K.M., & Williams, D.M. (1990). A comparison of the preoperative concerns of open heart surgery patients and their significant others. *The Journal of Cardiovascular Nursing, 5* (1), 43-53.

Brown, G.J. (1990). The prevalence of elderly abuse: A descriptive survey of case management records (Master's thesis, San Jose State University, 1989). *Masters Abstracts International, 28,* 570.

Calvert, M.M. (1989). Human-pet interaction and loneliness: A test of concepts from Roy's adaptation model. *Nursing Science Quarterly, 2* 194-202.

Eves, L.M. (1993). Support for parents of developmentally disabled children: Effect of adaptation (Master's thesis, D'Youville College, 1992). *Master's Abstracts International, 31,* 271.

Gardner, M.J. (1994). Spouse adaptation after the partner's open heart surgery. Unpublished master's thesis, Grand Valley State University.

Gibson, C.H. (1994). A study of empowerment in mothers of chronically ill children (Doctoral dissertation, Boston College, 1993). *Dissertation Abstracts International, 54,* 4078-B.

Grinspun, D. (1991). Factors influencing adaptation of spouses of head trauma patients. Unpublished master's thesis, University of Michigan, Ann Arbor.

Limandri, B.J. (1985). Help-seeking patterns of abused women: Self-esteem, role conflict and social support as influencing factors. Unpublished doctoral dissertation, University of California, San Francisco.

Perkins, I. (1988). An analysis of relationships among interdependence in family caregivers and the elderly, caregiver burden, and adaptation of the homebound frail elderly (Doctoral dissertation, The Catholic University of America, 1987). *Dissertation Abstracts International, 48,* 3250-3251-B.

Pruden, E.P.S. (1992). Roy Adaptation Model testing: Dyadic adaptation, social support, and loneliness in COPD dyads (Doctoral dissertation, University of South Carolina, 1991). *Dissertation Abstracts International, 52,* 6320-B.

Robinson, J.H. (1992). A descriptive study of widows' grief responses, coping processes and social support within Roy's adaptation (Doctoral dissertation, Wayne State University, 1991). *Dissertation Abstracts International, 52,* 6320-B.

Roy, C. (1988). Patient information processing and nursing research. In J. Fitzpatrick & R.L. Tauton (Eds.) *Annual Review of Nursing Research, 6,* New York: Springer.

Roy, C., & Andrews, H. (1991). *The Roy adaptation model* Norwalk, CT: Appleton & Lange.

Roy, C., & Roberts, S.L. (1981). *Theory construction in nursing: An adaptation model.* Englewood Cliffs, NJ: Prentice-Hall.

Short, J.D. (1994). Interdependence needs and nursing care of the new family. *Issues in Comprehensive Pediatric Nursing, 17,* 1-14.

Silva, M.C. (1987). Needs of spouses of surgical patients: A conceptualization within the Roy Adaptation Model. *Scholarly Inquiry for Nursing Practice, 1,* 29-44.

Smith, B.J.A. (1990). Caregiver burden and adaptation in middle-aged daughters of dependent elderly parents: A test of Roy's model (Doctoral dissertation, University of Pittsburgh, 1989). *Dissertation Abstracts International, 51,* 2290-B.

Smith, C.E., Mayer, L.S., Parkhurst, C., Perkins, S.B., & Pringleton, S.K. (1991). Adaptation in families with a member requiring mechanical ventilation at home. *Heart & Lung, 20,* 349-356.

Smith, C.E., Moushey, L., Ross, J.A., & Geiffer, C. (1993). Responsibilities and reactions of family caregivers of patients dependent on total parenteral nutrition at home. *Public Health Nursing, 10,* 122-128.

Bibliography

Pollock, S.E., Frederickson, K., Carson, M.A., Massey, V.H., & Roy, C. (1994). Contributions to nursing science: Synthesis of findings from Adaptation Model Research. *Scholarly Inquiry for Nursing Practice, 8*(4), 361-372.

Roy, C., & Andrews, H. (1999). *The Roy Adaptation Model.* Stamford, CT: Appleton & Lange.

Chapter 7

Adaptive Modes And Processes

In this chapter, we focus on 36 studies reported from 1970 through 1994 which examined adaptation in several modes or the adaptive processes as defined by the Roy Adaptation Model (RAM). These studies, published as articles, dissertations, and theses, used a variety of research designs other than the experimental or quasi-experimental designs which are reviewed in Chapter 9.

Purposes

In keeping with the purposes of the research monograph, this chapter aims to (a) critically analyze studies which include more than one adaptive mode or the adaptive processes, (b) evaluate the relationship of this research to the RAM, and (c) synthesize contributions of the studies to nursing science. Contributions to nursing science include applications for nursing practice, recommendations for research related to adaptive modes and processes, and suggestions for further theory and model development. The criteria developed and the processes used by the research team for analysis and synthesis of the studies are explained in Chapter 2.

Background

In viewing the person as an adaptive system, all adaptive modes and the adaptive processes were considered in research based on the RAM. Individual investigators often consider one adaptive mode or element of the model as the main focus of the research. Research on individual components of a model is useful both in the early stages of knowledge development and in studying the model components in greater depth. Studies focused primarily on particular adaptive modes and stimuli as defined by the RAM are reviewed in Chapters 3 through 6. However, in a number of studies the researcher focuses on multiple modes or on the adaptive processes of the individual or group. These studies are included in this chapter and are particularly useful for the purpose of synthesis of RAM-based knowledge.

The term "multiple modes" refers to use of more than one adaptive mode. According to the Roy Model, the adaptive modes are defined as physiologic, the needs and processes whereby a person maintains physiologic integrity; self concept, the physical and personal beliefs and feelings one holds about oneself for psychic integrity; role function, behavior related to interactive positions in a society that strives for social integrity; and interdependence, interactions in close relationships that maintain affectional adequacy (Roy & Andrews, 1991).

For the individual, the primary adaptive processes are inherent in the regulator subsystem—neural, chemical, and endocrine processes—and the cognator subsystem that uses perceptual/information processing, learning, judgment, and emotion to cope with a changing environment. The regulator processes are largely automatic, innate, and physiologic in nature. However, more is being learned about acquiring regulator coping processes, such as developing a deep muscle relaxation response to modify skin temperature, heart rate, and blood pressure. The cognator acts through cognitive and emotional channels. Many of these processes, such as learning how to act in a frightening situation are acquired. On the group level, organizations and communities act as adaptive systems, using subsystems parallel to the regulator and cognator to maintain stability and to deal with change. The primary adaptive subsystems of organized groups are known as the stabilizer and innovator (Roy & Anway, 1989).

Critical Analysis of Research on Adaptive Modes and Processes

As defined in this project, critical analysis includes a brief description of the reported research, followed by the use of established guidelines to critically analyze the research.

Description of Reported Research

The 36 studies selected for review are organized into five categories that occur naturally in the body of research. The five categories are: (a) adaptive mode assessment (n=9), (b) adaptive strategies (n=9), (c) perceptual information processing (n=7), (d) adaptation as an outcome (n=8), and (e) the nursing care group as an adaptive system (n=3). The nine studies that focused on adaptive mode assessment generally were designed to describe needs, problems, or experiences in more than one mode for selected samples. Studies in the category of adaptive strategies were all correlational studies that identified given cognator strategies as related to other variables. For clarity of presentation, nine studies are included in the broad category of adaptive strategies of the RAM, mainly originating in the cognator, and seven are examined in the subcategory of the cognator, perceptual information processing. The studies that examine adaptation as outcome are discussed together in one group. Finally, the studies focusing on the nursing care group as an adaptive system are described.

Adaptive mode assessment. Nine of the 36 studies focus on assessment in more than one adaptive mode (Table 7.1). Smith, Garvis, and Martinson (1983) did a secondary content analysis from interviews of parents with children diagnosed with cancer to describe the parents' needs

Table 7.1 – Description of Studies About Adaptive Mode Assessment (*N*=9)

Author(s) & Date	Purpose	Sample	Design	Findings
1. Smith, Garvis, & Martinson (1983)	To describe needs of parents adapting to the effect of children diagnosed with cancer and to demonstrate the potential for using nursing theory to review banked data	Parents within 6 weeks of the time a child had been diagnosed with cancer. (*N*=20)	Qualitative-descriptive	Interview questions that asked parents directly about themselves elicited mainly interdependence or self concept concerns. When asked questions about the child or effect of the diagnosis, their responses fit mainly into the self-concept and physiologic modes.
2. Farkas (1981)	To identify adaptation problems of elderly persons who applied to a nursing home by comparing them with elderly persons who had not made an application.	Subjects 75 years and over, with one significant other, who applied for admission to a nursing home (*n*=22) and a matched group who had not applied (*n*=22), *N*=44	Correlational	Waiting-list elderly had a greater mean percentage of disabilities in all four adaptive modes but perceived greater mean adaptation problems specific to the self concept and interdependence modes when compared with a matched group.
3. Varvaro (1991)	To describe adaptation in the four modes in women with coronary heart disease	Women who had experienced a coronary event over the past year (*N*=83)	Descriptive	Adaptation problems were identified in the physiologic mode, i.e., fatigue and decreased energy levels, and in the role function mode, i.e., role-related problems and serious role adjustment.
4. Gagliardi (1991)	To provide a detailed description of the family experience and social interactions of families having a child with Duchenne muscular dystrophy	Families having children with Duchenne muscular dystrophy (*N*=3)	Ethnographic	Six themes, reflecting all four adaptive modes, recurred in the common experiences of families: the erosion of hope for normalcy; society's confirmation of the impossibility of normalcy; the dynamics of the family; a smaller world; letting go or hanging on; and things must change.

(continued)

Table 7.1 (continued)

Author(s) & Date	Purpose	Sample	Design	Findings
5. Florence, Lutzen, & Alexius (1994)	To explore heterosexually infected HIV-positive women's experience of and adaptation to being infected	HIV-positive women (N=8)	Qualitative descriptive	Common themes emerged that indicated women's vulnerability, specifically in how they became infected, the manner in which they found out about their infection, and how they coped with their lives after receiving the diagnosis. Difficulties in all four adaptive modes were reported, particularly loneliness and isolation.
6. Thomas, Shoffner, & Groer (1988)	To assess gender differences in stress factors of adolescents, making comparisons in the four adaptive modes of the RAM	Freshman high school students (N=323)	Descriptive	Most frequently reported stressors for both boys and girls were hassling with parents and with siblings and making new friends. Significant gender differences in amount and types of stressors were identified.
7. Pittman (1992/1993)	To describe the enabling characteristics of chronically ill school-age children for the promotion of personal health.	Children in three chronicity category groups (N=75).	Descriptive	Four factors of enabling characteristics were identified by Q-sort methodology that represented the four adaptive modes. The most important enabling factors represented the self concept mode. Three patterns were identified by factor analysis; 92% of the children demonstrated positive

8. Kiikkala & Peitsi (1991)	To examine the content of nursing practice for preschool children with minimal brain dysfunction (MBD)	Patient charts (N=20)	Descriptive	Documented nursing practice focused mainly on the physiologic mode, especially exercise and sensory function. Nurses' descriptions of care for children with MBD included all four modes.
9. Trentini (1985/1986)	To describe patient problems selected by nurses as amenable to nursing interventions and the types of nursing actions selected in the care of patients with end-stage renal disease on dialysis	Registered nurses working with dialysis patients (N=46)	Correlational	The number of patient problems selected by nurses as amenable to nursing interventions was not significantly related to the number of years of nursing experience or type of education. The nurses' level of education was significantly related to number of nursing actions selected for solving problems in all four modes. Interdependent action was most often associated with interventions in the interdependence mode.

in each of the four adaptive modes. When asked about themselves, the parents tended to give answers that related mainly to interdependence or self concept.

Comparing subjects age 75 years and over who applied for admission to a nursing home with those who did not. Farkas (1981) also found interdependence and self concept adaptation problems prominent among the elderly waiting for admission. Differences between groups were found in worrying about health, repeatedly checking such things as clothing (ritualistic behavior), and preferring to have others take care of their affairs. However, the author provided evidence that adaptation problems in three of the modes arose from and were related to disabilities and difficulties in the physiologic mode for the waiting group. Role reversal was more frequently a problem for the significant other than for the elderly person.

In describing adaptation in the four modes among women who experienced a coronary event in the previous year, Varvaro (1991) noted adaptation problems in the physiologic mode—for example, "easily fatigued" (63%) and "decreased energy" (67%). However, measures of self-care activities and good health behaviors, such as eating and sleeping, showed physiologic adaptation. Role function problems were identified in 60% of the subjects with 28% reporting serious problems in role adjustment.

Using an ethnographic method for 10 weeks of observation and analysis, with a follow-up at 1 year, Gagliardi (1991) described the experiences of families having a child with Duchenne muscular dystrophy. A continuum of stages—recognition, working through, and resolution—emerged from six themes that were common in the experiences of the three families. The themes reflected all four adaptive modes.

In a pilot study done in Sweden, Florence, Lutzen, and Alexius (1994) used open-ended interview questions to explore the experience and adaptation of women infected with HIV. As in the study by Smith and colleagues (1983), the four adaptive modes provided the structure for analysis of each transcript. Again, difficulties were reported in all four adaptive modes, with considerable emphasis on interdependence. Issues of loneliness and isolation emerged with many women being unable to tell friends and acquaintances about their infection. Further, women who had supportive families seemed to be coping better than those who did not.

Thomas, Shoffner, and Groer (1988) did a survey study to describe gender differences in stress factors of adolescents, making comparisons in the four adaptive modes. Although the authors identified common stressors for both boys and girls, females were more concerned with self concept and interdependence issues, such as appearance changes and dating problems. Males identified stress factors related to role function, such as school performance and adjusting to a new job.

Pittman (1992/1993) used Q-sort methodology to describe enabling characteristics for the promotion of personal health of chronically ill school-age children. Using factor analysis, the author identified four factors that aligned with the four adaptive modes. The items selected by participants as indicating characteristics most like them represented the self-concept mode. Six enabling characteristics that were least like the subjects were associated with the physiologic mode. Such characteristics included identifying the relationship of cleanliness to health. Differences in behavior patterns among three groups were defined by key characteristics of chronic illness. Most of the children (92%) valued health behaviors.

Nursing care of children with minimal brain dysfunction (MBD) was the focus of a study by Kiikkala and Peitsi (1991). Data were gathered from nursing documents on 203 children treated in one hospital in Helsinki over a 4-year period. In addition, nurses working in the ward were asked to write descriptions of nursing care of children with MBD. Findings indicated that nursing practice focused on the physiologic mode—mainly exercise and sensory functions—and on the self concept mode. Nursing practice related to the role function and interdependence modes was supported to a lesser degree. The content of nursing care in the nurses' free-form reports was more vivid, useful, and comprehensive than in the nursing documents examined.

In the final study on assessment, Trentini (1985/1986) proposed to identify patient problems according to the four adaptive modes of the RAM. The investigator also aimed to identify the kind of nursing actions—dependent, independent, or interdependent–that nurses choose as the best alternatives for solving each selected problem. The hypotheses predicting the relationship of nurse variables, such as education and years of experience, to nurses' selections of problems in each mode of adaptation and to number of nursing actions chosen across all problems selected were not supported. However, the nurses' level of education was significantly related to number of nursing actions selected for solving problems. A combination of dependent and independent nursing actions was selected to solve problems in the physiologic mode. When dealing with self concept, role function, and interdependence modes, nurses also selected interdependent actions.

In summary, in studies in which the adaptive mode assessment was examined, all four modes were assessed in different samples in wellness, chronic, and acute illnesses; across age groups; and on individual and family levels. Investigators have studied data on assessment of adaptive modes from the perspectives of patients, significant others, and nurses. In some cases, the adaptive modes were used to design the study, while in other cases, they were used as post hoc categories for describing data.

Adaptive strategies. In the review of studies related to adaptive modes and processes, 16 of the 36 studies focused on strategies of the cognator adaptive subsystem. For clarity of presentation and for building knowledge, the nine studies that have direct relevance for understanding general adaptive strategies of the cognator and regulator are presented in this section (Table 7.2). Then seven studies are reviewed in a cognator subcategory of perceptual information processing.

Francisco (1989/1990) examined the extent to which the modes of adaptation and the use of humor predicted families' health as manifested in their level of functioning. Use of the strategy of humor to reduce tension, lessen anxiety, cope with difficult situations, and maintain a positive outlook on life was correlated at a significant level with the problem-solving dimension of family functioning. The investigator concluded that teaching the use of humor in transactional patterns of families may add to families' repertoire of coping patterns and raise the level of family functioning.

In two studies, Pollock (1986; 1989) investigated physiologic and psychosocial adaptation of adults with chronic illness. The author described adaptation to chronic illness as a complex process and studied some of the internal and external factors that influenced responses and consequent levels of adaptation. Pollock's (1986) construct of adaptation to chronic illness integrated the variables of chronicity, stress, adaptive behavior, and hardiness as key elements of the process. Hardiness was seen as a residual stimulus that was related to physiologic and psychosocial adaptation in patients with adult onset insulin-dependent diabetes mellitus (IDDM), but this relationship was not supported for patients with rheumatoid arthritis nor for those with hypertension. In a second study, Pollock (1989) found that 56% of the variance in predicting physiologic adaptation to IDDM was accounted for by five variables. These variables—outcome appraisal categories of harm and benefit, mixed-focus coping patterns, the hardiness characteristic, having been in a patient education program, and one of the emotion-focused coping strategies—provided insight into cognator adaptive strategies.

Barone (1993/1994) also studied Pollock's health-related hardiness factor and demographic characteristics to examine coping and the extent to which significant coping processes explained adaptation in adults with spinal cord injuries. Demographics and hardiness were found to be important. For example, subjects who were less hardy, who had less education, and whose injuries were more recent were more likely to use escape-avoidance coping strategies and less likely to use seeking of social support, problem solving based on planning, and positive reappraisal coping behaviors. Physiologic adaptation was accounted for by demographic factors. Overall psychosocial adaptation was related to younger age at time of injury and to an increased sense of control with less use of escape-avoidance, confrontive, and self-controlling coping behaviors.

Table 7.2 – Description of Studies About Adaptive Strategies of RAM (N=9)

Author(s) & Date	Purpose	Sample	Design	Findings
10. Francisco (1989/1990)	To describe the relationships and associations in family functioning, humor, and adaptation	Intact families of a mother, father, and one child between ages 13-19 years (N=36)	Correlational	The combined effect of adaptation and humor accounted for almost 70% of the variance of family functioning. The use of humor was positively associated with the dimension of problem solving. Physiologic, role function, and interdependence modes of adaptation were related to family functioning.
11. Pollock (1986)	To investigate physiologic and psychosocial adaptation of adults with chronic illness	Adults diagnosed with adult onset chronic illness (insulin-dependent diabetes mellitus, essential hypertension, or rheumatoid arthritis) (N=60)	Correlational	Hardiness among subjects with IDDM was related to physiologic and psychosocial adaptation, but this relationship was not supported for subjects with rheumatoid arthritis or for those with hypertension. Having attended a patient education program was related to physiological adaptation.
12. Pollock (1989)	To identify the relationships among physiologic adaptive responses, coping patterns, hardiness, and socioeconomic variables	Adults diagnosed with insulin-dependent diabetes mellitus (N=30)	Correlational	Fifty-six percent of the variance in predicting physiological adaptation to IDDM was accounted for by five variables: outcome appraisal categories of harm and benefit, mixed-focus coping patterns, the hardiness characteristic, having been in a patient education program, and one of the emotion-focused coping strategies. *(continued)*

Table 7.2 (continued)

Author(s) & Date	Purpose	Sample	Design	Findings
13. Barone (1993/ 1994)	To evaluate the extent to which demographic characteristics and hardiness explain coping and the extent to which coping processes explain adaptation	Adults with quadriplegia or paraplegia (N=243)	Correlational	For coping processes, two sets of variables indicated 73% of the variance, that is subjects with less education and with more recent injuries, who were less hardy in all three dimensions were more likely to use escape-avoidance coping strategies and less likely to use seeking of social support, planful problem solving, and positive reappraisal coping behaviors. For physiologic adaptation, subjects who had a lower level of spinal cord injury, who spent less time in rehab., and who had a greater sense of control had a higher total FIM score and experienced less frequent complications. For psychosocial adaptation, younger subjects who had an increased sense of control and who used less escape-avoidance, confrontive, and self-controlling coping behaviors were more likely to have higher overall psychosocial adjustment.

Study	Purpose	Sample	Design	Results
14. Grey, Cameron, & Thurber (1991)	To describe the influence of age, coping behaviors, and self-care behaviors on adaptation of preadolescents and adolescents with insulin dependent diabetes mellitus	Children with IDDM ages 8 to 18 years (N=103)	Correlational	Preadolescents and adolescents cope differently with diabetes mellitus. Preadolescents were significantly less depressed, less anxious, coped in more positive ways, had fewer adjustment problems, and were in better metabolic control than adolescents. Age and secondary sexual development was associated with psychosocial adaptation and metabolic control with 56% of variance explained.
15. Zhan (1993/1994)	To describe cognitive adaptation processing patterns used by hearing impaired elderly	Adults with manifested hearing loss (N=128)	Correlational	Results indicated a moderately strong positive correlation between cognitive adaptation processing and self consistency. Cognitive adaptation processing explained 42% of the variance in self consistency. Three patterns of cognitive adaptation processing–self perception, clear focus and method, and knowing awareness—significantly contributed to the maintenance of self consistency.

(continued)

Table 7.2 (continued)

Author(s) & Date	Purpose	Sample	Design	Findings
16. Roy (1977)	To compare the effects of varying degrees of decision-making on feelings of powerlessness and levels of adaptation, and to describe the relationship between levels of adaptation and indicators of wellness	Adult patients on medical-surgical units preparing for discharge within 24 hours (N=208)	Correlational	Decision-making is associated with levels of situational powerlessness in younger patients and those with short-term illness and with generalized powerlessness among middle-aged patients who had short-term illnesses. No relationship was demonstrated between powerlessness and physiologic adaptation or between levels of adaptation and indicators of wellness. There was a modest relationship between powerlessness and the two measures of psychosocial adaptation—anxiety and stress adaptation.
17. Dow (1992/1993)	To generate a mid-range model for adaptation after surviving cancer and describe the influence of having children; to develop and test the psychometric properties of the instrument Adaptation After Surviving Cancer; and to test differences in survival between case-matched comparison groups of women who had children and those who did not after breast cancer therapy	Phase I-Women who had children after breast cancer (n=20); Phase II-Cancer survivors (n=330); Phase III-Women who had children after cancer therapy (n=27) and those who did not (n=27)	Grounded theory; Instrument development; Correlational	Key elements in the process of surviving cancer and having children include: becoming and being a cancer patient, a cancer survivor, a mother, and transcending cancer. The instrument, Adaptation After Surviving Cancer, demonstrated reliability and validity. There was no difference in the number of recurrent breast cancers, metastatic cancers,

Author	Purpose	Sample	Design	Findings
				or deaths between the group of women who had children after breast cancer and the comparison group. Mothers had higher mean scores for total quality of life and for all subscales; and mothers scored in the higher range of total adaptation scores.
18. Phillips (1991)	To examine predictors of adaptation to shiftwork, predictors of injury status among shift workers, and whether differences in adaptation to shiftwork exist between injured and non-injured workers	Papermill workers who worked a permanent backward rotation schedule (N=239)	Correlational	Significant predictors of adaptation to shiftwork included: vigor/rest circadian factor, use of emotive and supportant coping styles, and work environment. The number of years on rotating shifts, age, and ability to wake before alarm predicted injuries. No significant difference was found in adaptation for injured and non-injured workers.

In describing the adaptation of preadolescents and adolescents diagnosed as having IDDM, Grey, Cameron, and Thurber (1991) also found that age was a factor. Preadolescents were significantly less depressed, were less anxious, coped in more positive ways, had fewer adjustment problems, and were in better metabolic control than adolescents. Adolescents were more likely to cope by employing avoidance behaviors that were associated with poorer adaptation and metabolic control.

Zhan (1993/1994) studied cognitive adaptation processing patterns used by the hearing impaired elderly to maintain self consistency. A purposive convenience sample of 128 adults aged 64 to 86 years with hearing-loss onset at or after age 40 was studied. Cognitive adaptation processing explained 42% of the variance in self consistency with the patterns of self perception, clear focus and method, and knowing awareness being the most prominent. Gender differences were found with men scoring higher on self consistency, cognitive adaptation processing, and perceived health status.

Roy (1977) looked at the effects on levels of adaptation of specific cognitive and emotional processes, degrees of decision-making, and feelings of powerlessness. As noted in studies described above by Barone (1993/1994) and Grey and colleagues (1991), age and length of illness affected adaptation levels. For example, levels of decision-making were associated with levels of situational powerlessness in younger patients and in those with short-term illnesses. Further, levels of decision-making were associated with generalized powerlessness among middle-aged patients with short-term illnesses. Two measures of psychosocial adaptation—anxiety and stress—were somewhat related to powerlessness and were not related significantly to measures of levels of wellness.

Dow (1992/1993) conducted a three-phase study analyzing the experience of surviving and having children after breast cancer. A grounded theory approach, based on interviews with 20 women, was used to generate a mid-range model and to develop an instrument, Adaptation After Surviving Cancer. The mid-range model described strategies of becoming and being a cancer patient, becoming and being a cancer survivor, becoming and being a mother, and transcending the cancer experience. The psychometric properties of the instrument on adapting to cancer were established using 330 cancer survivors, both men and women. The final phase of the study focused on a case match of women who had children after cancer therapy and those who did not. Significant findings included: no differences in the number of recurrent breast cancers, metastatic cancers, or deaths; mothers had higher mean scores for total quality of life and for all subscales, that is, health, social well-being, psychological well-being, and family; mothers consistently had higher scores of total adaptation; and when compared to normative data, mothers who had children after breast cancer had fewer stressors in the parent-child system.

In a study of adaptation and injury status of industrial workers on a rotating shift pattern, Phillips (1991) examined aspects of both cognator and regulator adaptive strategies. Using multivariate correlations for data from 239 shift workers, the author found that significant indicators of adaptation to shift work included: vigor/rest circadian factor (regulator subsystem), emotive and supportant coping styles defined by the instrument used (cognator subsystem), and work environment (stimuli). Differences between injured and non-injured workers could be found in demographic variables but not in adaptation. This is parallel to Roy's (1977) finding that there was little relationship between measures of adaptation and measures of wellness.

In the studies that dealt with general adaptive strategies, some strategies were more clearly defined within given populations. Reports of several studies showed that selection of adaptive strategies varies by age, illness, and social experience. However, significant evidence was not found to link adaptation strategies with health.

Perceptual information processing. Among the studies identified as focusing on strategies of the cognator adaptive subsystem, seven studies dealt with the cognator strategy of perceptual information processing (see Table 7.3). In two studies, nurses' perceptions were compared with patients'. Lynam and Miller (1992) compared self-perceived needs during labor of mothers of preterm infants with nurses' perceptions of these needs. Both mothers and nurses identified perceived needs in all four modes and the rank order for mothers and nurses by modes was the same; that is, self concept, interdependence, physiologic, and role function. However, mothers perceived the following needs as more important than the nurses perceived them: "to be asked opinions and preferences regarding type of delivery" (self concept mode) "to be assured of a safe outcome for my baby," and "to be informed of how my baby is tolerating the labor progress" (interdependence mode).

When Cohen (1980) compared nurses' and patients' perceptions of patient adaptation to hemodialysis there were more differences than agreements. Only 18 out of 75 items showed a significant relationship between the perceptions of nurses and their assigned patients. The total number of times nurses administered hemodialysis treatments to an assigned patient, as well as the level of education of the nurses, were significantly related to the number of perceptions nurses identified that were in agreement with patients' perceptions.

Using hospital observations, with interviews and drawings after discharge, Broeder (1985) explored school-age children's perceptions of isolation. Broeder combined the RAM with the stages described in Piaget's theory of cognitive development. Findings indicated that 9-year-olds had an understanding of the reason for isolation; 6- and 7-year-olds did not fully understand. Commonalities in these children's perceptions were iden-

Table 7.3 – Description of Studies About Perceptual Information Processing (N=7)

Author(s) & Date	Purpose	Sample	Design	Findings
19. Lynman & Miller (1992)	To describe and compare mothers' self-perceived needs during preterm labor and nurses' perception of these needs	Postpartum mothers of preterm neonates (n=14); registered nurses employed in labor and delivery (n=25)	Descriptive	Mothers' self-perceived needs included all four adaptive modes. There were no significant differences between mothers' and nurses' perceptions as measured by responses to the total number of items, however, five need statements showed significant group differences. The rank order of perceived needs by mode for both mothers and nurses was: self concept, interdependence, physiologic, and role function.
20. Cohen (1980)	To compare nurses' and patients' perceptions of patient adaptation to hemodialysis	Nurses assigned to hemodialysis patients (n=93) and patients receiving treatment (n=106)	Correlational	In comparing patients' adaptation as perceived by patients and nurses, there were more differences than agreements of perceptions between nurses and their assigned patients. This was particularly evidenced in investigating patient emotional reactions.
21. Broeder (1985)	To explore schcol-aged children's perceptions of isolation, after hospital discharge	Hospitalized children with isolation being part of the treatment regime (N=6)	Descriptive	Nine-year-olds indicated understanding of reason for isolation; 6- and 7-year old children did not fully understand reason. All children stated they felt scared when they saw illustration of nurse in isolation attire. All identified procedures as most stressful experience while in isolation.

22. Frederickson, Jackson, Strauman, & Strauman (1991)	To identify the relationship between perception and physiologic and psychosocial adaption in patients with cancer preparing to undergo aggressive chemotherapy	Subjects enrolled in Phase II clinical trials with Interleukin-2 cell therapy (N=45)	Correlational	Perception of symptoms was positively correlated with psychosocial adaptation and not with actual physiological status.
23. Wright (1993)	To assess parents' perceptions of quality of life after the diagnosis and treatment of cancer in their child	Parents of children at least 6 months after diagnosis of cancer (N=30)	Descriptive	The mean of the sample population's scores indicated a good or very good quality of life (QOL), but the sample perceived their QOL to be worse than before their child had cancer.
24. Scherubel (1985/ 1986)	To identify specific patient characteristics, in the self concept, role function, and interdependence modes, associated with an adaptive post hospital course; to identify the relationship of family environment to adaptation; and to examine the effect of cardiac classes on post hospital activities	Patients (n=54) and spouses (n=25) following myocardial infarction and coronary bypass surgery	Descriptive	Perceptions of self esteem, interpersonal behavior, and family relationships were lower than norms at the time of discharge. Findings included dissatisfaction with personal behavior, and increased interpersonal conflict. Subjects' perceptions and characteristics within families remained stable or improved slightly 3 to 6 months following discharge. Families exhibiting cohesion, achievement orientation, and strong moral-religious values were associated with positive adaptive responses in subjects.

(continued)

Table 7.3 *(continued)*

Author(s) & Date	Purpose	Sample	Design	Findings
25. Dobratz (1990/ 1991)	To examine the interrelationships and to explain the effects of the person-environment variables upon psychological adaptation in the process of dying	Recipients of hospice care services (N=97)	Correlational	Subject responses included patterns of self-transactions which represented higher and lower levels of death aware-ness, i.e., transcending; becoming; reconciling; anguishing; avoiding; relinquishing; and regressing. Predictor variables accounted for 38% of the adjusted variance in psychological adaptation. The significance of social support, pain, and age were confirmed as direct predictors of the outcome.

Table 7.4 – Description of Studies About Adaptation as an Outcome (*N*=8)

Author(s) & Date	Purpose	Sample	Design	Findings
26. Dobratz (1993)	To examine effects of selected person-environment variables as they influenced psychological adaptation in home hospice patients	Home hospice patients (*N*=97)	Correlational	All variables explained 38% of adjusted variance for adaptive psychological processes as compared with 20% of the adjusted variance for psychological well being. Social support and age were indicators of psychological adaptation. Pain was inversely associated with the outcome of adaptation.
27. Phillips & Brown (1992)	To examine to what extent adaptation to shiftwork is predicted by selected variables and whether there is a difference in adaptation to shiftwork between workers on a rotating shift schedule who were injured compared to those who have not been injured	Mill workers (*N*=239)	Correlational	Ten variables accounted for 51% of the variance in adaptation scores. Eight of the ten were considered accurate predictors of adaptation, the most important being the vigor/rest factor, with increased scores being related to positive adaptation. There was no statistically significant difference in adaptation to shiftwork between those who were injured and those who have not been injured.

(continued)

Table 7.4 *(continued)*

Author(s) & Date	Purpose	Sample	Design	Findings
28. Jackson, Strauman, Frederickson, & Strauman (1991)	To evaluate the biopsychosocial effects of Interleukin-2 therapy (IL-2), the short- and long-term emotional effects of the therapy, and effect of the treatment regimen on the patient's quality of life	Patients receiving IL-2 treatment (N=45)	Correlational	Physiological toxicities were experienced in all treatment regimens, but altering the schedule was somewhat successful in decreasing toxicities. Emotional concerns and symptom distress increased during treatment but returned to baseline by the 1-month time point. Patients who reported less physical and psychological distress before treatment were more likely to survive.
29. Strohmyer, Noroian, Patterson, & Carlin (1993)	To describe the overall level of adaptation, the relationships between functional and psychosocial adaptation levels, and demographic factors predictive of positive psychosocial adaptation of survivors of multiple trauma 6 months after discharge from a tertiary trauma center	Survivors of multiple trauma (N=18)	Descriptive	Most of the sample reported positive functional adaptation. All reported problems with worry; over 70% had severe problems in self-devaluation, guilt, depression, hostility, body image distortion, and anxiety. Employment status was the best single predictor of psychosocial adaptation.
30. Shuler (1990)	To examine the relationships among social isclation, loneliness, self concept, and physical and psychosocial adaptation in patients with cancer	Patients being treated in rural outpatient cancer centers (N=65)	Correlational	There was a significant positive relationship between loneliness and social isolation and between loneliness and self concept.

Study	Purpose	Sample	Design	Results
31. Collins (1992/1993)	To determine if there are relationships among functional health, social support, and the level of morale of older women living alone.	Women living alone for at least 2 years in Appalachian counties in Western Kentucky ($N=60$)	Correlational	Significant associations were found between functional health and morale and between social support and morale. Age was negatively correlated with both morale and functional health. A model containing age and social support was found to account for 27.1% of the variance in morale.
32. O'Brien (1991)	To assess elderly clients, with mentors, perceived social adaptation in nursing homes	New residents of a nursing home ($n=5$) and mentors who had been in the nursing home for at least 1 year ($n=5$)	Qualitative-descriptive	All mentees reacted to the mentorship program in a positive manner. The results of comparing the mentees' interview responses to an outcomes checklist based on the RAM showed a majority of responses reflecting positive adaptation in all four modes.
33. Selman (1989)	To examine the impact of having a total hip replacement (THR) on physiologic function, self concept, role function, and interdependence	Adults who had a THR in the past 12-24 months ($N=46$)	Descriptive	Based on positive scores in all areas and enthusiastic comments, it was concluded that quality of life as represented by the four adaptive modes was positively affected by having a THR. A common theme of written comments was that having a THR restored a normal life.

tification of nursing procedures as the most stressful experience while hospitalized in isolation, being scared during the interviews when they saw an illustration of a nurse in isolation attire, and reflecting feelings of deprivation from the experience.

Frederickson, Jackson, Strauman, and Strauman (1991) studied patients enrolled in Phase II clinical trials with Interleukin-2 cell therapy to identify the relationship between perception and physiologic and psychosocial adaptation. In keeping with propositions derived from the RAM, the authors found evidence of a positive but nonsignificant relationship between actual physiologic status and perceived physiologic adaptation; a positive but nonsignificant correlation between physiologic status and psychosocial adaptation; a positive and significant relationship between perceived physiologic adaptation and psychosocial adaptation. Further analyses showed that actual physiologic status was not linked to survival. Rather, those patients who were still alive at 6 months had better physiologic and psychosocial adaptation. Measures in this study focused on patient perceptions, which was different from the measures of illness and injury in studies by Phillips(1991) and Roy (1997).

Wright's (1993) study of parents of children diagnosed with cancer differs from that of Smith and colleagues (1983) in that it is a primary analysis of quantitative data, using a tool specifically based on the adaptive modes of the RAM. The outcome variable was perceptions of quality of life (QOL) for parents who had a child at least 6 months after the time of diagnosis. While the parents' scores indicated a good or very good QOL, the sample perceived QOL to be worse than before their children had cancer.

Scherubel (1985/1986) described adaptation patterns in patients and spouses following an acute cardiac event. The investigator concluded that perceptions of self esteem, interpersonal behavior, and family relationships were lower than norms at the time of discharge. Subjects' perceptions and relationship characteristics remained stable or improved slightly three to six months following discharge. Interpersonal styles significantly influenced return to work and social activities. Families that exhibited cohesion, achievement orientation, and strong moral-religious values were associated with positive adaptive responses in subjects.

Recipients (N=97) of hospice care were studied by Dobratz (1990/1991) to examine the interrelationships and to explain the effects of the person-environment variables upon psychological adaptation in the process of dying. She described a central construct of hierarchical process patterns related to death awareness. These self-transactions were interpreted as levels of self perception: transcending, becoming, reconciling, anguishing, avoiding, relinquishing, and regressing. The dying people whose scores reflected patterns of self-transactions to the right of the continuum, interpreted meaning, connected with others, accepted and adjusted expectations, and managed symptoms. In the patterns to the left of the continuum, the dying people agonized in suffering and avoided or repressed cognitions. Demographics, health, and social factors were predictors of outcome, and this aspect of Dobratz' work (Dobratz, 1993) is reported in the following section on adaptation as an outcome.

These seven studies highlighted the significance of perceptual information processing as one particular component of cognator strategies, and provided descriptions of the perceptual processes in specific situations. In addition, common influencing factors—age, experience, and education—were noted among the studies.

Adaptation as an outcome. In several of the studies on the adaptive modes and processes described earlier, adaptation as an outcome has been included. However, the next eight studies (see Table 7.4) show investigations in which adaptation as an outcome is the particular research focus. For example, after Dobratz' dissertation work, which was described above as uncovering perceptual processes through grounded theory, the investigator (Dobratz, 1993) specifically reported the effects of selected person-environment variables as they influence psychosocial adaptation in home hospice patients. Dobratz formulated and tested a causal model of psychological adaptation as an outcome variable. All variables explained 38% of adjusted variance for adaptive psychological processes, with social support and age emerging as predictors of the outcome.

Similarly, a publication by Phillips and Brown (1992) reported the outcome of adaptation as predicted by the adaptive strategies described above (Phillips, 1991). The authors noted that inability to adapt to the effects of shiftwork could contribute to a worker's risk of injury. One outcome, adaptation, looked at the physiologic and psychosocial health consequences of shiftwork. Data on injury status of participants was also collected. Eight of ten variables were considered accurate predictors of adaptation, and these accounted for 51% of the variance in adaptation scores. There was no significant difference in adaptation to shiftwork between those who were injured and those who were not injured.

Extending the analysis of the study on perceptual processes reported above, Jackson, Strauman, Frederickson, and Strauman (1991) evaluated the biopsychosocial outcome effects of Interleukin-2 therapy with 45 patients. Although patients were in good physical condition at the start of therapy, physiologic toxicities were experienced in all treatment regimens. The need for nursing care increased during treatment, and altering the schedules could decrease toxicities. Symptom distress also increased during treatment, but returned to baseline by one month following treatment. Patients who reported less physical and psychological distress before treatment were better adapted and were more likely to survive.

Strohmyer, Noroian, Patterson, and Carlin (1993) described the overall level of adaptation and the relationships between functional and psychosocial adaptation levels and the effects of demographic factors in survivors of multiple trauma 6 months after discharge. Although the sample was small and the generalizability not established, the report of this pilot study contained a vivid description of adaptive outcomes. Most of the sample reported functional adaptation: independence in self-care, sphincter control, and mobility. However, all reported problems with worry; over 70% had severe problems in self-devaluation, guilt, depression, hostility, body image distortion, and anxiety. Subjects who were employed at 6 months following discharge reported significantly better psychosocial adaptation scores than those not employed.

In a sample of patients being treated in rural outpatient cancer centers, Shuler (1990) used multivariate correlational methods to describe factors that accounted for physical and psychosocial adaptation to illness. Physical and psychological adaptation was theoretically defined as an individual's ability to respond to and cope with stimuli using physiologic, psychologic, and sociologic modes. The author found a significant positive relationship between loneliness and social isolation and between loneliness and self concept. A small but nonsignificant percentage of the variance in adaptation was accounted for by these variables.

In another rural setting, Collins (1992/1993) studied older women living alone in Appalachia. The outcome variable studied was morale, defined as an internal manifestation of adaptation characterized by positive self-regard and satisfaction with self, a sense of place for oneself within the environment, an acceptance of reality of what cannot be changed, and freedom from distressing symptoms of anxiety. Multiple regression analysis revealed that both functional health and social support were significant predictors of morale. The findings were interpreted as reflecting the vulnerability of older women living alone in rural areas.

O'Brien (1992) conducted a pilot study of social adaptation of the elderly to the nursing home environment wherein a mentorship program was used. The author noted that interview responses of the new residents of the nursing home, who were mentored by another resident, showed positive adaptation in 11 of 12 responses in the physiologic mode; in 4 of 6 responses in the role function mode; and in 4 of 6 responses in the interdependence mode.

In the final study on adaptation as an outcome, Selman (1989) examined the effect of total hip replacement on physiologic function, self concept, role function, and interdependence. This study measured change in the four adaptive modes in the 12 to 24 months following surgery. The results showed a positive change in all four modes and overall satisfaction with the hip replacement surgery.

In this section, adaptation as an outcome has been defined in differing ways, and studies were reported that had a variety of samples. Investigators found adaptation as an outcome an important variable and have derived implications from their findings that are discussed in the synthesis section of this chapter.

The nursing care group as an adaptive system. Two different organizational models of the nursing care group as an adaptive system were derived by Lutjens (1990/1991; 1991) and by Rich (1991/1992) (Table 7.5). Lutjens (1990/1991; 1991) examined the relationships among predictor variables conceptualized as environmental stimuli, and the criterion variable length of stay conceptualized as a manifestation of the organizational coping mechanisms of stabilizer and innovator. Based on data from 973 charts, and using multiple linear regression analysis, she found that length of stay was better predicted by the patients' projected need for nursing intensity than by the cumulative frequency of nursing condition, medical intensity, and medical condition. The combination of all four variables was the best predictor of length of stay. Lutjens concluded that the study provided new knowledge relative to the ability of nursing intensity to influence length of stay and suggested further development and refinement of patient classification systems.

Using data collected for her dissertation, Lutjens (1991) specifically reported on the use of nursing theory for the conduct of nursing research. She focused on deriving the framework for the study from the theory of social organizations and from Roy and Anway's (1989) application of the model to theories for nursing administration. The management information system was conceptualized as a stabilizer structure, while the innovator structure was conceptualized as the structure and processes for change. Lutjens used both the process and the content of her dissertation study and concluded that the RAM provided a useful framework to guide and design studies that will contribute to the study and practice of nursing administration.

A theoretically derived Stress-Transformational Coping Model of Burnout Prevention was tested by Rich (1991/1992). This model was derived from integration of the RAM, stress and coping theory, and a hardiness model. The independent variables used to empirically examine the proposed pathway to burnout were: commitment, control, challenge, optimism, self-esteem, the organizational resources of peer and supervisory support, and the preferred transformational coping style. The dependent variable was the degree of burnout. Results suggested that two separate paths to burnout exist, one through stress and coping and the other through the organizational climate. The original model was replaced by a new model which showed that all the resources are equally important and can work comprehensively to promote well-being and prevent burnout among staff nurses.

Table 7.5 – Description of Studies About the Nursing Care Group as an Adaptive System (N=3)

Author(s) & Date	Purpose	Sample	Design	Findings
34. Lutjens (1990/ 1991)	To determine the explanatory power of nursing condition, nursing intensity, medical condition, & medical intensity on length of stay	Patients' charts (N=973)	Correlational	The length of stay was better predicted by patients' projected need for nursing intensity than by the cumulative frequency of nursing condition, medical intensity, and medical condition. The combination of all four variables was the best predictor of length of stay.
35. Lutjens (1991)	To determine the explanatory power of environmental stimuli on length of stay (LOS)	Patients' charts (N=973)	Correlational	The theory of social organizations as adaptive systems derived from the RAM provided a framework to guide and design studies in nursing administration.
36. Rich (1991/1992)	To test a stress transformational coping model of burnout prevention and to assess the goodness of fit of the proposed model from the data	Registered nurses employed in an acute care setting (N=246)	Correlational	The proposed model did not adequately fit the data. A revised model was constructed indicating a direct path between organizational resources and burnout. There was a significant negative relationship between personal and organizational resources and perceived work stress. Organizational resources had a significant negative relationship to burnout, but was positively associated with emotional focused coping. The new model revealed that burnout is prevented through social resources of the organization, the personal resources of nurses, and coping responses when stress is encountered.

Fewer studies focus on the nursing care group as an adaptive system than on the individual and families as adaptive systems. However, the three studies provide direction for research that can be done in the complex organizational environments in which many nurses practice.

Critical Analysis of the Reported Research

The 36 studies on adaptive modes and processes described in this chapter are critically analyzed using accepted criteria for the quality of the research. In applying the criteria, it was recognized that for a given manuscript editors may have limited what was published for reasons of space or style. In the current chapter, however, nearly 50% of the studies were dissertations (n=16), or theses (n=1). Thus some investigators may have had the advantage of explaining their frameworks, methods, and findings in greater detail than others. In each case, the reports were evaluated as presented without the advantage of dialogue with the investigators.

Quantitative studies (n=32) were primarily descriptive and correlational. The qualtitative studies (n=4) included descriptive and ethnographic designs.

Critical analyses of quantitative studies. The critical analyses of research on adaptive modes and processes that used quantitative methods are summarized in Table 7.6. The analysis of the 32 studies is based on criteria established by the research team and explained in Chapter 2.

Investigators of the quantitative studies mainly manifested an objective effort to control for threats to internal and external validity. There were no studies that did not address these issues to some extent, only three studies had partial control in both validity categories, with 88% achieving most of the criteria. Awareness of methodologic issues may have been heightened for the large number of researchers who were doctoral students or recent holders of the degree. While the quality of the studies was generally good, many investigators acknowledged the limitations of descriptive and correlational studies. For example, sample selection was largely by convenience to maximize the variables under study, but limited by lack of random selection or assignment. However, in most studies the criteria for selection of subjects was clearly stated, the sample used in the analysis was described, and subject attrition was not a major problem. History and maturation were less likely to affect many of the studies done on the strict time schedules of graduate students and in carefully selected settings.

One study that provides examples of control of threats to validity is Dobratz' (1991/1992) study of the causal influences of psychological adaptation in home hospice patients. Subjects met the criteria for being a dying patient as defined by the National Hospice Association, as well as the other inclusion criteria: recipient of hospice services, 30 years of age or older, English-speaking, absence of impaired cognition, and willing to

Table 7.6 – Critical Analysis of Quantitative Adaptive Modes and Processes Research (*N=32*)

Criteria	Evaluation		
	Yes	*Partially*	*No*
Design			
Threats to Internal Validity Controlled	2, 6, 7, 9, 10, 11, 12, 13, 14, 15, 16, 17, 18, 19, 20, 21, 22, 23, 25, 26, 27, 28, 29, 30, 31, 33, 34, 35, 36	3, 8, 24	
Threats to External Validity Controlled	2, 6, 7, 8, 9, 11, 12, 13, 14, 15, 16, 17, 18, 19, 20, 21, 22, 23, 25, 26, 27, 28, 30, 31, 33, 34, 35, 36	3, 8, 9, 10, 24, 29	
Measurement			
Reliability of Instruments Addressed	6, 7, 9, 11, 12, 13, 14, 15, 17, 18, 19, 20, 22, 23, 25, 26, 28, 29, 30, 31, 33, 34, 35, 36	3, 8, 10, 16, 21, 24, 27	2
Validity of Instruments Addressed	6, 7, 9, 10, 11, 12, 13, 14, 15, 16, 17, 18, 19, 20, 22, 23, 24, 25, 26, 27, 28, 29, 30, 31, 33, 34, 35, 36	3, 8, 21	2
Data Analysis			
Appropriate	2, 7, 8, 9, 10, 11, 12, 13, 14, 15,16, 17, 18, 20, 21, 22, 24, 25, 26, 27, 28, 31, 33, 34, 35, 36	6, 19, 24, 29, 30,	3
Interpretation of Results			
Consistency of Findings with Conclusions	2, 6, 7, 8, 9, 10, 11, 12, 13, 14, 15, 16, 17, 18, 19, 20, 25, 26, 27, 30, 31, 33, 34, 35	21, 23, 24, 28, 29	3

(continued)

Key: 2= Farkas (1981); 3= Varvaro (1991); 6=Thomas, Shoffner, & Groer (1988); 7= Pittman (1992/1993); 8= Kiikkala & Peitsi (1991); 9= Trentini (1985/1986); 10= Francisco (1990); 11= Pollock (1986); 12= Pollock (1989); 13= Barone (1993/1994); 14= Grey, Cameron, & Thurber (1991); 15= Zhan (1992/1993); 16= Roy (1977); 17= Dow (1992/1993); 18= Phillips (1991); 19= Lynam & Miller (1992); 20= Cohen (1980); 21= Broeder (1985); 22= Frederickson, Jackson, Strauman, & Strauman (1991); 23= Wright (1993); 24= Scherubel (1985/1986); 25= Dobratz (1990/1991); 26= Dobratz (1993); 27= Phillips & Brown (1992); 28= Jackson, Strauman, Frederickson, & Strauman (1991); 29= Strohmyer, Noroian, Patterson, & Carlin (1993); 30= Shuler (1990); 31= Collins (1992/1993); 33= Selman (1989); 34= Lutjens (1990/1991); 35= Lutjens (1991); and 36= Rich (1992).

---

participate. The investigator spent considerable time orienting the staff to the research study and worked part-time as a research associate at one of the two data collection sites. She received full support and sponsorship of the research from the agencies. Of the 114 subjects, 3 required second sessions to complete the tools, 2 had a rapid physical decline before a second session could be scheduled, 10 were assessed as being unable to participate due to physical fatigue or cognitive impairment, and 5 patients refused to sign the consent form after initial agreement. Thus the final sample was 97 subjects.

In contrast, investigators (Strohmyer et al., 1993) in a pilot study of multiple trauma patients were able to control only partially for threats to internal validity. Inclusion criteria were carefully stated and 76 of 120 multiple trauma survivors who were discharged 6 months before the study met the criteria. However, 26 of these were lost to follow-up, 8 declined to participate, and 6 were unable to answer questionnaires. Of the 36 who agreed to participate, 2 were in litigation and received legal advice not to participate; an additional 4 believed the questionnaires did not apply to them; and 10 did not return the questionnaires. Of the 20 subjects who returned the questionnaires, 2 did not complete them. The study provided interesting findings, but for the purpose of knowledge building, they were limited by questions about how representative the sample was of the population of survivors of multiple trauma.

Random selection was possible for one study. Lutjens (1990/1991) used a computer-generated random sample of records of 1,000 patients discharged under medical-surgical Diagnostic Related Categories (DRGs). In addition, she conducted a pretest that reflected a high degree of similarity in length-of-stay between patients whose hospital care was paid for under DRG payments and those who were not. Lutjens recognized that correlational designs conducted in naturalistic settings have the advantage of being stronger in realism, thus the possibility exists that the findings are generalizable to similar settings. On the other hand, she noted that retrospective studies are not strong because the conditions under which the data were collected were not known entirely, and the occurrence of more than one phenomenon at the same time does not necessarily infer causation, thereby limiting generalizability. The issue of inferred causality is relevant for the large number of studies using correlational design to investigate adaptive modes and processes.

A study by Kiikkala and Peitsi (1991) also used chart review–for a different purpose–and showed only partial control of threats to internal and external validity. The investigators proposed to describe the components of nursing care for preschool children with MBD by examining nursing documents from every patient treated in a given unit over a 4-year period. They also used descriptions of nursing care of children with MBD written by nurses working in the ward. Threats to internal validity were partially controlled, since all patient records were used to avoid problems of selection and of attrition. However, the investigators did not discuss possible changes on the unit or in the staff over those 4 years, thus allowing the possibility of threats related to history and maturation. Further, the environment and possible extraneous variables were not well described, thus limiting generalizability. Information was not given about the nurses who provided the accounts of nursing care nor was there a description of the conditions of collection of this data. However, some internal validity can be assumed from the fact that the accounts were from the nurses caring for children with the particular condition and this unit was the major unit for this population in the capital of Finland.

The descriptive study of adaptation in the four modes among women with coronary heart disease by Varvaro (1991) provided examples of threats to external validity. The sample of women was described according to coronary event experienced (coronary bypass surgery, myocardial infarction, and angina), age, ethnicity, and religion. However, the subjects were part of a larger study and this report did not provide data on other factors, such as health status and family or social situation, that may have affected adaptation.

Barone (1993/1994) provided an example of a study in which both internal and external threats to validity were well controlled. The sample was a nonprobability purposive sample with clear inclusion criteria which included proportional regional representation from members of the National Spinal Cord Injury Association. Power analysis indicated that a sample size of 190 participants was sufficient for the purpose of the study. One thousand questionnaire packets were mailed nationally, and a 29% response rate was obtained, considerably above the usual return rate of 10% or less for mailed self-administered questionnaires (Williamson, Karp, Dalphin, & Gray, 1982). A toll-free telephone number was used to assist participants—particularly those with quadriplegia—in filling out the questionnaire and to promote adequate sampling. In all, 243 subjects were included in the data analysis. Barone designed her study to take into account key influencing factors. In her analysis, she measured and used sociodemographic characteristics of age, gender, marital status, educational level, time post-injury, level and grade of injury, and time in rehabilitation; Health-Related Hardiness; coping strategies; physiologic adaptation; and psychosocial adaptation.

Measurement issues of reliability and validity of instruments were not addressed as well as issues of design, although 75% of the studies adequately addressed reliability of instruments. Similarly, validity of instruments was addressed adequately in 88% of the studies. Farkas (1981) published a study in which measurement issues were not addressed. The investigator reported using two interview schedules, as well as developing scales for powerlessness and knowledge/utilization of services. There was no description of the interviews or scales, and no validity or reliability data on either one were provided.

The study by Grey and colleagues (1991) is an example of adherence to scientific criteria regarding measurement. The investigators reviewed literature on the reliability and validity of all instruments and also evaluated their own data for consistency with the reports. The authors convincingly discussed the rationale for measuring physiologic adaptation by assessing metabolic control using glycosylated hemoglobin. Measures of self-care and recent stressors were likewise reported as both reliable and valid. Notably, the Life Events Checklist (LEC) was developed by one of the researchers for children and adolescents. Still, the same standards for valid and reliable measurement were applied. All items were evaluated for face and content validity by experts in pediatrics and stressful life events research.

Wright (1993) also revised an instrument and addressed reliability and validity, but less completely than the previous authors. Good content and construct validity, as well as good internal consistency were reported for the scale. In the parent version of the scale, the wording of each item was changed to indicate the subject was the parent of a child with cancer. Two items were omitted because their content was deemed inappropriate for the subjects. The revised instrument was submitted to content validity evaluation by experts in pediatric oncology nursing. However, the investigator argued that, considering the nature of the changes to the instrument, the estimates of reliability and validity of the children's scale can be assumed for the parent's scale. While this may be the case, at the current stage of development of knowledge in nursing, and particularly with instruments to measure variables of the RAM, scientific rigor would be enhanced by reporting reliability and validity data on the form of the instrument used in the study. Wright's approach to using the subjects as their own controls contributed to reliability of the measurement.

Francisco (1989/1990) is another investigator who changed a scale without reporting revised reliability data. However, she carefully attended to validity issues. It may be noted that her use of the adaptive modes of the model contributed to establishing the validity of her instrument, as was the case in a number of other studies analyzed.

In a creative study of school-age children's perceptions of isolation after hospital discharge, Broeder (1985) used observations during hospitalization and interviews at home that included children's drawings. The investigator reviewed the literature on children's communication through drawing and there is evidence that she used this instrument appropriately. However, the data collection by observation was only vaguely described and a discussion of the validity and reliability of the data collected with this approach was not given. On the other hand, Cohen (1980) reported on the construction and testing of interview guides and questionnaires for her study comparing perceptions of patient adaptation as viewed by nurses and patients undergoing hemodialysis.

The next criterion used in the critical analysis related to the appropriateness of the data analysis. Appropriateness addressed whether the statistic chosen can answer the research question, and if the assumptions for the use of the statistic were met. In all but one study, data analysis was judged to be appropriate, or partially so. A wide range of data analysis methods were used, including descriptive statistics, such as frequencies, means, and standard deviations. Various tests of differences and correlation, such as analysis of variance, chi-square, Pearson's Product Moment Correlation, Spearman's Rho, and Kendall's Tau; as well as several multivariate measures, including multiple regression analysis, causal modeling, and path analysis were also used.

The one study where the data analysis was judged not appropriate was that conducted by Varvaro (1991). In this descriptive study, data were taken from a sample of women with coronary heart disease who had volunteered for a larger study. The investigator used a combination of reporting numbers of subjects with tables of mean scores and standard deviations for items on instruments. Ranges of scores were not given. In a related issue, Varvaro had difficulty interpreting her results and was not consistent in discussing data, findings, and conclusions. Scores on self care activities were reported as a measure of physiologic mode adaptation, whereas in the discussion of findings on the self concept mode, the author reported concern for self-care activities by 40 subjects.

Investigators for two studies compared nurses' perceptions to patients' perceptions (Lynam & Miller, 1992; Cohen, 1980). One provides an example of appropriate data analysis. The other was partially appropriate, although both met the established criterion for interpretation of results. Lynam & Miller effectively used means and rank orders to describe and compare needs of women experiencing preterm labor as perceived by the nurse and by the patient. However, when no differences were found in responses to the total number of questionnaire items, then a Spearman's r was computed on each item and probabilities of differences computed. Assumptions related to correlational measures include normality of distribution of scores in both groups and approximate equal variability (Munro & Page, 1993). When each item was made a variable these assumptions were jeopardized and the risk of a Type I error was increased, particularly with the low sample size.

Cohen, on the other hand, appropriately used descriptive statistics, comparing her sample to published reports of descriptions of the national hemodialysis population. In addition, the investigator used cross-tabulation tables with a nonparametric statistic, chi square, to identify differences. The study comparisons were further strengthened by the fact that each nurse in the study had cared for a patient(s) in the study.

Several dissertations provided evidence of appropriate and sophisticated use of data analyses and careful interpretation of results. Phillips (1991) tested predictors of adaptation to shiftwork by entering all variables into a regression analysis with stepwise entry and removal. Ten variables, several of which related to circadian type, accounted for 51% of the variance in adaptation scores; therefore the null hypothesis was rejected. Similarly, Dobratz (1990/1991) appropriately used causal modeling and path analyses. She established the meeting of assumptions for each statistical procedure. For example, the investigator calculated low interrelationships among the variables and did residual analysis using scatterplots before determining multiple prediction. Conclusions were carefully discussed in relation to the limitations of using a convenience sample of dying patients receiving hospice care.

Critical analyses of qualitative studies. Among the 36 studies examining multiple adaptive modes and processes, four were classified as using qualitative designs. Descriptive content analysis was used in two studies (Florence et al., 1994; Smith et al., 1983); ethnographic method was used by Gagliardi (1991); and in a pilot study master's thesis, O'Brien (1991) summarized the content of audiotaped interviews with five new nursing home residents who had been assigned a mentor. The critical analyses of these studies are summarized in Table 7.7.

To ensure validity, Smith and colleagues (1983) used at least three of the five strategies: descriptive vividness, methodologic congruence, analytical preciseness, theoretical connectedness and heuristic relevance. They clearly described how they selected messages as their unit of analysis and defined them as an idea, theme, or expression in a single content area. The messages were classified within the four adaptive modes. Reliability was addressed in terms of calculating interrater reliability to determine consistency in interpreting the transcribed parent interviews. The investi-

Table 7.7 – Critical Analysis of Qualitative Adaptive Modes and Processes Research (N=6)

Criteria	Evaluation		
	Yes	Partially	No
Design			
Strategies to ensure			
validity used	1, 4, 5		32
Strategies to ensure			
reliability used	1, 4, 5	32	
Data Analysis			
Appropriate method	1,4, 5		32
Interpretation of Results			
Consistency of findings			
with conclusions	1, 4, 5		32

Key: 1 = Smith et al. (1983); 4 = Gagliardi (1991); 5 = Florence, Lutzen, & Alexius (1994) and 32 = O'Brien (1991).

gators appropriately presented the data in bar graphs that showed percentage of responses that indicated messages in each of the adaptive modes when parents were asked four subjective and four objective questions.

Similarly, Florence and colleagues (1994) used transcribed interviews to identify themes that were categorized according to the four adaptive modes. The investigators in this study addressed reliability by critiquing initial themes during debriefing sessions to minimize individual biases. Descriptive vividness contributed to validity. Direct quotations and summaries of the interview content were used effectively to present the data. In analyzing the intepretation of results, the authors reached important conclusions from their data about the experience and adaptation of women who were infected with the HIV virus. However, in some cases, it was unclear how interpretations were obtained. For example, themes in the self concept mode were idenfitied and emotional symptoms ranged from mild worry to delusions and paranoia. This may be so, but not enough information was given to judge whether this conclusion was consistent with the data.

O'Brien's (1991) study differed from the others in that no single approach to qualitative design and analysis was used. Rather, the study provided a description of tape-recorded interviews with newly admitted elderly residents of a nursing home. The subjects had participated in a mentorship program with another elderly resident who had lived at the nursing home for 1 year or more. This was intended to be a pilot study and may not be expected to meet all the criteria outlined in Chapter 2. However, the researcher encountered more threats to internal and external validity than was anticipated. Whereas the study was intended for five subjects with mentors, one subject withdrew and one was not interviewed because of deterioration in mental status. Thus, only three subjects were interviewed. Further, their length of stay varied from 2 months to 1 year, which was similar to the mentors' length of stay in the institution. The investigator noted that the questionnaire was pretested by a panel of judges, but no information about the pretest was provided. Finally, there was some lack of clarity in the appropriateness of the data analysis method, and in the consistency of the data with the findings and conclusions, the latter based on some confusion regarding the purpose of the study.

When Gagliardi (1991) used an ethnographic approach to study experiences of families having a child with Duchenne muscular dystrophy, she included naturalistic inquiry with participant observation. The investigator met all criteria for ensuring validity and reliability in the design of the study. Methodologic congruence was particularly notable, as the investigator carefully documented each step of the procedure. Further, the author used analytical preciseness effectively in describing themes with both quotations and pictorial illustrations. External auditors and support group members validated the content and themes. Data analysis included multiple techniques that met the criteria of being appropriate for the design and data. In addition to constant comparison, the analysis included examination of transcripts and analytic memos, validation of the content codes, and identification of interrelated themes among the codes. Presentation of the data under three themes was precise and effective. Conclusions were insightful and consistent with the findings.

Evaluation of Relationships to the RAM

The 33 studies on adaptive modes and processes that met the basic criteria established for critical analysis were evaluated for linkages to the RAM. Based on the critical analysis of the research, both descriptive and analytical, and on the evaluation to the linkages of the RAM, results from the 33 studies were used to test RAM propositions.

Linkages to the Roy Adaptation Model

Evaluation of the linkages between studies on the adaptive modes and processes, and the basic tenents of the Roy Adaptation Model, is summarized in Table 7.8. Linkages of research variables, empiric measures, and findings to the RAM are identified as explicit, implied, or absent.

Table 7.8 – Evaluation of Linkages to the RAM (N=33)

Linkages to RAM	Evaluation		
	Explicit	Implicit	Absent
Research Variables	1, 2, 3, 4, 5, 6, 7, 8, 9, 10, 11, 12, 13, 14, 15, 16, 17, 18, 20, 22, 23, 24, 25, 26, 27, 28, 29, 30, 31, 33, 34, 35, 36	19, 21	
Empiric Measures	1, 2, 3, 4, 5, 6, 7, 8, 9, 10, 11, 12, 13, 14, 15, 16, 17, 18, 19, 20, 21, 22, 23, 24, 25, 26, 27, 28, 29, 30, 31, 33, 34, 35, 36		
Findings	1, 2, 3, 4, 5, 6, 7, 8, 9, 10, 11, 12, 13, 14, 15, 16, 17, 18, 19, 20, 21, 22, 23, 24, 25, 26, 27, 28, 29, 30, 31, 33, 34, 35, 36	21	

Key: 1 = Smith, Garvis, & Martinson (1983); 2 = Farkas (1981); 3 = Varvaro (1991); 4 = Gagliardi (1991); 5 = Florence, Lutzen, & Alexius (1994); 6 =Thomas, Shoffner, & Groer (1988); 7 = Pittman (1992/1993); 8 = Kiikkala & Peitsi (1991); 9 = Trentini (1985/1986); 10 = Francisco (1990); 11= Pollock (1986); 12 = Pollock (1989); 13 = Barone (1993/1994); 14 = Grey, Cameron, & Thurber (1991); 15 = Zhan (1992/1993); 16 = Roy (1977); 17 = Dow (1992/1993); 18 = Phillips (1991); 19 = Lynam & Miller (1992); 20 = Cohen (1980); 21 = Broeder (1985); 22 = Frederickson, Jackson, Strauman, & Strauman (1991); 23 = Wright (1993); 24 = Scherubel (1985/1986); 25 = Dobratz (1990/1991); 26 = Dobratz (1993); 27 = Phillips & Brown (1992); 28 = Jackson, Strauman, Frederickson, & Strauman (1991); 29 = Strohmyer, Noroian, Patterson, & Carlin (1993); 30 = Shuler (1990); 31 = Collins (1992/1993); 32 = O'Brien (1991); 33 = Selman (1989); 34 = Lutjens (1990/1991); 35 = Lutjens (1991); and 36 = Rich (1992).

Most of the studies on adaptive modes and processes made explicit linkages of the research variables, empiric measures, and findings to the RAM. This is contrary to findings in the evaluating studies in other chapters and to what was usually reported in the literature (Silva, 1986; Silva & Sorrell, 1992). One factor that may have influenced this positive evaluation is the large number of dissertations. One case in point is Collins' study (1992/1993) in which she carefully described how the Roy model served as a guiding framework in choosing appropriate variables and methods of measurement to assess the adaptation level of older women living alone in Appalachia.

A selection of examples of the variables related to the model from the dissertations are cited. Collins (1992/1993) used morale as an outcome variable. She defined it as an internal manifestation of adaptation characterized by positive self-regard and satisfaction with self, a sense of place for oneself within the environment, an acceptance of reality or what cannot be changed, and freedom from distressing symptoms of anxiety. The conceptualization of the research variable, and the measurement of it, with the Philadelphia Geriatric Center Morale Scale, is consistent with Roy's descriptions of person and environment (Roy, 1977, Roy & Andrews, 1999).

Zhan (1993/1994) explicitly reported that she used the RAM as a framework because of the emphasis on cognitive adaptation processing and self consistency as a component of the self concept adaptive mode. Dow (1992/1993) related her work to both the philosophic and scientific assumptions of the RAM. She investigated adaptation and becoming a mother after having breast cancer as both a process and an outcome. Dow described each of these perspectives on adaptation in the qualitative, instrument development, and quantitative phases of her research. Lutjens (1990/1991) provided discussion of the evolution of a predictive model related to the nursing care system, as it was linked to the RAM, and the use of the RAM in theorizing for nursing administration (Roy & Anway, 1989).

Examples of the explicit relationships between research variables and measurement and the RAM are found in journal articles as well as dissertations. Pollock (1986) focused in particular on the stimuli affecting physiologic and psychosocial adaptation in chronic illness. The variables were linked to the RAM throughout the study and relevant measurements were used. Frederickson and colleagues (1991) studied the cognator process of perception as it relates to adaptation. The two variables were explicitly linked to the model, as were the empiric measures selected. Lynam and Miller (1992) also looked at perceptions, and compared mothers' self perceived needs during preterm labor with nurses' perception of these needs. A rating of an implicit link was given because there was a lack of clarity in understanding the RAM concept of the cognator process of perception.

Two of the qualitative studies (Gagliardi, 1991; Kiikkala & Peitsi, 1991) did not link the RAM explicitly in the initial design of the study, but as data were collected, variables were identified and linked. Further, the qualitative research process outlined for both studies was consistent with the RAM and with methods used to study the model as described by Roy and Barone (1996).

All studies either explicity or implicitly linked findings to the RAM. The studies went beyond identification of the RAM as the framework of the study and discussed the model in some detail. These discussions were consistent with the literature on the RAM. The relationships to the RAM included linkages of variables to major model concepts, efforts to select appropriate empiric measures, and relating findings of the research to the model. In the one study which implicitly related the findings to the model, Broeder (1985) discussed the significance of identifying stressors for the child in isolation. In general, the model served well in the design, implementation, and analyses of adaptive modes and processes research.

Testing RAM Propositions

Criteria used to select studies for testing of propositions from the RAM were derived from the analysis and evaluation of the research. Studies were excluded if there was serious threat to internal and external validity of the design, problems with instrument validity and reliability, inappropriate analysis of data, lack of consistency between findings and conclusions, and if the major study variables were not explicitly or implicitly related to the RAM. Thirty-three of the 36 studies are used to test propositions from the RAM. Nine of the general propositions listed in Chapter 2 were tested by the BBARNS authors using the 33 research reports. Under each general proposition, more specific propositions related to adaptive modes and processes were derived (Table 7.9). These are referred to as ancillary and practice propositions.

The RAM shows central processes by which the individual or group adapts to the environment. At the individual level, these are the regulator and the cognator processes; at the group level the processes are the stabilizer and innovator. Two generic propositions state that these processes affect innate and acquired ways of adapting. Five ancillary propositions are derived from the evidence of the studies on adaptive modes and processes.

Six studies sought to identify patterns of unique cognator processing in given patient groups. Vivid descriptions of the cognator processes of adapting are given for families with children with muscular disease, women tested as HIV-positive, chronically ill children, hearing impaired elderly, women who became mothers after breast cancer, and patients in hospice care. The results of the studies provide clear support for the first ancillary proposition.

A second ancillary proposition notes that cognitive processing specifically affects self concept. Examples from the research show that cognitive adaptation processing affected self consistency (Zhan, 1992/1993) and decision-making affected levels of perceived powerlessness in some patients (Roy, 1977). However, decision-making did not always affect powerlessness, and the proposition was not supported by this additional data.

Table 7.9 – Testing of Propositions from the Roy Adaptation Model. (N=33)

Propositions from the RAM	Ancillary and practice propositions	Supported by results	Not supported by results
1. At the individual level, regulator and cognator processes affect innate and acquired ways of adapting.	a. Patterns of unique cognator processing can be identified in given patient groups.	Gagliardi (1991); Florence, Lutzen, & Alexius (1994); Pittman (1993); Zhan (1993/1994); Dow (1992/1993); Dobratz (1990/1991)	
	b. Cognitive processing affects self concept and self concept may affect cognitive processing.	Pittman (1994/1993); Zhan (1993/1994); Roy (1977); Scherubel (1985/1986); Strohmyer, Noroian, Patterson, & Carlin (1993)	Roy (1977)
	c. Perception affects adaptation.	Frederickson, Jackson, Strauman, & Strauman (1991); Jackson, Strauman, Fredericksn & Strauman (1991)	
2. At the group level, stabilizer and innovator processes affect adaptation.	a. A combination of nursing and medical factors best predicts patients' length of stay.	Lutjens (1990/1991); Lutjens (1991)	
	b. Organizational resources have a negative relationship to the phenomenon of nurse burnout.	Rich (1991/1992)	

(continued)

Table 7.9 (continued)

Propositions from the RAM	Ancillary and practice propositions	Supported by results	Not supported by results
3. The characteristics of the internal and external stimuli influence adaptive responses.	a. Serious medical diagnoses in children affect adaptation in all modes for their parents.	Smith, Garvis, & Martinson (1983); Gagliardi (1991); Wright (1993); Farkas (1981); Varvaro (1991)	
	b. The adaptive modes are differentially affected by varying stimuli.	Florence et al. (1994); Thomas, Shoffner, & Groer (1988); Kiikkala & Peitsi (1991)	
	c. Education can affect adaptation.	Pollock (1986)	Pollock (1986)
	d. Intensity of the stimulus affects adaptive response.	Broeder (1985)	
	e. The quality of the stimulus affects the adaptive response.	Selman (1989)	
	f. Age and gender influence adaptation.	Grey, Cameron & Thurber (1991); Zhan (1993/1994); Roy (1977); Broeder (1985); Collins (1992)	
4. The characteristics of the internal and external stimuli influence the adequacy of cognitive and emotional processes.	a. Social support affects coping.	Florence et al. (1994); Collins (1992/1993)	
	b. Acquired ways of coping are affected by type of chronic illness, particularly related to characteristics of control, predictability, and hardiness.	Pittman (1993); Pollock (1986); Barone (1993/1994); Roy (1977)	

Proposition		
c. Perceptions of patients' needs by nurses and patients are more similar in some situations than in others.	Lynam & Miller (1992); Cohen (1980)	
d. Nurses' judgments about nursing problems and actions are affected by experience and education.	Trentini (1985/1986)	Trentini (1985/1986)
5. The adequacy of cognator and regulator processes will affect adaptive responses		
a. Patterns of unique cognator processing identified in given patient groups are related to effective adaptive behavior.	Gagliardi (1991); Florence et al. (1994); Pittman (1992/1993); Zhan (1993); Dow (1992/1993); Dobratz (1990/1991)	
b. Specific cognator strategies such as humor, outcome appraisal, mixed-focus coping, hardiness, emotion-focused coping, self perception, clear focus and method, knowing awareness, cohesion, achievement orientation, and strong moral-religious values are related to effective adaptive behavior.	Francisco (1989/1990); Pollock (1989); Zhan (1993/1994); Scherubel (1985/1986)	
c. Cognitive strategies may change under stress.	Scherubel (1985/1986); Roy (1977)	
d. Circadian factors affect adaptation to changing time schedules.	Phillips (1991); Phillips & Brown (1992)	
e. Adaptative processes relate to health.	Dow (1992/1993); Frederickson et al. (1991); Jackson et al. (1991)	Phillips (1991); Phillips & Brown (1992); Roy (1977)

(continued)

Table 7.9 (continued)

Propositions from the RAM	Ancillary and practice propositions	Supported by results	Not supported by results
6. Adaptation in one mode is affected by adaptation in other modes through cognator and regulator connectives.	a. Positive role changes affect physiologic well-being and quality of life.	Dow (1992/1993)	Shuler (1990)
	b. Interdependence behavior affects role function.	Scherubel (1986)	
7. The pooled effect of focal, contextual, and residual stimuli determines the adaptation level.	a. Stimuli contribute different weights to the outcome of adaptation.	Strohmyer et al. (1993); Shuler (1990)	
	b. Common focal stimuli can be identified through statistical techniques such as predictive modeling.	Collins (1992/1993); Phillips (1991); Dobratz (1990/1991); Lutjens (1990/1991)	
8. Adaptation is influenced by the integration of the person with the environment.	People adjust their answers to questions based on norms of what is socially acceptable.	Smith et al. (1983)	
9. The variable of time influences the process of adaptation.	Adaptive responses change over the duration of a health-illness experience.	Barone (1993/1994); Roy (1977); Dow (1992/1993); Dobratz (1990/1991)	

Further, a reciprocal relationship of self concept influencing cognitive processing was noted in several studies. The issue of two-way relationships in the propositions is discussed in one of the final chapters. Roy has highlighted the significance of perception to adaptation in several publications (Roy, 1988; Roy & Roberts, 1981). Using the same sample of patients, two studies supported the proposition that perception affects adaptation (Frederickson et al., 1991; Jackson et al., 1991).

Two authors addressed group level adaptive processes. Lutjens' (1990/1991; 1991) study supported the general proposition by specifying and testing an explanatory model for how various factors in the health organization contributed to patient length of stay, viewed as a manifestation of an adaptive system. Similarly Rich (1991/1992) found specific relationships between decreased organizational resources and increased burnout in nurses.

The next general proposition is that the characteristics of internal and external stimuli influence adaptive responses. In the studies on adaptive modes and processes that were reviewed, several specifications of stimuli characteristics were identified. For example, three investigators noted the effects of serious illness in a child upon adaptation of parents (Gagliardi, 1991; Smith et al., 1983; Wright, 1993). Another three studies showed which modes are more affected by given stimuli (Florence et al., 1994; Thomas et al., 1988; and Kiikkala & Peitsi, 1991). For example, Thomas and colleagues (1988) studied high school freshmen and found that the adaptive modes were affected differently based on gender. Pollock's (1986) study found that education affected physiologic adaptation but not psychosocial adaptation. Thus the related proposition is both supported and not supported by the same study.

According to the RAM, characteristics of internal and external stimuli also influence adequacy of cognitive and emotional processes. The general proposition received support through the identification of four ancillary propositions among the studies on adaptive modes and processes. Two studies found a relationship between social support and coping (Collins, 1992/1993; Florence et al., 1994). In patients with a variety of chronic illnesses, four investigators found type of chronic illness, and personal characteristics— control, predictability, and hardiness—affected the acquired ways of coping (Barone, 1993/1994; Pittman, 1992/1993; Pollock, 1986; Roy, 1977).

Lynam and Miller (1992) found that the rank order of perceived needs by mode for mothers of preterm neonates and for nurses was the same: self concept, interdependence, physiologic, and role function. On the other hand, Cohen (1980) found more differences than agreements between nurses and their assigned patients in perceptions of patient adaptation. However, both studies support the notion that it is the characteristics of the stimuli, both internal and external, that affect cognitive processes. In another study in which nurses made judgments about patients' problems, and also about types of nursing action, Trentini (1985/1986) found mixed results. Education and years of experience did not affect the number of patient problems identified by the nurse, but level of education was significantly related to number of nursing actions selected for solving problems.

A key proposition of the RAM is that the adequacy of the cognator and regulator processes will affect adaptive responses. In the six studies that identified patterns of unique cognator processing for given patient groups, the investigators also related these patterns to a vivid description of adaptive behavior. In another set of studies, the investigators found relationships between specific cognitive strategies and adaptive behavior. For example, Zhan (1992/1993) found that in adapting to hearing loss, the elderly used cognitive adaptation processing strategies such as self perception, clear focus and method, and knowing awareness.

In another study by Scherubel (1985/1986), families exhibiting cohesion, achievement orientation, and strong moral-religious values were associated with positive adaptive responses. Further, two studies found that cognitive strategies change under stress. Phillips (1991) and Phillips and Brown (1992) examined regulator processes and found that circadian factors, such as vigor and rest and the ability to waken before the alarm clock sounds, affected adaptation to shift work.

The ancillary proposition that adaptive processes relate to health has been a long time assumption of the RAM (Roy, 1970). However, the studies reviewed showed mixed findings related to support of this proposition. Support is noted in two sets of data. In a carefully matched sample, Dow (1992/1993) found that women who have children, and higher adaptation, after breast cancer treatment are not at greater risk of developing recurrent or metastatic disease as a result of hormonal changes of pregnancy. In the two reports drawn from one data set, Frederickson and colleagues (1991) and Jackson and colleagues (1991) cited evidence for the effect of perception of health. Conversely, Roy (1977) was unable to demonstrate a relationship between adaptation and level of wellness in adult medical surgical patients who were about to be discharged from the hospital. Phillips (1991) likewise did not find a significant difference in adaptation between injured and non-injured workers.

Among the studies reviewed which met the critical standard for analysis there are at least two examples that relate to the general proposition that adaptation in one mode is affected by adaptation in other modes through cognator and regulator connectives. Dow (1992/1993) found a relationship between becoming a mother after having breast cancer (role function), and both physiologic well-being (physiologic) and quality of life (self concept and interdependence). The proposition was not supported by Shuler (1990), who found a small nonsignificant percentage of physical and psychosocial adjustment (physiologic and psychosocial modes) to illness was accounted for by social isolation, loneliness (interdependence), and self concept. Scherubel's (1985/1986) data demonstrated one adaptive mode affecting another by identifying that interpersonal styles (interdependence) significantly influenced return to work and social activities (role function).

The seventh general proposition addresses the pooled effect of focal, contextual, and residual stimuli as determining adaptation level. Three studies supported the ancillary proposition that the stimuli contribute different weights to the outcome of adaptation. For example, Strohmyer and colleagues (1993) examined factors predictive of positive psychosocial adaptation of survivors of multiple trauma and found that employment status was the best single predictor. Based on data from five studies (Collins, 1992/1993; Dobratz, 1990/1991; Lutjens, 1990/1991; Lutjens, 1991; Phillips, 1991), another ancillary proposition is derived—that the effect of common stimuli can be calculated. For example, Dobratz (1990/1991) calculated that the variables of social support, pain, and age were direct predictors of psychological adaptation in the process of dying.

The general proposition that adaptation is influenced by the integration of the person with the environment is illustrated by the work of Smith and colleagues (1983). The authors interpret their data on parents of children with cancer to indicate that parents initially respond with socially acceptable answers, such as needs for information about the child's condition or treatment, and concerns about financial matters.

The final proposition tested in the chapter on adaptive modes and processes relates to the observation that the passing of time influences the process of adaptation. This was supported by data from four studies (Barone, 1993/1994; Dobratz, 1990/1991; Dow, 1992/1993; Roy, 1997) which indicated that adaptive responses change over the duration of a health-illness experience. Barone found that adapting to spinal cord injury varied by the length of time since injury. Likewise, Dow and Dobratz both described changes over time in the process of adaptation to cancer and to dying.

In summary, most of the studies supported the general propositions of the RAM, and instances of the propositions not being supported were identified. The ancillary propositions derived from the general propositions and the findings of specific studies provide new insights into the meaning of the general propositions and potential for practice. An integration of testing the propositions in studies of adaptive modes and processes with the tests in other chapters is discussed in Chapter 11 which covers contributions to nursing knowledge related to the propostions derived from the RAM.

Synthesis of Research on Adaptive Modes and Processes: Contributions to Nursing Science

A synthesis of the 33 studies that met methodologic and model linkage criteria is used to identify contributions of the research on adaptive modes and processes to nursing science. Contributions are discussed in three sections: applications to clinical practice, directions for future research, and development of the Roy Adaptation Model.

Applications to Nursing Practice

The primary goal of model-based research is to affect the quality of nursing practice (Barone & Roy, 1996). The studies on adaptive modes and processes are used to derive applications to practice (Table 7.10). For purposes of this review, applications to practice are placed in three categories as described in Chapter 2.

Several of the studies that examine adaptive mode assessment provide findings that have high potential for implementation, because they identify the significance of given assessment factors for nursing practice. Based on results from an analysis of interviews with parents adapting to the effect of childhood cancer, Smith and colleagues (1983) recommend that nurses continue to pose questions that allow parents to identify their needs related to the adaptive modes. Further, nurses can help parents realize that they can identify what would meet their child's physiologic, self concept, role function, and interdependence needs, because when parents are engaged in meeting their child's needs their own adaptive strengths are enhanced. Similarly, Wright's (1993) findings indicated that nurses will be aware of the changing quality of life of parents after the diagnosis and treatment of cancer in their child. The study by Gagliardi (1991) also had implications for assessment that can be implemented without risk.

The vivid qualitative description of the experiences of families having a child with Duchenne muscular dystrophy can sensitize nurses to the losses experienced by the family and child. They can be made aware of the families' needs in all four adaptive modes as the boys evolve through physical, social, and educational changes. Community education related to destigmatizing the disability is also warranted, as are programs that increase contact between disabled and nondisabled children.

Nurses who care for children with diabetes need to plan their care with knowledge of the findings of Grey and colleagues (1991) that age and secondary sexual development explained a large percentage of the variation in psychosocial adaptation and metabolic control. Although nurses cannot change developmental level, they can be aware of the significant adjustment problems of adolescents compared to preadolescents and assess for signs of such difficulties so that appropriate interventions can be planned.

Table 7.10 – Potential for Implementation from Adaptive Mode and Processes Research (*N*=33)

Category One: High potential for implementation

Smith, Garvis, Martinson (1983)	Wright (1993)
Varvaro (1991)	Gagliardi (1991)
Grey, Cameron, & Thurber (1991)	Selman (1989)
Dow (1992/1993) —Phases II and III	Scherubel (1985/1986)
Strohmyer, Noroian, Patterson, & Carlin (1993)	
Broeder (1985)	Barone (1993/1994)
Dobratz (1993)	Francisco (1990)
Kiikkala & Peitsi (1991)	Rich (1992)
Collins (1992/1993)	

Category Two: Needs further clinical evaluation before implementation

Florence, Lutzen, & Alexius (1994)	Pittman (1992/1993)
Dobratz (1990/1991)	Zhan (1992/1993)
Dow (1992/1993) —Phase II	Frederickson, Jackson,
Jackson, Strauman, Frederickson,	Strauman, & Strauman (1991)
& Strauman (1991)	

Category Three: Further research indicated before implementation

Thomas, Shoffner, & Groer (1988)	Pollock (1986;1989)
Trentini (1985/1986)	Phillips (1991)
Roy (1977)	Shuler (1990)
Phillips & Brown (1992)	

Two phases of Dow's (1992/1993) study have implications for clinical application in their current form. The Adaptation After Surviving Cancer Profile was demonstrated to be psychometrically sound and can be used in both practice and research to assess patients' adaptive processes and outcomes. Further, Dow's findings in the third phase of her study suggested that cancer survivors have led more satifying, fuller, and rewarding lives after treatment ended, thus challenging the prevailing notion that cancer survivors have major hurdles and difficulties in adapting to cancer. In particular, nurses who counsel women considering having a child can use the findings that women who have children after breast cancer are not at greater risk for developing recurrent or metastatic disease. Because of the controlled case matching with an appropriate sample, the findings were published as a definitive work by the National Cancer Institute (Dow, Harris, & Roy, 1994). Sellman (1989) also provides helpful findings that nurses can use in counseling people making decisions related to their lives and health. Patients having total hip replacement surgery had an increased quality of life, as represented by the four adaptive modes, and a common theme reported was that the surgery restored a normal life.

The finding from Scherubel's (1985/1986) study that can be immediately useful to nurses in clinical practice was the relationship found between family environment and the post hospital course of adaptation for patients following coronary bypass surgery. Families exhibiting cohesion, achievement orientation, and strong moral-religious values were associated with positive adaptive responses. Although descriptive correlational studies do not immediately indicate intervention strategies, they do identify positive factors that can be assessed and supported by nurses.

The works by Broder (1985), Strohmyer and colleagues (1993), Barone (1993/1994), and Dobratz (1993) all identify factors affecting the process of adaptation that nurses can use in planning nursing care. Broder described how children felt scared by illustrations of a nurse in isolation attire and all identified procedures as the most stressful experience while in isolation. Although nurses cannot change these factors, they can help children become familiar with the environment, and help them express and cope with misunderstandings, fears, and stressors. In caring for patients with multiple trauma, the 6 month follow-up descriptive data by Strohmyer and colleagues can be useful to nurses in helping patients anticipate and plan for management of problems that occurred in most of the patients studied—self-devaluation, guilt, depression, hostility, body image distortion, and anxiety.

Barone's work highlights the importance of rehabilitation nurses assisting patients' use of escape-avoidance coping strategies and maintaining hope of recovery shortly after sustaining a spinal cord injury. Furthermore, nurses can predict that the older the person with a spinal cord injury, the longer the time and greater the intervention required for psychosocial adaptation. Nurses can also realize that patients with paraplegia may achieve greater physiologic adaptation than those with quadriplegia. Similarly, Dobratz (1993) identified contextual stimuli that affect psychosocial adaptation in hospice patients. Invaluable for both the nurse and family caregiver is the knowledge that social support and pain can be managed.

The finding from Francisco's (1989/1990) study that can be applied in practice is that humor was positively related to problem solving and that the combined effect of adaptation and humor account for a large percent of the variance of family functioning. The nurse can help people consciously link the use of humor to cognitive coping strategies such as problem-solving. For example, when a family faces a dilemma, each person can be asked to create a fanciful solution of a family on Mars facing this dilemma. After the fun of sharing fanciful stories, the family can approach their own problem-solving in a possibly more effect way.

Interestingly, an outcome of the study by Kiikkala and Peitsi (1991) was to recommend implementation of the Roy Adaptation Model in practice. The recommendation was based on finding a need to improve nursing assessment beyond physiologic function, and to improve nurses' documentation of nursing care. Rich's (1991/1992) study found a significant negative correlation between organizational resources of the institution and burnout in nurses. The immediate application of this finding is that the institution can provide increased organizational resources such as regular staffing patterns to decrease burnout. Similarly, Collins (1992/1993) identified the importance of social support for morale of older women living alone. Nurse can be creative in finding ways of connecting older women with new support systems as older women lose customary sources of social support.

In category two—studies needing further evaluation before implementation—parts of three studies were based on qualitative data and four on quantitative data. The qualitative data collected by Dobratz (1990/1991), Zhan (1992/1993), Dow (1992/1993—Phase II), and Florence and colleagues (1994) provide vivid accounts of the process of adaptation using cognator strategies. The patterns presented from the findings represent plausible representations of patients' situations. However, because the observations were made on a limited number of subjects, these patterns need to be subjected to further evaluation by clinicians and/or researchers, to judge their appropriateness for describing cognitive processing to achieve adaptation in the populations that they represent. Similarly, the issue of representativeness of the sample places Pittman's (1992/1993) study in category two. Enabling characteristics of chronically ill school-age children are identified in a sample of children in three groups, defined by characteristics of the chronic illnesses, who regularly attended federally funded, community-based children's clinics. Further clinical and empiric investigations can reveal if these characteristics are sufficiently generalizable to warrant their use in planning nursing interventions.

The last two studies in category two raise a different issue related to further evaluation before implementation. Frederickson and colleagues (1991) and Jackson and colleagues (1991) found that patients' perceptions before radical chemotherapy were predictive of outcomes, including mortality at 6 months. They emphasized that nurses need to design assessment protocols that emphasize the clients' views of their physical states as well as the degree of distress their symptoms produce. Further, such nursing assessments may have implications for clinical judgments related to whether a client is a good candidate for aggressive medical interventions.

The remaining studies were judged to need further testing before implementation. Thomas and colleagues (1988) found gender differences in stress factors for adolescents. Despite a fairly large sample size, however, the only variable controlled was rural, urban, and suburban schools. Thus further testing is indicated before accepting as a basis for practice that the differences noted were based solely on gender and not on other characteristics that occur with both boys and girls.

Trentini (1985/1986) found relationships between nurses' backgrounds and decisions the nurses made about patients' problems and appropriate nursing actions. The sample was limited to nurses working with dialysis patients and to apply this finding to all nurses or even to all nurses in this clinical area would be premature. Further testing is recommended to understand these variables and to ascertain their generalizability.

Pollock's (1986) model of adaptation to chronic illness was partially supported and warrants further testing to make it useful in applications to clinical practice. Similarly, Roy's (1977) hypothesized relationships among degrees of decision-making, feelings of powerlessness, and levels of adaptation, and the relationship between levels of adaptation and indicators of wellness was partially supported. The author suggested intervening variables that might clarify these relationships, but the proposed changes have not been tested for support of these relationships and for the use of such findings in practice.

The lack of a statistically significant relationship between adaptation to shiftwork and injury is the finding from Phillips (1991) and Phillips and Brown (1992) that needs further investigation before the nurse can relate it to practice. Although the sample was fairly large, the number of injuries was small, limiting the possibility of demonstrating a relationship with the data collected and thus indicating further testing. Likewise, Shuler (1990) found a small but nonsignificant percentage of the variance in physical and psychosocial adjustment to illness was accounted for by social isolation, loneliness, and self concept. Given the weakness of the relationships and vagueness of the variables, the study cannot be the basis for implementations in practice without further concept analysis and testing.

Finally, category three includes two reports in which Lutjens (1990/ 1991; 1991) found that a combination of effects of nursing condition, nursing intensity, medical condition, and medical intensity on length of stay was the best predictor of length of stay. The investigator discussed the limitations of the use of patient charts as the only source of data and particularly recommends further work on designing tools to clinically measure nursing intensity. Thus instrument development and research expanding the sources of data collection are warranted.

Recommendations for Model-based Research

Recommendations for research based on the RAM are identified in all of the 33 studies used to synthesize the research on adaptive modes and processes. Although studies that need further testing before implementation in practice have readily apparent implications for future research, other studies also are sources for recommendations for model-based research. This is particularly the case when findings were equivocal or unexpected based on previous theoretic or empiric evidence. In some cases, concept clarification is recommended, as discussed in considering theory development, before further empiric work.

The seven adaptive mode assessment studies contribute to understanding assessing of the adaptive modes of the RAM. However, within each of the studies there are additional questions to be asked. Further, taken together these studies represent only a beginning of the needed systematic empiric investigation of understanding the clinical manifestations and factors influencing the adaptive modes and processes. The need for thorough nursing assessment in all adaptive modes was evident in several studies. In addition, a need exists for assessment tools for the cognator and regulator adaptive processes. Thus designing and validating assessment tools for practice can be a focus for research.

Smith and colleagues (1983) highlighted the issue of parents of children with cancer giving socially acceptable answers to questions about their needs. This finding leads to the recommendation that the nurse and patient interaction in assessing the adaptive modes will be a topic for research. What factors affect the timing of the assessment of the four adaptive modes? Are there some modes that are assessed best early in the relationship? What are the approaches to establishing trusting relationships to obtain clinically useful assessments within all four adaptive modes given the time and resource constraints of the practice setting?

Studies that showed adaptive strategies in general, and perceptual information processing in particular, prompt further research. Findings of several studies demonstrated the usefulness of qualitative methods in describing adaptive processes. Studies describing adaptive processes, such as children and adults adapting to chronic illness, becoming a mother after breast cancer, elders adapting to hearing loss, people being heterosexually infected with HIV, and hospice patients going through life closure, can serve as models for examining the central adaptive processes in other populations considered priority for study. For example, qualitative descriptive researchers doing studies based on the RAM can focus on the frail elderly, long-term care givers, mothers and children who are victims of various types of abuse, people migrating internationally or regionally, those dealing with natural disasters, and others who suffer the stresses of a fast-paced technocratic world.

The processes that have been described in the reported studies can be subjected to verification and tested for generalizability. Furthermore, all studies on the adaptive processes were correlational. Intervention studies are a high priority for further research. Intervention studies to promote the patterns identified as healthy adaptation are recommended.

Based on the literature identified for this review, it is recommended that studies be systematically designed to cover all cognator and regulator processes. Only one study included regulator processes and this resulted in positive findings. Much more, however, needs to be done. Studies on the congruence of patients' and nurses' perceptions of patients' needs provided differing results. The topic needs further research to determine key characteristics of congruent nurse and patient perceptions that are conducive to promoting patient adaptation. From this understanding, interventions to achieve such congruence in the clinical situations already studied, that of mothers of preterm infants and patients having dialysis, and of patients in other clinical situations, can be designed and tested.

The need to find ways to measure patients' perceptions was recommended by many investigators. Barone (1993/1994) raised the significant issue of development of instruments to measure cognator coping and adaptation for spinal cord patients. She notes that the most appropriate instruments available were selected, however, they lacked sensitivity and specificity for the patient population.

Dow's (1992/1993) instrument, Adaptation After Surviving Cancer Profile, provides an example of developing a psychometrically sound tool that authentically deals with adaptation as a process. Zhan (1992/1993) developed a tool on self-consistency (Zhan, 1994) and modified a tool in process of development, Cognitive Adaptation Processing Scale (CAPS) in the Elderly (Roy & Kazanowski, in preparation). Psychometric evaluation in the study sample provides promise, but the tool needs further testing on larger samples.

Several key concepts for further research were identified in the investigations reviewed. Hardiness, humor, family cohesion, and moral-religious values all may be effective in promoting adaptation and this can be confirmed with replication studies and new designs. Based on mixed findings in two studies (Roy, 1977) clinical investigations to identify the effect of powerlessness as an intervening variable between cognator processes and adaptation are recommended. Influencing factors such as age, gender, and time also were identified as needing further clarification and clinical investigation.

Finally, an important recommendation for model-based research comes from the mixed findings in relating adaptation to health outcomes. Better measurement tools are needed for both concepts. The nature of the relationship between the two variables needs to be clarified and intervention studies to promote health through adaptation is a major field for future research.

Directions for Theory and RAM Development

Studies in which adaptive modes and processes were investigated can be used to identify directions for further theory and model development. In the context of this chapter, theory development relates to derivation of concepts, formation of propositions, and interrelation of propositions. In addition, theory development requires creative and rigorous structuring of ideas that (a) project a tentative, purposeful, and systematic view of phenomena (Chinn & Kramer, 1995) and that (b) provide plausible explanatory descriptions. Model development relates to the insights, understandings, and potential changes among the key elements indicated by the RAM.

Four major areas for theory and model development are identified from the 36 studies that were critically analyzed. Further conceptual and theoretic development needed includes (a) further descriptive refinement of cognator processes, (b) concept analysis of specific cognitive strategies, (c) understanding the relationship of cognator processes to the self-concept mode, and (d) understanding the role of perception in cognator and regulator processes.

Based on testing of the propositions, patterns of unique cognator processing were identified in six groups of patients. Researchers need to compare and contrast processes to find any commonalities that might be integrated into higher level conceptualization among patient groupings. This additional level of synthesis can contribute to the conceptual description of cognator processes. Furthermore, specific cognator strategies were identified as noted in proposition 5b (Table 7.9). Careful concept analysis of each of these strategies, such as defining characteristics for humor and knowing awareness, is the first step to new theoretic formulations. The resulting concepts can be used to revise existing statements and relational propositions.

An interesting relationship between cognitive processing and self concept was noted in several studies and indicates that this may be a reciprocal relationship (Pittman, 1993; Roy, 1977; Scherubel, 1986; Strohmyer et al., 1993; Zhan, 1993). Although one's self concept over time can influence judgment, learning, emotion, and perceptual information processing—the reverse can also happen. This two-way relationship is implied in the discussion of influences on the development of self concept (Roy & Andrews, 1999). However, it has not been clearly articulated before. Furthermore, this insight raises questions about the direction and nature of all the propositional statements. A broad theoretic issue identified for future exploration is that of the relationship between cognator and regulator processes and the adaptive modes.

Some evidence was provided to show that perception affects adaptation. From a theoretic perspective, the concept should be clarified in order to reach new understandings. The evidence is not clear about whether support exists for assuming that a connector for the cognator and regulator is provided by perceptual information processing. Researchers who study the brain and information processing need to re-examine the concept of perception and its place in the RAM.

Summary

In use for more than 25 years, the RAM is a holistic approach to patient care that is useful in practice, research, and education. The model has lived up to the promise of nursing model development in the 1970s through extensive use and has evolved through continued growth and refinement. Out of the 163 nursing studies included in this monograph, 36 specifically focused on adaptive modes and processes. These studies generally meet the criteria for quantitative and qualitative research. In addition, links to the RAM were particularly strong in this set of studies.

Based on the critical analysis and on the evaluation of linkages to the model, 33 studies were used to synthesize the research and to describe contributions to nursing science. Both general and specific applications for practice and recommendations for future research were developed based on the findings of the studies. Finally, possibilities for future theory and model development were discovered.

References

Barone, S.H. (1994). Adaptation to spinal cord injury (Doctoral dissertation, Boston College, 1993). *Dissertation Abstracts International, 54,* 3547-B.

Barone, S.H., & Roy, C. (1996). Application of the Roy Adaptation Model in nursing research: An example from rehabilitation nursing. In B. Neuman & P. Walker *Blueprints for nursing models in action.* (pp. 64-87). New York: National League for Nursing.

Broeder, J.L. (1985). School-age children's perceptions of isolation after hospital discharge. *Maternal Child Nursing Journal, 14,* 153-174.

Chinn, P.L., & Kramer, M.K. (1995). *Theory and nursing: A systematic approach.* St. Louis: Mosby.

Cohen, B.J. (1980). The perception of patient adaptation to hemodialysis: A study of registered nurses and hemodialysis patients (Doctoral dissertation, Columbia University Teachers College, 1980). *Dissertation Abstracts International, 41,* 129-130-B.

Collins, J.M. (1993). Functional health, social support, and morale of older women living alone in Appalachia (Doctoral dissertation, University of Alabama at Birmingham, 1992). *Dissertation Abstracts International, 51,* 1781-B.

Dobratz, M.C. (1991). Patterns of psychological adaptation in death and dying: A causal model and exploratory study (Doctoral dissertation, University of San Diego, 1990). *Dissertation Abstracts International, 51,* 3320-B.

Dobratz, M.C. (1993). Causal Influence of psychological adaptation on dying. *Western Journal of Nursing Research, 15,* 708-729.

Dow, K.H. (1993). An analysis of the experience of surviving and having children after breast cancer (Doctoral dissertation, Boston College, 1992). *Dissertation Abstracts International, 53,* 5641-B.

Dow, K.H., Harris, J.R., & Roy, C., (1994). Pregnancy after breast-conserving surgery and radiation therapy for breast cancer. *Journal of National Cancer Institute Monographs,* No. 16, 131-137.

Farkas, L. (1981). Adaptation problems with nursing home application for elderly persons: An application of the Roy adaptation nursing model. *Journal of Advanced Nursing, 6,* 363-368.

Florence, M.E., Lutzen, K., & Alexius, B. (1994). Adaptation of heterosexually infected HIV-positive women: A Swedish pilot study. *Health Care for Women International, 15,* 265-273.

Francisco, S.M. (1990). Roy's modes of adaptation and use of humor related to family functioning (Doctoral dissertation, University of Pittsburgh, 1989). *Dissertation Abstracts International, 50,* 2843-2844.

Frederickson, K., Jackson, B. S., Strauman, T., & Strauman, J. (1991). Testing hypotheses derived from the Roy Adaptation Model. *Nursing Science Quarterly, 4,* 168-174.

Gagliardi, B.A. (1991). The impact of Duchenne muscular dystrophy on families. *Orthopedic Nursing, 10*(5), 41-49.

Grey, M., Cameron, M. E., & Thurber, F. W. (1991). Coping and adaptation in children with diabetes. *Nursing Research, 40,* 144-149.

Jackson, B.S., Strauman, J., Frederickson, K., & Strauman, T. (1991). Long-term biopsychosocial effects in interleukin-2 therapy. *Oncology Nursing Forum, 18,* 683-690.

Kiikkala, I., & Peitsi, T. (1991). The care of children with minimal brain dysfunction: A Roy adaptation analysis. *Journal of Pediatric Nursing, 6,* 290-292.

Lutjens, L.R.J. (1991). Relationships between medical condition, nursing condition, nursing intensity, medical severity and length-of-stay in hospitalized medical-surgical adults using the theory of social organizations as adaptive systems (Doctoral dissertation, Wayne State University, 1990). *Dissertation Abstracts International, 52*, 1354-B.

Lutjens, L.R.J. (1991). Derivation and testing of tenets of a theory of social organizations as adaptive systems. *Nursing Science Quarterly, 5*, 62-71.

Lynam, L.E., & Miller, M. A. (1992). Mothers' and nurses' perception of the needs of the women experiencing preterm labor. *Journal of Obstetric, Gynecologic, & Neonatal Nursing, 21*, 126-136.

Munro, B.H., & Page, E.B. (1993). *Statistical methods for health care research.* (2nd ed.). Philadelphia: Lippincott.

O'Brien, C.S. (1992). A pilot study of perceived social adaptation of the elderly to the nursing home environment utilizing a mentorship program. (Master's thesis, D'Youville College, 1992). *Masters Abstracts International, 30*, 1297.

Phillips, J.A. (1991). Adaptation and injury status of industrial workers on a rotating shift pattern. (Doctoral dissertation, University of Alabama at Birmingham, 1991). *Dissertation Abstracts International, 52*, 2995-B.

Phillips, J.A., & Brown, K.C. (1992). Industrial workers on rotating shift pattern: Adaptation and injury status. *AAOHN Journal, 40*, 468-476.

Pittman, K.P. (1993). A Q-analysis of the enabling characteristics of chronically ill school-age children for the promotion of personal wellness (Doctoral dissertation, University of Alabama in Birmingham, 1992). *Dissertation Abstracts International, 53*, 4593-B.

Pollock, S.E. (1986). Human response to chronic illness: Physiologic and psychosocial adaptation. *Nursing Research, 35*, 90-95.

Pollock, S.E. (1989). Adaptive responses to diabetes mellitus. *Western Journal of Nursing Research, 11*, 265-280.

Rich, V.L. (1992). The use of personal, organizational, and coping resources in the prevention of staff nurse burnout: A test of a model (Doctoral dissertation, University of Pittsburg, 1991). *Dissertation Abstracts International, 52*, 3532-B.

Roy, C. (1977). Decision-making by the physically ill and adaptation during illness (Doctoral dissertation, University of California, Los Angeles, 1977). *Dissertation Abstracts International, 38*, 5060-A.

Roy, C. (1988). Human information processing. In J.J. Fitzpatrick, R.L. Tauton, & J. Q. Benoliel (Eds.) *Annual review of nursing research.* (Vol. 4, pp. 237-262). New York: Springer.

Roy, C., & Anway, J. (1989). Roy's Adaptation Model: Theories and propositions for administration. In B. Henry, C. Arndt, M. DiVincenti, & G. Marriner-Tomey (Eds.) *Dimensions and issues in nursing administration.* St. Louis: Mosby.

Roy, C., & Roberts, S. (1981). *Theory construction in nursing: An adaptation model.* Englewood Cliffs, NJ: Prentice-Hall.

Scherubel, J.C.M. (1986). Description of adaptation patterns following an acute cardiac event (Doctoral dissertation, University of Illinois at Chicago, Health Sciences Center, 1985). *Dissertation Abstracts International, 46,* 2627-B.

Selman, S.W. (1989). Impact of total hip replacement of quality of life. *Orthopedic Nursing, 8*(5), 43-49.

Shuler, P.J. (1990). Physical and psychosocial adaptation, social isolation, loneliness, and self concept of individuals with cancer (Doctoral dissertation, The Catholic University of America, 1990). *Dissertation Abstracts International, 51,* 2289-B.

Silva, M.C. (1986). Research testing nursing theory: State of the art. *Advances in Nursing Science, 9,* 1-11.

Silva, M.C., & Sorrell, J. M. (1992). Testing of nursing theory: Critique and philosophical expansion. *Advances in Nursing Science, 14,* 12-23.

Smith, C.E., Garvis, M.S., & Martinson, I. M. (1983). Content analysis of interviews using a nursing model: A look at parents adapting to the impact of childhood cancer. *Cancer Nursing, 6,* 269-275.

Strohmyer, L.L., Noroian, E. L., Patterson, L. M. & Carlin, B. P. (1993). Adaptation six months after multiple trauma: A pilot study. *Journal of Neuroscience Nursing, 25,* 30-37.

Trentini, M. (1996). Nurses' decisions in dialysis patient care: An application of the Roy Adaptation Model (Doctoral dissertation, The University of Alabama in Birmingham, 1995). *Dissertation Abstracts International, 47,* 575-B.

Thomas, S.P., Shoffner, D.H., & Groer, M.W. (1988). Adolescent stress factors: Implications for the nurse practitioner. *Nurse Practitioner, 13*(6), 20-29.

Varvaro, F.F. (1991). Women with coronary heart disease: An application of Roy's adaptation model. *Cardiovascular Nursing, 27* (6), 31-35

Wright, P.S. (1993). Parents' perceptions of their quality of life. *Journal of Pediatric Oncology Nursing, 10,* 139-145.

Zhan, L. (1994). Cognitive Adaptation Processing and Self Consistency in the Hearing Impaired Elderly (Doctoral dissertation, Boston College, 1993). *Dissertation Abstracts International, 54,* 4086-B.

Bibliography

Burns, N., & Grove, S.K. (1993). *The practice of nursing research* (2nd ed.) Philadelphia: Saunders.

Dow, K.H., Harris, J., & Roy, C. (1994). Pregnancy after breast conserving surgery and radiation therapy for breast cancer. *Journal of the National Cancer Institute, 16,* 131-137.

Fawcett, J., & Downs, F. (1992). *The relationship of theory and research* (2nd ed.). Philadelphia: F.A. Davis.

Lynn, M. (1986). Determination and quantification of content validity. *Nursing Research,. 35,* 382-385.

Roy, C. (1970). Adaptation: A conceptual framework for nursing. *Nursing Outlook, 18,* 42-45.

Roy, C. (1990). Response: Conceptual clarification. *Nursing Science Quarterly, 3,* 64-66.

Roy, C., & Andrews, H. (1991). *The Roy Adaptation Model* Norwalk, CT: Appleton & Lange.

Roy, C., & Andrews, H. (1999). T*he Roy Adaptation Model: The definitive statement* (2nd ed.). Stamford, CT: Appleton & Lange.

Roy, C., & Kazanowski, M. (in preparation). Cognitive adaptation processing scale: Conceptual development and psychometric testing.

Williamson, J., Karp, D., Dalphin, J., & Gray, P. (1982). *The research craft.* Boston: Scott, Foresman, and Company.

Woods, N.F., & Catanzaro, M. (1988). *Nursing research: Theory and practice.* St. Louis: Mosby.

Zhan, L., & Shen, C. (1994). The development of an instrument to measure self-consistency. *Journal of Advanced Nursing, 20,* 509-516.

Chapter 8

Studies Focusing on Stimuli

This chapter includes research reported between 1970 and 1994 that was focused primarily on stimuli as described in the Roy Adaptation Model (RAM). Nineteen studies based on the RAM were classified as focusing on stimuli and included 11 articles, 5 dissertations, and 3 theses. All studies by researchers investigating environmental stimuli who used either an experimental or quasi-experimental design are included in Chapter 9 except two (Cottrell & Shannahan, 1986; Cottrell & Shannahan, 1987). As part of a program of research on a given stimulus, these two studies are included in this chapter.

Purposes

The purposes in this chapter are to (a) critically analyze research focusing on stimuli, (b) evaluate the relationship to the RAM of research focusing on stimuli, and (c) synthesize contributions of the reported studies to nursing science. Contributions to nursing science include applications for nursing practice, recommendations for model-based adaptation research, directions for further theory and RAM development of the concept of stimuli.

Background

Stimuli are inputs that evoke a response. Roy notes that people and groups are adaptive systems affected by their internal and external environment. According to the RAM, elements of the environment at the individual level are considered stimuli. The three classes of stimuli are focal, contextual, and residual (Roy & Andrews, 1991). Helson (1964) first named and described these classes of stimuli in psycho-physical research. The focal stimulus is the one most immediately confronting the person or receiving the person's primary attention. The focal stimulus calls for an adaptive response. Many stimuli may never become focal unless they become more intense such as minor pain, or unless the situation changes as with a sudden lack of interesting stimuli, leading the person to become aware of the pain. Contextual stimuli include all internal and external inputs that surround and influence the focal stimulus, but are not the center of attention. Since they are present in the same situation as the focal stimulus, contextual stimuli contribute to the behavior initiated by the focal stimulus. Background music may be comforting but unnoticed unless a lull in the immediate activity takes place. Finally, residual stimuli are background factors that affect the situation but cannot be validated or measured directly at the time. They often include underlying beliefs, attitudes, traits, and cultural factors.

Stimuli are closely related to the adaptation process itself and to the modes, with behavior in one mode sometimes acting as a stimulus to another mode. Review of research based on the RAM identified 19 studies that specifically focused on given stimuli such as technologic environments, specialized treatment procedures, or health status.

Critical Analysis of Research Focusing on Stimuli

Critical analysis includes a brief description of the reported research followed by critical analyses of the studies using guidelines previously established for all content areas (see Chapter 2 for description). Criteria were modified for quantitative and qualitative studies.

Description of Reported Research

Studies focusing on stimuli derived from the model were examined for common themes. Three main categories of stimuli were environment ($n=4$), health status ($n=10$), and treatment ($n=5$). Health status was further subdivided into (a) pregnancy and childbirth, (b) stress and health, and (c) illness.

Environment. In 4 of the 19 studies categorized as stimuli related to environment, researchers focused on a particular setting or situation as the stimulus (Table 8.1).

Armer (1988/1989) examined adjustment to congregate living of 50 rural community-based elderly. The investigator used the RAM as the theoretic rationale for predicting the relationships among the variables. Using a cross-sectional, descriptive correlational design, Armer examined a number of stimuli. The focal stimulus was identified as relocation. Contextual stimuli were perception of relocation choice, predictability in post-location environment, perceived social support, perception of choice in the post-location environment, appraisal of the move as a challenge as compared to a threat, variability in the environment, use and helpfulness of coping strategies, and self-rated health. The dependent variable was post-relocation adjustment. Findings included a number of stimuli significantly and positively related to relocation adjustment. These were perception of choice in relocation, perception of choice and predictability in the post-location environment, appraisal of the relocation event as a challenge, and perception of social support from family and neighbors. The regression of independent variables on the dependent variable of relocation adjustment revealed that 51% of the variation was accounted for by perception of choice to relocate, predictability, perception of social support, cognitive appraisal, and coping strategies. Cognitive appraisal of viewing the move as a challenge accounted for the largest amount of variation. Using the same regression on the variable of relocation adjustment, the appraisal of threat contributed the most to the equation.

In an exploratory study of adaptation of medical-surgical patients to technologic stimuli, the focal stimulus was identified as attachment to invasive (intravenous) or noninvasive (telemetry) bedside technology, and manual (IV gravity system or continuous attachment to telemetry) versus automated (IV pumps or intermittent attachment to telemetry units) devices (Campbell-Heider, 1988). Results of a structured interview supported the hypothesis that patients attached to invasive devices are more likely to report the occurrence of technologic stimuli and adaptive responses than are those patients attached to noninvasive instruments. Also, patients with manual technologies were more likely to report the presence of the stimuli and responses. Anxiety was reported by only 16% of the sample, less than anticipated. Other study variables such as the number of other attachments or the number of days attached were not significantly related to adaptation.

Using the theoretic framework, instrumentation, sample, procedure, and data from the previous study, Campbell-Heider (1993) published additional analyses. Results indicated that patients connected to invasive attachments most frequently reported their awareness of limitations on their mobility, threats to their self-esteem, increased dependence, and increased surveillance of machines. Patients attached to only one invasive device for less than 3 days reported more stimuli and more need for behavioral responses.

In a qualitative study, Munn and Tichy (1987) interviewed 10 staff nurses with more than a year of full-time experience in a pediatric intensive care unit (PICU). Using a semistructured interview guide, nurses were asked to identify factors they perceived as stressful to school-aged children and adolescents in the PICU. Identified from the literature and the findings were four major categories: environmental, physical, psychological, and social. The most common themes related to equipment and procedures, (invasive and noninvasive), and to separations from family.

Health status. In the category of health status, the researchers focused on stimuli related to specific health or illness conditions. The 10 studies in this category were further subdivided into pregnancy and childbirth ($n=5$), stress and health ($n=2$), and illness ($n=3$) (Table 8.2). In five studies a variety of components were examined in the category of pregnancy and childbirth. In three studies, use of birth chairs were compared to traditional delivery tables. In one study, attitudes and perceptions of nurses and clients experiencing abortion were compared, and in the fifth study, factors that influence the use of contraception were examined.

Table 8.1 – Description of Studies that Were Focused on Stimuli: Environment (*N*=4)

Author(s) & Date	Purpose	Sample	Design	Findings
1. Armer (1988/1989)	To examine factors that affect adjustment of elderly to congregate living	Rural community elderly (*N*=50)	Correlational	Perception of choice in relocation, perception of choice and predictability in the post-location environment, appraisal of the relocation event as a challenge, and perception of social support from family and neighbors were significantly related to relocation adjustment. The strongest contributor to relocation adjustment was appraisal of the event.
2. Campbell-Heider (1988)	To explore adaptation of patients to invasive versus non-invasive technological stimuli	General adult medical-surgical patients (*N*=75)	Correlational	Patients attached to invasive devices (IVs) were more likely to report technologic stimuli and adaptive responses than those attached to non-invasive equipment (telemetry). Patients connected to manually controlled equipment were more likely to report their presence than those connected to automated equipment.

Study	Purpose	Sample	Design	Findings
3. Campbell-Heider (1993)	To explore behavioral adaptation to invasive versus noninvasive technological stimuli	General adult medical-surgical patients (N=75)	Correlational	Patients connected to invasive (IVs) attachments reported more awareness of limitations on mobility, threats to self-esteem, more dependence, and an increase in surveillance of the machines than those connected to noninvasive equipment (telemetry).
4. Munn & Tichy (1987)	To identify staff nurses' perceptions of stressors for children in a PICU	Staff nurses with 1 year PICU experience (N=10)	Qualitative	The most frequently mentioned stressor was equipment, including cardiac monitors, ventilators, and intravenous pumps. Equipment and invasive and noninvasive procedures were stressors in all modes; children "monitor their monitors." Only a separation from family was identified to be as stressful as equipment and procedures.

(continued)

Table 8.2 – Description of Studies that Were Focused on Stimuli: Health Status (N=10)

Author(s) & Date	Purpose	Sample	Design	Findings
		Pregnancy and Childbirth		
5. Blain (1993)	To compare the attitude of staff nurses toward abortion with those of women who had undergone an abortion and to describe the women's perception of nursing care	Staff nurses (n=11) and women after an abortion (n=41); N =52	Correlational	No relationship was found between nurses' attitudes toward abortion and the women's attitude toward abortion or the relationship between the nurses' attitude toward abortion and the women's perception of nursing care that they received.
6. Shannahan & Cottrell (1985)	To compare the effect of the birth chair on length of second stage of labor, fetal outcome, and maternal blood loss	Term birth mothers (N=60)	Correlational	Second stage labor using the birth chair was not significantly different than using the traditional delivery table. There was a trend toward a more lengthy labor with the birth chair. In addition, use of the birth chair resulted in longer time pushing in both the labor and delivery rooms, and there was significantly more blood loss with the birth chair than with the traditional delivery table.

7. Cottrell & Shannahan (1986)	To compare the effects of the birth chair with the delivery table in relation to fetal outcome, the duration of second stage labor, perineal swelling, maternal blood loss, and frequency of lacerations and episiotomies	Term birth mothers using birth chair (*n*=33) using delivery table (*n*=22); *N*=55	Quasi-experimental	There was a difference only in greater perineal swelling for those women using the birth chair as compared to those using the traditional delivery table and no significant difference between the two groups in maternal blood loss.
8. Cottrell & Shannahan (1987)	To compare the effect of the birth chair on fetal outcome when compared to delivery table	Term birth mothers using birth chair (*n*=33) using delivery table (*n*=22); *N*=55	Quasi-experimental	When the birth chair or delivery table was elevated to 30° the neonate's Apgar score in the first minute was significantly higher than when the chair or table were not elevated. Also, umbilical cord oxygen saturation was significantly higher and carbon dioxide saturation was significantly lower when the birth chair was at a 45° angle.
9. Kromer (1993/ 1994)	To determine factors affecting postpartum adolescents' use of contraceptives	Postpartum adolescent mothers (*N*=30)	Descriptive	Postpartum adolescents with high peer pressure and a higher level of knowledge about birth control were more likely to report use of contraceptives. The relationship between perception of barriers to obtaining contraceptives and their use was not significant.

(continued)

Table 8.2 *(continued)*

Author(s) & Date	Purpose	Sample	Design	Findings
		Stress and Health		
10. Pollock (1981/ 1982)	To categorize the primary stress factors that affect health status and to operationalize concepts of the RAM	Experts in RAM (*N*=3)	Qualitative- theory development	Forty stressors were catego- rized according to the RAM modes; stress measurements were identified to measure each of the three classes of stimuli. Two modifications of the RAM were suggested to expand the model for measurement: include dimension of effectiveness in the definition of level of adaptation; and create three modes: physiologic, psychologic, and sociologic integrity.
11. Preston & Dellasega (1990)	To assess the relationships among health status, stress, marital status and gender among the elderly	Non-institutionalized elderly over 65 (*N*=900)	Correlational	Among the elderly, the health status of older married men was unrelated to level of reported stress. Older married women experienced the poorest level of health and the highest levels of reported stress.

12. Bean (1987/1988)	To compare the needs of patients newly diagnosed with cancer with those of patients with recurrent cancer	Newly diagnosed cancer patients (n=15), diagnosed with recurrent cancer (n=15); N=30	Descriptive	Patients newly diagnosed with cancer reported more needs in the self-concept mode, and those with recurrent cancer reported more needs related to the interdependence mode. Those with recurrent disease reported more needs overall and in every mode than those with newly diagnosed disease.
13. DeRuvo (1992/1993)	To compare the needs of patients with head and neck cancer to those with cancer of the digestive system undergoing radiation and to compare the categories of needs of both according to the RAM and nursing diagnosis system	Patients with cancer of the head and neck (n=15) and patients with cancer of the digestive system (n=15); N=30	Descriptive	Patients with head and neck cancer experienced more needs than patients with cancer of the digestive system. Results also indicated that there was a core of needs common to selected cancer patients undergoing external beam radiation therapy.
14. Leech (1982)	To determine the psychosocial and physiologic needs of patients with arterial occlusive disease (AOD) before reconstructive surgery	Patients with AOD before surgery (N=60)	Correlational	Patients reported physiologic needs based on lack of knowledge associating smoking with AOD (85% were currently smoking) and the benefits of dietary management and regular foot care. Psychosocial needs were related to the effects of the disease on patients' self-concept and role function (83%). Generally, patients felt they were not in control during their hospitalization (96%). Patients identified specific needs for information and for support.

Blain (1993) compared attitudes and perceptions of 11 staff nurses in the United Kingdom toward abortion, to attitudes toward abortion and expectations regarding nursing care of 41 clients who had undergone abortion or termination of pregnancy. No significant correlations were identified between the attitudes toward abortion and perceptions of the nurses regarding nursing care and the attitudes and perceptions of the clients.

A series of studies were focused on the effects of a birth chair on labor and fetal outcome (Shannahan & Cottrell, 1985; Cottrell & Shannahan, 1986; Cottrell & Shannahan, 1987). Using the RAM as the conceptual framework, researchers identified the birth chair as a contextual stimulus and labor as the focal stimulus. In the first study (Shannahan & Cottrell, 1985), a retrospective chart audit of 60 births was used to compare the effect of the birth chair on the length of second-stage labor, fetal outcome, and maternal blood loss. Results were contrary to prediction. The authors found that second-stage labor using the birth chair was not significantly different. However a trend toward longer labor was noted. In addition, those patients using the birth chair had longer times pushing in the labor and delivery rooms, and had significantly more blood loss than those using the traditional delivery table.

Based on the investigators' results of the first study, they undertook a second, prospective, quasi-experimental study (Cottrell & Shannahan, 1986) to compare the effects of the birth chair with the delivery table relative to fetal outcome, the duration of second-stage labor, perineal swelling, maternal blood loss, and frequency of lacerations and episiotomies. The sample included 33 women using the birth chair and 22 using the delivery table. Although the sample size was small, results indicated differences only in greater perineal swelling using the birth chair and, unlike the previous study, no significant difference was noted in maternal blood loss.

The purpose of the third study (Cottrell & Shannahan, 1987), was to determine the effect of the birth chair on fetal outcome compared to the effect of the traditional delivery table. Using the same sample of 55 women, the findings indicated that when either the birth chair or delivery table was elevated to a 30 degree angle, the Apgar score in the first minute was significantly higher. Additionally, when the birth chair was at a 45° angle, umbilical cord oxygen saturation was significantly higher, and carbon dioxide saturation was significantly lower.

Kromer (1993/1994) examined factors affecting postpartum contraceptive use among 30 adolescent mothers in a descriptive, comparative study. Peer pressure and peer norms were identified as focal stimuli, and barriers to obtaining contraceptives and knowledge about birth control were the contextual stimuli. Findings indicated that postpartum adolescents with high peer pressure and a higher level of knowledge about birth control were more likely to report the use of contraceptives. The relationship between perception of barriers to obtaining contraceptives and the use of contraceptives was not significant.

In the next subcategory, two studies were focused on the relationship between stress and health. In a qualitative, theory development study, Pollock (1982) expanded the concepts within the RAM by categorizing primary stress factors that affect health status. The researcher identified valid and reliable instruments to measure any part of the stress concept and evaluated the relationship among the three stimuli—focal, contextual, and residual. She developed the theoretic and operational definitions for each stimulus and identified interactions among the stimuli. Links with the RAM were, in part, put into operation through development of the Nursing Health Assessment that provided parameters for using the model.

Preston and Dellasega (1990) interviewed 900 noninstitutionalized elderly persons over age 65 to assess relationships among health status and stress, marital status, and gender. Findings indicated that of the four possible variables, health status of elderly married men was unrelated to stress and that married women experienced the poorest level of health and the highest stress levels.

In the subcategory of illness, studies were focused on specific illnesses that served as the stimulus for needs or adaptation or both. Bean (1987/1988) compared the needs of newly diagnosed adult cancer patients ($n= 30$) undergoing chemotherapy with those of adult recurrent-cancer patients undergoing chemotherapy. The focal stimulus was identified as the cancer experience; contextual stimuli were reported as primarily nausea and vomiting, loss of appetite, and fatigue; and residual stimuli were religiosity and transcendence, past experience with others with cancer, inactivity, and wasting time. The findings indicated that patients newly diagnosed with cancer reported more needs in the self-concept mode, particularly related to hope. Patients with recurrent cancer identified more needs related to the interdependence mode. Overall, those with recurrent disease reported more needs (134) in general, as well as in every mode, than those who were newly diagnosed (60). In addition, a significant relationship existed between an increasing number of interdependence needs and the increasing number of disease recurrences.

DeRuvo (1992/1993) studied nursing diagnoses and needs of cancer patients. She identified the focal stimulus as the administration of external beam radiation therapy. She compared the needs of those with cancers of the head and neck to those with cancers of the digestive system. The needs of 30 adult cancer patients were classified according to the RAM adaptive modes, nursing diagnoses, and associated defining characteristics. Major findings indicated that patients with cancers of the head and neck had 30 nursing diagnoses and those with cancers of the digestive system experienced 25 nursing diagnoses. Patient needs were evident in three modes: physiologic, self-concept, and role function, with the frequency of needs in the same order. No needs were reported in the interdependence mode, and discussion followed regarding concern over interrater reliability and specificity of the model. In addition, reported adaptive needs were compared to Gordon's functional health patterns. The results indicated that, regardless of conceptual framework, a core of common nursing diagnoses was common to cancer patients receiving external beam radiation. These common diagnoses were altered nutrition and self- concept, and high risk for infection, although they varied in priority depending on the location of the cancer.

Leech (1982) explored the psychosocial and physiologic needs of patients with arterial occlusive disease (AOD) preceding reconstructive surgery. Data were obtained from 60 patients, 1 to 2 days prior to surgery, using a 48-item interview schedule, body cathexis questionnaire, and chart review. Findings related to the physiologic mode indicated that 74% smoked. More than 80% did not relate perceived benefits of dietary management or of regular foot care to their health status. The primary hospital discomfort was from the aortographic procedures. Related to the self-concept and role function modes, 83% were unhappy with the progression of the disease and felt frustration, depression, and feelings of uselessness. Only 4% felt they were in control; however, a sense of control was important to these subjects. Although subjects wanted to make decisions about their health, few understood the relationship between preventive behaviors and the pathophysiologic processes of the disease. Negatively perceived changes in self-concept and role relationships were associated with negative body cathexis, low levels of adaptation to the disease, and perception of illness as severe disease.

Therapies. The final category of studies were focused on therapies (N=5). Researchers examined stimuli specific to medical therapies or surgical treatments such as chemotherapy, parenteral therapy, or surgery (Table 8.3).

Cornell (1990) investigated patterns of anxiety in a longitudinal panel study among 30 adult clients receiving 3 weeks of home parenteral antibiotic therapy. The focal stimulus was home parenteral antibiotic therapy, and the contextual stimuli were gender, marital status, socioeconomic status, education, and opportunity for hands-on experience with the equipment prior to discharge. Findings indicated that anxiety levels decreased over time but were greatest between weeks two and three. Significant levels of anxiety were experienced by females, married subjects, white collar workers, less educated adults, and those who did not have the opportunity for hands-on experience with the equipment prior to discharge.

Dahlen (1980) examined the adaptive responses to visual prostheses of 99 elderly patients who had undergone cataract surgery. Using eight pretested, researcher-designed instruments and the Attitude to Blindness Scale, clients were evaluated prior to cataract surgery, 1 month after surgery, and 6 to 8 weeks following fitting for visual prosthesis. Findings revealed significant relationships between adaptation to the visual prosthesis and the following predictor variables—level of education, knowledge score, attitude toward blindness, attitude toward cataract/cataract surgery, presence of other eye pathology, presence of other physical handicap, physicians' health rating, preoperative central visual acuity in the operated eye, and self-assessment of reading change.

Data from chart reviews, telephone interviews, and hospital and home care bills were used by Hazlett (1989) to assess a program of home ventilator management for 15 children with chronic respiratory insufficiency. Data were collected following intensive discharge preparation of the family which averaged 2.9 months, and subsequent discharge. The results indicated a substantial reduction (78%) in overall cost of care—the decrease often diminished by insurance companies limiting reimbursement of home care costs. Members of five families, particularly mothers, reported a reduction in stress with the child at home; while three families were overwhelmed by the home care needs of the child, five families reported they were burdened because of the lack of help from family members and other resources, and two families felt trapped since they viewed home care as the only alternative to prolonged hospitalization.

Leuze and McKenzie (1987) conducted a pilot study to evaluate nurses' knowledge of patient's physiologic and psychosocial needs (n=20 patients). Preoperative nurses knew more about their patients when the preoperative assessment was based on the RAM than nurses whose patients were assessed using the traditional form.

Takahashi and Bever (1989) compared 48 preoperative assessments of ambulatory care patients by 24 nurses to observations of preoperative nurse assessments, chart audits, and self-reported questionnaires. Preoperative assessment was identified as the focal stimulus. Findings indicated nurses reported performing more preoperative nursing assessment activities than the number of preoperative nursing assessment activities observed by investigators. Viewed as a contextual stimulus, education was the only factor accounting for differences in the quality and quantity of assessment. Baccalaureate prepared nurses performed significantly better on two patient teaching items than did diploma graduates. Of the nine nursing assessment activities most consistently observed, the majority were related to medical-legal requirements such as documentation, while none were in the psychological category.

Critical Analyses of Reported Research

Each of the 19 studies focusing on stimuli was critically analyzed with respect to the quality of the research. Seventeen of the 19 studies were quantitative, and two were qualitative.

Table 8.3 – Description of Studies that Focused on Stimuli: Therapies (N=5)

Author(s) & Date	Purpose	Sample	Design	Findings
15. Cornell (1990)	To determine patterns of anxiety among patients receiving three weeks of home parenteral antibiotic therapy	Adult patients (N=30)	Correlational	Anxiety levels significantly decreased over time but most significantly between 2nd and 3rd weeks. Significant levels of anxiety were experienced by female, married, white collar workers, and those who did not have an opportunity for hands-on experience with the equipment before discharge.
16. Dahlen (1980)	To examine adaptive responses to visual prosthesis of patients who had undergone cataract surgery	Elderly patients who had undergone cataract surgery of one eye (N=99)	Descriptive	There was a significant relationship between the following predictor variables and adaptation to visual prosthesis: level of education, knowledge about vision and surgery, attitude toward blindness, attitude toward cataract/cataract surgery, presence of pathology in the other eye, presence of other physical handicap, physician's health rating, preoperative central visual acuity in the operated eye, and self assessment of reading change.

Study	Purpose	Sample	Design	Findings
17. Hazlett (1989)	To determine financial and psychosocial adaptation of families to a child on home ventilator management	Families of children with chronic respiratory insufficiency on home ventilator management (N=15)	Descriptive	There was a substantial reduction in overall costs of care. One-third of the families reported a reduction in stress with the child at home. However, three families were overwhelmed by the needs of the child, five felt burdened because of the lack of help from other family members and other resources, and two viewed home care as the only alternative but felt trapped by the level and degree of care required.
18. Leuze & McKenzie (1987)	To evaluate differences between circulating nurses' knowledge of patients when the preoperative assessment was based on the RAM compared to the control preoperative assessment	Nurses of patients undergoing elective surgery: control (n=10), experimental (n=10)	Quasi-experimental	Circulating nurses' knowledge of the patients whose preoperative assessment was based on the RAM was significantly higher than nurses' knowledge of patients whose preoperative assessment utilized the traditional assessment method.
19. Takahashi & Bever (1989)	To compare nurses' perceptions of their preoperative assessments to observed assessments	Perioperative nurses in an ambulatory care setting (n=24), preoperative patients (n=48)	Descriptive	Nurses reported performing more preoperative assessments than were observed or located through chart audit. Education was the only factor accounting for differences in level of assessment.

Critical Analysis of Quantitative Research

Critical analyses of the 17 quantitative studies are shown in Table 8.4. In over 80% of the studies, measures were taken to control for the threats to internal and external validity. More than 90% of the researchers analyzed the data appropriately and addressed the reliability and validity of the instruments. Consistency of findings with conclusions was found in all studies.

In 16 of the studies investigators attempted to control for threats to internal validity. History and maturation represented threats to internal validity, particularly when dealing with the elderly. In three studies (Armer, 1988/1989, Dahlen, 1980, Preston & Dellasega, 1990), the age ranges of the sample were wide. However, this problem was addressed through statistical methods such as analysis of covariance or multiple regression. Cornell (1990) collected minimal data regarding history or maturation during the 2-week period of data collection, which might also account for the changes in the dependent variable of anxiety. Preston and Dellasega (1990) did not describe data on their elderly subjects that might have contributed to the findings.

Leech (1982) addressed potential problems with instrumentation and selection by personally visiting surgical ward patients who were 1 to 2 days preoperative. Armer (1988/1989) also collected all data herself; however, her instrument required recalling of previous relocations by elderly subjects between the ages of 61-98. She used regression analysis to control for age, gender, and length of residency in the congregate dwelling, but was unable to tape record the responses of all subjects. Blain (1993) had respondents return questionnaires by mail and stated that most responses were obtained this way but gave no indication of how many nor how the others were returned. On the other hand, Campbell-Heider (1988; 1993) carefully controlled for threats to instrumentation by training research assistants to collect data, conducting a pilot study, and developing a standardized protocol for data collection.

In a study of the elderly and adaptation to cataract surgery, Dahlen (1980) partially controlled for history and maturation through the use of pre- and post-tests over time. She administered a total of nine instruments and used appropriate statistical techniques to determine the effect of other variables.

Blain (1993) acknowledged problems with mortality by indicating that less than 16% of clients attended their scheduled follow-up clinic appointment. Hazlett (1989) was unable to control for mortality of children with chronic respiratory insufficiency on a home ventilator management program. Five of the 15 subjects in her study withdrew because of readmission, termination of the program, or death.

Table 8.4 – Critical Analysis of Quantitative Stimuli Research (N=17)

Criteria	Evaluation		
	Yes	*Partially*	*No*
Design			
Threats to internal validity controlled	1,2,3,6,12,13, 14,15,16 17,18,19	5,7,8,11	9
Threats to external validity controlled	1,2,3,6,11,12, 13,14,15,16,17	8,18,19	5,7,9
Measurement			
Reliability of instruments addressed	1,2,3,6,11,12, 13,15,16,17	7,8,9,14, 18,19	5
Validity of instruments addressed	1,2,3,6,7,8,9, 11,12,13,14,15, 16,17,18,19		5
Data Analysis			
Appropriate	1,2,3,6,7,8,9, 11,12,13,14,15, 16,17,18,19		5
Interpretation of Results			
Consistency of findings with conclusions	1,2,3,5,6,7,8,9, 11,12,13,14,15, 16,17,18,19		

Key: 1=Armer, 1988/1989; 2=Campbell-Heider,1988; 3=Campbell-Heider,1993; 5=Blain, 1993; 6=Shannahan & Cottrell,1985; 7=Cottrell & Shannahan,1986; 8=Cottrell & Shannahan,1987; 9=Kromer,1993/1994; 11=Preston & Dellasega, 1990; 12=Bean,1988; 13=DeRuvo,1992/1993; 14=Leech,1982; 15=Cornell,1990; 16=Dahlen,1980; 17=Hazlett,1989; 18=Leuze & McKenzie,1987; 19=Takahashi & Bever,1989.

Armer (1988/1989) addressed issues of selection through identification of extensive inclusion criteria for subjects. Although 75% were female, the gender proportion was representative of the population. Blain (1993) provided little descriptive data on the 11 nurses and their care for patients undergoing abortion, although data were collected on age, sex, religious beliefs, and professional experience. Likewise, no data were reported on the demographics of the patients. The report, however, did indicate the demographics were representative of patients attending the clinic but made no mention of the criteria or characteristics.

In a convenience sample of postpartum adolescents, Kromer (1994) was unable to successfully control for threats to either internal or external validity. She failed to request any information about demographics or evidence that participants could read and write. This was particularly disappointing since the conceptual and empiric findings could have provided unique contributions to testing of RAM propositions.

In 14 studies, evidence indicated attempts to control for external validity. Cornell (1990) attempted to control environment during the second and third phases of data collection through telephone reminders to return their questionnaires. In a program of research, Cottrell and Shannahan (1985; 1986; 1987) improved each subsequent design. For example, in the first study, external validity was in question since no controls or recordings of the angles of either the birth chair or the delivery table were found, although the hypotheses were based in part on the effects of gravity on second stage and outcome of labor. However, in the third study, angles were controlled and/or verified using a protractor. Takahashi and Bever (1989) examined the preoperative assessments completed by 24 nurses at two sites which posed a threat to environment control. The sample size was large, and the variability of nurses was also high. The use of an additional site further jeopardized the findings.

Campbell-Heider (1988; 1993) addressed the representativeness of the sample through attempts to equalize the numbers of subjects in each of four types of technology attachments. Preston and Dellasega (1990) controlled for the representativeness of their sample through a combination of stratification, quota, cluster, and probability sampling to select sites and telephone numbers, as well as through random digit dialing. Their 24% refusal rate represented a combination of subject refusals and family-member refusals on behalf of the subject. Armer (1989) pilot-tested the order of instruments to reduce the effects of fatigue.

Participants in the study by Leuze and McKenzie (1987) were made aware of their placement in either the experimental or control group when they found a special questionnaire on the chart or an evaluation checklist after the patient's surgery. This procedure increased the risk of the Hawthorne effect as a contributor to the significance of their findings.

Most authors addressed instrument reliability and validity and included enough information to determine the appropriateness of the measures. Blain (1993) reported no data on instrument reliability or validity, although a tool was adapted for the study. Preston and Dellasega (1990) included minimal reliability information and subsequently combined the concepts of self-concept and interdependence, further reducing validity. However, DeRuvo (1992/1993) used a panel of three nurse experts on the RAM, nursing diagnosis, and oncology nursing. The experts classified symptoms according to the general category of modes and demographics as contextual stimuli. A second panel with similar qualifications classified and validated each of the symptoms to a specific mode. This panel encountered some difficulty and, following discussion, attained 100% agreement on 68% of the items.

Bean (1987/1988) had five experts on the RAM review the semi-structured questionnaire for content validity and three additional nurse experts on the model evaluate categorization of responses according to needs. They established content analysis and reported interrater reliability of 83%. The experts reported a repetition of needs between the self-concept and interdependence modes. Campbell-Heider (1988; 1993) reported using "the gold standard" for content validity and included a review and validation of the structured interview schedule by the author of the model.

All but one author appropriately analyzed data. Blain (1993) reported the use of a Pearson's correlation on a 12-item attitude questionnaire. Most statisticians are forgiving of treating ordinal data as interval/ratio when there are more than 25-30 items on the scale. A Kendall's Tau statistic would have been more appropriate.

All studies drew conclusions consistent with the statistical analyses and findings. For example, based on the research, Dahlen (1980) recommended preoperative teaching for the elderly that will contribute to adaptation following cataract surgery in this population.

Critical analyses of qualitative research. Critical analyses of the two qualitative studies are presented in Table 8.5.

Investigators for the two qualitative studies used strategies to ensure validity: descriptive vividness, methodologic congruence, analytical preciseness, theoretic connectedness, and heuristic relevance. Pollock (1981/ 1982) used strategies such as extensive descriptions of the literature review; descriptions of the connections between the conceptual, theoretic, and empiric measures of the major RAM concepts and stress; and consultation with the model author. Munn and Tichy (1987) addressed threats to validity through describing contextual conditions, criteria for participant selection, and procedural stages for data collection. In addition, they used a semi-structured interview guide. One researcher collected all data to further enhance reliability. The two qualitative studies used appropriate methods of data analysis such as content analysis. Both studies demonstrated consistency of data with the findings and conclusions. Pollock (1982) provided operational definitions for the three categories of stimuli and correlated the definitions with specific instruments measuring stress.

Table 8.5 – Critical Analysis of Qualitative Stimuli Research (N=2)

Criteria	Evaluation		
	Yes	Partially	No
Design			
Strategies to ensure validity used	4, 10		
Strategies to ensure reliability used	4,10		
Data analysis			
Appropriate method	4,10		
Interpretation of results			
Consistency of data with findings and conclusions	4,10		

Key: 4=Munn & Tichy,1987; 10=Pollock,1981/1982

Evaluation of Relationships to the RAM

Sixteen studies focusing on stimuli were evaluated for linkages to the RAM. Based on adequacy in meeting the criteria for critical analysis of the research and the evaluation of linkages to the RAM, the studies were used to test propositions from the RAM.

Evaluation of Linkages to the RAM

Evaluation of the linkages between elements of the 16 studies focusing on stimuli and the Roy Model is summarized in Table 8.6. Most authors explicitly identified the model and linked research variables, empiric measures, and findings to the model.

Bean (1987/1988) used the model to conceptualize the study and discussed the cancer experience as the focal stimulus. Contextual stimuli were the related symptoms such as nausea. Reported needs were identified as adaptation and assigned to the appropriate modes. Empiric measures were derived from the model. Findings were related to the model and confirmed that invasive technologic stimuli required more adaptive responses than did noninvasive technology.

The weakest area relating research to the model was in the discussion of the findings. Ten studies were explicit, four implied, and two made no linkages.

Table 8.6 – Evaluation of Linkages to the RAM (N=16)

Linkages to RAM	Evaluation		
	Explicit	*Implicit*	*Absent*
Research variables	1,2,3,4,6,8, 10,12,13,14, 15,16,17,18	11,19	
Empirical measures	2,3,4,6,8, 10,12,13,14, 17,18,19	1,11,15,16	
Findings	2,3,4,10,11, 12,13,15, 17,18	1,14,16,19	6,8

Key: 1=Armer, 1988/1989; 2=Campbell-Heider,1988; 3=Campbell-Heider,1993; 4=Munn & Tichy,1987; 6=Shannahan & Cottrell,1985; 8=Cottrell & Shannahan,1987; 10=Pollock,1981/1982; 11=Preston & Dellasega, 1990; 12=Bean,1988; 13=DeRuvo,1993; 14=Leech,1982; 15=Cornell,1990; 16=Dahlen,1980; 17=Hazlett,1989; 18=Leuze & McKenzie,1987; 19=Takahashi & Bever,1989

Testing of Propositions from the RAM

Criteria were developed to determine if the results of research using the RAM supported the propositions derived from the model. Findings from five studies relating to stimuli were used to test the RAM propositions listed in Chapter 2. Nine propositions were represented in this research, as noted in Table 8.7.

Nine propositions from the RAM were supported or not supported by studies focused on stimuli. One study supported the first proposition that the regulator and cognator processes affect innate and acquired ways of adaptating at the individual level. Takahashi and Bever (1989) found education the only factor accounting for differences in the agreement between actual nursing assessment activities and validation of those activities by observation or chart audit. Baccalaureate prepared nurses performed significantly better on teaching patients than did diploma graduates. Thus, level of education attained affects cognator activity.

The third proposition states that characteristics of the internal and external stimuli influence adaptive responses. Findings from five studies supported this proposition. Pollock (1981/1982) distinguished between the degree of intensity for each category of stimuli (focal, contextual, and residual) and proposed the intensity of adaptive responses from high to low.

Table 8.7 Testing of Propositions from the RAM (N=15)

Propositions from the RAM	Ancillary and practice propositions	Supported by results	Not supported by results
1. At the individual level, regulator and cognator processes affect innate and acquired ways of adapting.	The educational level of nurses affects nursing assessments and actions.	Pollock (1981/1982)	Takahashi & Bever (1989)
3. The characteristics of the internal and external stimuli influence adaptive responses.	a. Some external stimuli place greater demands on the adaptive system.		
	(1) Invasive therapies place more demands upon the adaptive system than do noninvasive therapies.	Campbell-Heider (1988;1993); Munn & Tichy (1987)	
	(2) A child at home on a ventilator places greater demands on the family than when the child is in the hospital.	Hazlett (1989)	
	(3) The reoccurrence of cancer places greater demands upon the adaptive system than does newly diagnosed cancer.	Bean (1987/1988)	
	b. Adaptation level is affected by the magnitude of exposure to focal stimuli.	Pollock (1981/1982)	
	(1) Adaptation in more than one mode is affected by the magnitude of the focal stimuli.	Campbell-Heider (1988;1993); Munn & Tichy (1987); Hazlett (1989)	

(continued)

4. The characteristics of the internal and external stimuli influences the adequacy of cognitive and emotional processes.	Parents' adaptation to their child on ventilators at home are determined by the number and use of resources.	Hazlett (1989)
6. Adaptation in one mode is affected by adaptation in other modes through cognator and regulator connectives.	a. Visual adaptation is enhanced by knowledge, visual status, attitudes, and educational level.	Dahlen (1980)
	b. Happiness and physical health affect each other and are modified by gender and marital status.	Preston & Dellasega (1987)
7. The pooled effect of focal, contextual, and residual stimuli determines the adaptation level.	a. Good previous experience and personal resources facilitate adjustment to relocation.	Armer (1988/1989)
	b. Recurrence and site of cancer alters priority of needs in the modes.	Bean (1987/1988) DeRuvo (1992/1993)
	c. Age affects perceptions of health needs and gender affects self-concept and physiologic needs in pre-operative vascular patients.	Leech (1982)
8. Adaptation is influenced by the integration of the person with the environment.	a. Use of the birth chair modifies outcomes of labor and delivery.	Cottrell & Shannahan (1986;1987)
	b. Relocation adaptation is influenced by sense of prediction and control.	Armer (1988/1989)

Table 8.7 (continued)

Propositions from the RAM	Ancillary and practice propositions	Supported by results	Not supported by results
	c. Parents adapt better if they utilize contextual resources such as family members.	Hazlett (1989)	
	d. Adaptation to eye surgery is influenced by actual and perceived vision.	Dahlen (1980)	
9. The variable of time influences the process of adaptation.	a. Focal stimuli become contextual stimuli over time as an indicator of effective adaptation.		
	(1) Patients with invasive and noninvasive therapies become less vigilant over time.	Campbell-Heider (1988;1993)	
	(2) Anxiety decreases with home IV therapy over time.	Cornell (1990)	
	(3) Parents who focus only on the child at home on a respirator report greater burden.	Hazlett (1989)	
	b. The needs are greater for patients with recurrent cancer than those with newly diagnosed cancer.	Bean (1987/1988)	

10. The variable of perception influences the process of adaptation.	a. Perception of an event is a stronger predictor of adaptation than is the focal stimuli.	Armer (1988/1989) Dahlen (1980)
	b. Perception of an event and contextual stimuli are the strongest combined predictors of adaptation.	Armer (1988/1989)
11. Perception influences adaptation through linking the regulator and cognator subsystems.	Self-concept and role affect actual and perceived severity of illness.	Leech (1982)
12. Nursing assessment and interventions relate to identifying and managing input to adaptive systems.	a. Nurses manage input through environmental, physical, psychological, and social stimuli.	Leuze & McKenzie (1982)
	b. Nurses identified stressors for children in a Pediatric Intensive Care Unit corresponding to focal, contextual, and residual stimuli in the RAM.	Munn & Tichy (1987)

Based on the proposition that characteristics of the internal and external stimuli influence adaptive responses, one group of studies confirmed that some external stimuli place greater demands on the adaptive system than others. Campbell-Heider (1988; 1993) found that invasive therapies place more demands on the adaptive system than noninvasive therapies. Patients connected to invasive equipment reported more awareness of limited mobility, more threats to their self-esteem, and an increase in feelings of dependence. Munn and Tichy (1987) found that nurses perceive children's stress in the PICU as primarily the result of fears related to PICU equipment and to invasive and noninvasive procedures. Hazlett (1989) reported that parents felt a greater burden when children on ventilators were at home as compared to when children were in the hospital. Bean (1988) found that patients with recurrent cancer reported more needs than those with newly diagnosed cancer.

Based on the same proposition, another group of studies supported confirmation that adaptation level is affected by the magnitude of exposure to the focal stimuli. Pollock (1981/1982) proposed statements based on the literature and theoretic development indicating that adaptation level can be quantified by measuring the magnitude of the stimuli. Three studies confirmed that the magnitude of the focal stimuli can result in adaptation in more than one mode. Campbell-Heider (1988; 1993) found that patients attached to invasive equipment were more likely to report that adaptation was required in all four modes than were patients using noninvasive equipment. Hazlett (1989) found that parents who focused only on caring for their ventilator-dependent child at home were more likely to report adaptive needs in all modes than those who had support systems that allowed the parents to engage in other activities. Munn and Tichy (1987) found that children in the PICU reported stressors in all four modes.

The fourth proposition states that the characteristics of internal and external stimuli influence the adequacy of cognitive and emotional processes and was supported by Hazlett (1989). Related to their adaptation, parents reported they did not feel excessively burdened by the needs of the ventilator-dependent child at home, depending on ability to acknowledge and use resources such as family and financial support.

Investigators in two studies supported the sixth proposition that adaptation in one mode is affected by adaptation in other modes through cognator and regulator connectives. Dahlen (1980) found that the adjustment of patients to cataract surgery and visual prosthesis was determined by cognator function such as level of education and knowledge about the surgery. She also found that adaptation to the surgery on only one eye was influenced by physiologic factors such as vision and pathology in the other eye and by self-assessment of reading change. Preston and Dellasega (1987) noted that among the elderly, happiness and physical health were related and that gender and marital status also affected happiness and physical health.

The seventh proposition—that the pooled effect of focal, contextual, and residual stimuli determine adaptation level—was supported by four studies. Armer (1988/1989) found that previous positive experiences with moving, self-rated health, a positive attitude, and personal resources eased the adjustment of the elderly to congregate living. Bean (1988) found that the needs of patients with recurrent cancer were greater than those of patients with newly diagnosed cancer. The contextual and residual stimuli related to a decrease in hope were viewed as contributing factors. DeRuvo (1993) found that when comparing patients with either cancer of the digestive tract or cancer of the head and neck who were undergoing beam radiation, the needs were similar. Leech (1982) studied preoperative patients with arterial occlusive disease. She found that age and gender affected perceptions of health, self-concept, and physiologic needs.

Researchers in four studies supported the eighth proposition—that adaptation is influenced by integration of the person with the environment. Cottrell and Shannahan (1986; 1987) found that the use of the birth chair improved oxygenation of the fetus and increased perineal swelling in the mother. Armer's study (1988/1989) provided support that positive adjustment of the elderly who relocated to congregate living was determined by a sense of predictability, perceived social support, and the appraisal of the move as a challenge. Findings from the study by Hazlett (1989) revealed that parents of a ventilator-dependent child at home adapted better to the experience if they were able to use contextual resources such as other family members' help. Elderly patients adapted better to cataract surgery and visual prosthesis when they gave high ratings to their actual and perceived vision (Dahlen, 1980). In other words, vision allows the individual to better relate to the environment, thereby enhancing adaptation.

Investigators in four studies supported the ninth proposition—that the variable of time influences the process of adaptation, though not always in the same way. A stimulus may become more or less burdensome over time. Results of three studies supported the statement that the focal stimulus becomes a contextual stimulus over time as an indicator of effective adaptation. Campbell-Heider (1988; 1993) found that patients with invasive and noninvasive therapies who report fewer adaptive needs become less aware of their equipment over time. Likewise, patients receiving IV therapy at home became less anxious over time, particularly between the second and third week of treatment (Cornell, 1990). However, parents of a ventilator-dependent child who focus only on the care of their child, reported that caring for the child at home was a burden (Hazlett, 1989). Bean's study (1988) found that living with cancer and experiencing a recurrence elicited more adaptive needs than did a new diagnosis of cancer.

The 10th proposition—that the variable of perception influences the process of adaptation—was supported by researchers in two studies. Armer (1988/1989) and Dahlen (1980) found that the perception of the event is a stronger predictor of adaptation than is the focal stimuli. Dahlen (1980) reported that elderly patients adapted better to cataract surgery and visual prosthesis when they perceived they had good reading ability. Armer found that the elderly who perceived their move to congregate living as positive and challenging reported more positive adaptation to the move than those who did not perceive the move as positive and challenging. The researcher also found that perception of an event and contextual stimuli are the strongest combination of predictors of adaptation. The elderly who adapted best to the move were those who had a positive outlook toward the move and reported previous positive experiences with a move.

The proposition that perception influences adaptation through linking the regulator and cognator subsystems was supported by one study. Leech (1982) found that in patients with AOD, self-concept and role affected actual and perceived severity of the disease.

Investigators in two studies supported the 12th proposition that nursing assessment and interventions relate to identifying and managing input to adaptive systems. Leuze and McKenzie (1982) found that preoperative nurses managed input through environmental, physical, psychological, and social stimuli. Nurses' knowledge of the patient was higher when the preoperative assessment of the patient was based on the RAM than when nurses did not use the RAM. Nurses identified stressors for children in the PICU that corresponded to the focal, contextual, and residual stimuli in the RAM in the study by Munn and Tichy (1987).

In summary, results of 15 studies focusing on stimuli were used to test nine propositions of the RAM. The propositions evaluated here and those tested in the other content chapters are synthesized in Chapter 11 in which contributions to nursing science are viewed from the perspective of testing propositions in studies reported in all reserach review chapters.

Studies Related to Stimuli: Contributions to Nursing Science

Of the studies that were focused on stimuli, 16 were synthesized to derive contributions to nursing science. These studies are discussed in relation to their contributions to clinical practice, research, and theory. Many of the findings have relevance in each of the three areas.

Applications to Nursing Practice

Nursing knowledge can be developed through testing model concepts and proposing nursing interventions which can be implemented in the practice setting (Pollock, Frederickson, Carson, Massey & Roy, 1994). Specifically, interventions can be posed that promote or maintain adaptation to various stimuli in diverse populations and settings. Interventions need to be tested and refined before implementation in the practice setting. Studies reviewed in the chapter were examined for applications to practice within three categories established by project criteria described in Chapter 2 (Table 8.8).

Of the 16 studies evaluated for implications for nursing practice, 11 were included in Category 1. The studies contained support for empiric relationships from which to derive effective interventions that did not pose harmful risks to subjects. Three studies met the criteria for Category 2, which indicated the need for further clinical evaluation before implementation. Two studies met the criteria for Category 3, which indicated no current application existed for practice, but potential existed for relevancy after additional testing.

Applications for practice are presented according to the three categories. Within each category, studies are organized and presented according to the three main content areas of stimuli: (a) environment, (b) health status, and (c) therapies.

Table 8.8 – Application to Nursing Practice: Studies Related to Stimuli (*N*=16)

Category One: High potential for implementation
Armer (1988/1989)
Campbell-Heider (1988)
Campbell-Heider (1993)
Pollock (1981/1982)
Preston & Dellasega (1990)
Bean (1987/1988)
DeRuvo (1992/1993)
Leech (1982)
Cornell (1990)
Dahlen (1980)
Leuze & McKenzie (1987)

Category Two: Needs further clinical evaluation before implementation
Munn & Tichy (1987)
Hazlett (1989)
Takahashi & Bever (1989)

Category Three: Further research indicated before implementation
Cottrell & Shannahan (1986)
Cottrell & Shannahan (1987)

The findings from three of the studies in Category 1 were related to individuals who experienced stressful stimuli in their external environment (Armer, 1988/1989; Campbell-Heider, 1988; 1993). Nurses can assess the attitudes and fears of individuals confronted with stressful alterations in their external environment. Education about a move and the functioning of equipment can allay some anxiety. In addition, nurses can be supportive by encouraging their clients to express their fears and to reinforce the understanding that the nature of the stressors are time limited. Enlisting the assistance of family and friends has also been found important for promoting clients' adaptation to external stimuli.

In two studies, the relationship between stress and health was examined. Pollock (1981/1982) explored the theoretic relationship between primary stress factors and health. She proposed quantifiable levels of stress according to the specific magnitude of the stimuli. Preston and Dellasega (1990) found that older married women had the poorest health status and highest stress levels compared to older single women and single or married men. Nurses can counsel clients about the effects of stress. In particular, married older women appear to experience more stress than other groups of elderly. Stress-management programs are needed for clients exposed to experiences identified as stressful.

In three studies, the effects of illnesses on adaptation were examined (Bean, 1988; DeRuvo, 1993; and Leech, 1982). Patients with illnesses need information about their condition. They become more aware of the presence and progression of their disease during procedures and treatments. Support from nurses and family members needs to be planned based on assessment and timing of the stressors that confront the clients.

In three studies, therapies as specific stimuli were examined (Cornell, 1990; Dahlen, 1980; Leuze & McKenzie, 1987). Patients need to know details about the therapy—such as what it is, what it does, what the side effects are, and how long they will be receiving it. In addition, nurses can counsel patients about anxiety the patients may experience during procedures and what might be done to reduce uncomfortable feelings over time. The use of the RAM as a structure for organizing nursing assessments of patients has been found useful in a variety of studies.

Based on criteria established, three studies were judged to require further clinical evaluation before implementation. Based on results from Munn and Tichy (1987), the most significant stressors for children in the PICU were equipment, procedures, and separation from family. While these stressors were consistent with the literature on children's hospitalization experience, nurses need to confirm the significant stressors with the children and their families. For example, experience of unpredictability is possibly more stressful than the procedure itself. Hazlett (1989) found that for families with children on ventilators at home, the experience was generally stressful. While it often appears preferable for children to be at home rather than in the hospital, the findings of this study indicated a number of problems such as the experience of family burden and costs not reimbursable outside the hospital. Nurses can assess and determine characteristics of families able to manage a child at home on a ventilator, and may assess health policy issues related to reimbursement to the families for home care costs. Takahashi and Bever (1989) found that nurses reported performing more preoperative assessments than could be confirmed through chart audit or observation. Nurses need to be concerned about documenting both assessment and outcomes of the care they provide.

Two studies were assigned to Category 3, indicating that further testing is warranted before implementation. Cottrell and Shannahan (1986; 1987) compared the birth chair to the traditional delivery table in relation to maternal and fetal outcome. The findings for use of the birth chair were an increase in maternal perineal swelling, and for the fetus, a higher Apgar score, higher oxygen saturation, and lower carbon dioxide saturation levels in the umbilical cord. Further study needs to be done using an experimental design with a larger sample to evaluate the effects of the birth chair. This is particularly important because researchers in an earlier study (Shannahan & Cottrell, 1985) indicated an increase in maternal bleeding with the birth chair, raising concerns about its use.

Recommendations for Model-Based Research

Future directions for model-based research were identified from all studies that had applications to nursing practice, but were most obvious in the studies where further testing was indicated (Category Three). In addition, studies where findings were unclear or differed from previous research are priority areas for further research.

Instrument development is needed for studies using the RAM and focusing on stimuli. Instruments are needed to measure all three stimuli (focal, contextual, and residual), as conceptualized in the RAM. Most researchers used instruments (primarily structured or semi-structured interviews) that they designed. While developing instruments specific to numerous and varied stimuli is not possible, developing general guidelines for measuring adaptation to a group of health problems such as chronic illnesses is possible.

Further research is indicated to develop more specificity to the operational definition of the modes. Researchers often "collapsed" self-concept, role development, and interdependence modes into a single category labeled psychosocial (Hazlett, 1989; Leech, 1982; Munn & Tichy, 1987; Pollock, 1982; Takahashi & Bever, 1989). The authors expressed confusion about the categories, particularly between the self-concept and interdependence modes or between the self-concept and role function modes (DeRuvo, 1993; Preston & Dellasega, 1990). In addition, Bean (1988) identified the lack of specificity in the descriptions of the modes as the primary factor for low interrater reliability.

Studies that were focused on stimuli specific to the environment (Armer, 1988/1989; Campbell-Heider, 1988, 1993; Munn & Tichy, 1987) documented the stressful aspects of relocation and of technologic environments such as a PICU, or of attachment to equipment. Further exploration is needed to determine interventions that will promote adaptation to these environments in both adults and children. Interventions should include factors within each mode as well as consideration of the presence or absence of related contextual stimuli.

Results from studies using the birth chair indicated that maternal and fetal outcomes may be altered (Cottrell & Shannahan, 1986, 1987). Further research is needed to confirm the effectiveness of the birth chair and, particularly, to examine the possibility of negative side effects. Further information is also needed to determine the effects of demographics such as age, number and type of previous deliveries, and personal preferences for the delivery experience.

In studies pertaining to the relationship of stress to health and illness, results indicated that contextual stimuli such as type of cancer, severity of illness, gender, and marital status affected adaptation (Bean, 1987/1988; DeRuvo, 1992/1993; Leech, 1982; Pollock, 1981/1982; Preston & Dellasega, 1990). Further research is indicated to isolate the specific contributions various stimuli make to adaptation. Intervention studies need to be designed using nursing strategies that promote adaptation in healthy and ill individuals by managing stimuli.

Directions for Theory and RAM Development

Directions for further theory and model development of stimuli were identified from the testing of RAM propositions. All 15 studies supported the propositions partly because of the nondirectional nature of the propositions. For the propositions to be of more value, direction should be provided for deriving hypotheses. For example, one proposition is that the characteristics of the internal and external stimuli influence adaptive responses. A derived ancillary proposition is that some external stimuli place greater demands on the adaptive system than do others. Future studies can be designed to test directional statements building on the five studies related to stimuli which support the RAM propositions.

Considering further the proposition that the characteristics of the internal and external stimuli influence adaptive responses, researchers have indicated that the magnitude of exposure to the focal stimulus affects adaptation and that some stimuli place greater demands on the adaptive system than do others. However, the magnitude of exposure can be mediated by other variables and affect adaptation. The direction adaptation will take is unclear when more demanding external stimuli are present. For example, Hazlett (1989) found that all parents did adapt to providing home care for their child on a ventilator. However, some used resources and adapted better, while others experienced the care as a burden and felt trapped.

The second proposition—that the pooled effect of focal, contextual, and residual stimuli determines the adaptation level—was supported by studies of Bean (1987/1988) and DeRuvo (1992/1993). The pooled effect of the stimuli was examined and appeared linear. The effect of the stimuli on adaptation level indicated the result of interaction among the stimuli. Future model developers should consider interaction among the stimuli.

The findings of many studies suggest that the proposition—the variable of time influences the process of adaptation—merits further development. Investigators of four studies indicated that over time focal stimuli become more contextual as an indicator of adaptation (Campbell-Heider, 1988, 1993; Cornell, 1990; Hazlett, 1989). However, Bean (1987/1988) found that patients with recurrent cancer reported more needs that represented every mode, as compared to patients with newly diagnosed cancer. Further development of the model is needed to identify types of focal stimuli that become contextual as an indicator of effective adaptation. Likewise, further development of the model needs to clarify the role and importance of the concept of time. Based on these five studies, the concept of time is potentially important.

Summary

Studies which were focused primarily on stimuli according to the RAM were reviewed in this chapter. Of the 163 studies included in this monograph, 19 were identified for inclusion in research concentrating on stimuli. Studies were critically analyzed, the relationships of the studies to the RAM were evaluated, and the contributions of the studies to nursing science were synthesized. Findings from the studies supported the use of the RAM in guiding nursing practice and research on stimuli and strengthen the interrelationships among theory, research, and practice. Contributions to nursing science from all model research, including the studies focusing on stimuli, will be discussed in Chapter 11.

References

Armer, J.M. (1989). Factors influencing relocation adjustment among community-based rural elderly (Doctoral dissertation, University of Rochester, 1988). *Dissertation Abstracts International, 50,* 1321-B.

Bean, C.A. (1988). Needs and stimuli influencing needs of adult cancer patients (Doctoral dissertation, University of Alabama in Birmingham, 1987). *Dissertation Abstracts International, 48,* 2259-B.

Blain, S. (1993). Attitudes to women undergoing TOP. Nursing Standard, 7(37), 30-33.

Campbell-Heider, N. (1988). Patient adaptation to the hospital technological environment. (Doctoral dissertation, The University of Rochester, 1988) Dissertation Abstracts International, 49, 1618-B.

Campbell-Heider, N. (1993). Patient adaptation to technology: An application of the Roy model to nursing research. Journal of the New York State Nurses Association, 24(2), 22-27.

Cornell, D.L. (1990). Patterns of anxiety with home parenteral antibiotic therapy (Master's thesis, University of Nevada, Reno, 1990). Masters Abstracts International, 28, 572.

Cottrell, B.H., & Shanahan, M. (1986). Effect of the birth chair on duration of second stage labor and maternal outcome. Nursing Research, 35, 364-367.

Cottrell, B. H., & Shanahan, M.O. (1987). A comparison of fetal outcome in birth chair and delivery table births. Research in Nursing & Health, 10, 239-243.

Dahlen, R. A. (1980). Analysis of selected factors related to the elderly person's ability to adapt to visual prostheses following senile cataract surgery (Doctoral dissertation, The Catholic University of America, 1980). Dissertation Abstracts International, 41, 389-B.

DeRuvo, S. L. S. (1993). Nursing diagnoses using Roy's adaptation model for persons with cancer receiving external beam radiation (Master's thesis, The University of Arizona, 1992). Masters Abstracts International, 31, 270.

Hazlett, D.E. (1989). A study of pediatric home ventilator management: Medical, psychosocial, and financial aspects. Journal of Pediatric Nursing, 4, 284-294.

Helson, H. (1964). Adaptation level theory. New York: Harper Row Publishers.

Kromer, E.A. (1994). A descriptive study of factors affecting postpartum adolescent contraceptive use from a Roy framework (Master's thesis, D'Youville College, 1993). Masters Abstracts International, 32, 228.

Leech, J.L. (1982). Psychosocial and physiologic needs of patients with arterial occlusive disease during the preoperative phase of hospitalization. Heart & Lung, 11, 442- 449.

Leuze, M. & McKenzie, J. (1987). Preoperative assessment using the Roy Adaptation Model. AORN Journal, 46, 1122-1134.

Munn, V.A., & Tichy, A.M. (1987). Nurses' perceptions of stressors in pediatric intensive care. Journal of Pediatric Nursing, 2(6), 405-411.

Pollock, S.E. (1982). Level of adaptation: An analysis of stress factors that affect health status (Doctoral dissertation, The University of Texas at Austin, 1981). Dissertation Abstracts International, 42, 436-B.

Pollock, S.E., Frederickson, K., Carson, M.A., Massey, V.H., & Roy, C. (1994). Contributions to nursing science: Synthesis of findings from Adaptation Model Research. *Scholarly Inquiry for Nursing Practice, 8*(4), 361-372.

Preston, D.B., & Dellasega, C. (1990). Elderly women and stress: Does marriage make a difference? *Journal of Gerontological Nursing, 16*(4), 26-31.

Roy, C., & Andrews, H. (1991). *The Roy Adaptation Model: The definitive statement.* Norwalk, CT: Appleton & Lange.

Shannahan, M. D., & Cottrell, B. H. (1985). Effect of the birth chair on duration of second stage labor, fetal outcome, and maternal blood loss. *Nursing Research, 34,* 89-92.

Takahashi, J. J., & Bever, S. C. (1989). Preoperative nursing assessment: A research study. *AORN Journal, 50,* 1022-1035.

Bibliography

Woods, N.F., & Catanzaro, M. (1988). *Nursing research: Theory and practice.* St. Louis: Mosby.

Chapter 9

Intervention Research

This chapter includes information about nursing intervention research reported between 1970 and 1994 which used the Roy Adaptation Model (RAM). Information about a few intervention studies was included in previous chapters when they were either part of a larger program of research or a pilot study in a specific area. The 28 studies in this chapter include 14 journal publications, seven dissertations and seven theses.

Purposes

The purposes of the chapter are to (a) critically analyze nursing intervention studies which have utilized the RAM, (b) evaluate the relationships of the research to the RAM, and (c) synthesize the contributions of the research to nursing science. Included in the contributions to nursing science are applications for nursing practice, recommendations for model-based intervention research, and directions for theory and RAM development. The criteria developed and the processes used by the BBARNS investigators for analysis and synthesis of the studies are explained in Chapter 2.

Background

Nursing intervention as described in the RAM focuses on the methods by which a patient's goals are to be attained (Roy & Andrews, 1991; 1999). A person as an adaptive system is confronted by stimuli from the internal and external environment which trigger the coping mechanisms to produce behaviors. Roy suggests that ineffective behaviors result when the stimuli exceed the person's ability to cope. The nursing process involves assessing behaviors and related stimuli and synthesizing this information into the nursing diagnosis. Goal setting is related to the desired behavioral outcomes of nursing care which in turn are related to identified problem areas. Nurses then intervene to modify the stimuli which promote effective behaviors.

Identification of approaches for nursing intervention includes selecting which stimuli to change. Roy and Andrews (1991) state that whenever possible, the focal stimulus should be the focus of nursing interventions. If the focal stimulus cannot be managed, the contextual stimuli should be changed in an attempt to enhance the adaptation level. The adaptation level includes the effectiveness of cognator and regulator processes that may be a direct focus of intervention. A combination of approaches can be used to achieve the desired outcomes. The intervention of nurses can be considered contextual stimuli for patients' adaptation. Finally, nurses evaluate the effectiveness of nursing interventions in relation to a person's outcome behavior and the goal.

Outcome behaviors indicate the adaptation status. Roy and Andrews (1991) label output behavior as either adaptive or ineffective. Responses are a person's behavior as an adaptive system. Behaviors can be observed in four adaptive modes: physiologic, self-concept, role function, and interdependence. Responses are carried out through these four modes, and the adaptation level can be observed. Adaptive responses promote the integrity of the person in relation to the goals of adaptation: survival, growth, reproduction, and mastery. Conversely ineffective responses do not promote integrity nor facilitate adaptation goals.

Investigators for studies included in this chapter used either an experimental or quasi-experimental design. A study met the criteria for experimental design if: (a) an independent variable was manipulated by the investigator to observe dependent variables for effect; (b) a control group was used for comparison; and (c) the subjects were randomly assigned to either an experimental or control group (Beck, 1991). In four studies, researchers used an experimental design; in 23, a quasi-experimental design; and in one an ex post facto design.

Critical Analysis of Intervention Research

The 28 studies described in this chapter will be critically analyzed using previously established guidelines—see Chapter 2 for description. Criteria were modified for use with experimental and quasi-experimental designs.

Description of Reported Research

Intervention studies derived from the model were conducted to investigate a number of nursing interventions—for example, small nebulizer inhalation treatments and animal visitation therapy. Studies were divided into three categories of interventions: (a) cognator ($n=10$); (b) physiologic ($n=11$); and (c) interdependence ($n=7$).

Cognator intervention research. In 10 of the 28 studies, the focus of the research was on the cognator coping subsystem (see Table 9.1). The cognator subsystem is a major system of coping processes described in the RAM. The cognator responds through four cognitive-emotive channels: perceptual and information processing, learning, judgment, and emotion. Eight intervention studies were focused on learning; judgment or emotional components were examined in two studies. No investigators reported studies of perceptual and information processing components.

In two studies, investigators recorded the effects of a structured education program on adult patients' anxiety and knowledge levels after myocardial infarction (MI). Guzzetta (1979) evaluated the relationship between level of learning, anxiety, and three teaching periods in 45 men with post-acute transmural or subendocardial myocardial infarction. The three teaching periods, or contextual stimuli, were initiated according to the number of days following MI. At level one, the treatment variable consisted of educating patients during the third, fourth, and fifth days after transfer from the CCU to telemetry; at level two patients were educated during the seventh, eighth, and ninth days after transfer; and at level three, patients were educated during the 11th, 12th, and 13th days after transfer. The teaching intervention was a component of the cognator learning coping process which was empirically measured with a written pre-, post-teaching test developed by the investigator. Anxiety was evaluated with the Anxiety Depression scale for medically ill patients. Physiologic effect of anxiety was measured with a 24-hour urine specimen tested for cortisol level.

The formal cardiac teaching program significantly improved patients' knowledge of their illnesses and related health care issues. A significant inverse correlation between learning and psychological anxiety was found. Cardiac teaching was most effective 1 week after the patient's transfer from the CCU. No correlation was found between learning and physiologic anxiety.

Zonca (1980) investigated the effects of a formal in-hospital patient education program on psychological and physiologic anxiety in 60 adults admitted to the coronary care unit with a diagnosis of acute MI. Subjects were assigned to three groups. The control-group subjects received conventional informal teaching by staff on the unit. The first experimental group participated in a formal, one-to-one educational program and the second experimental group received the same educational program but attended each session with a spouse or significant other. Results indicated statistically significant improvement on knowledge tests and changes in health behavior for the experimental groups receiving the formal education program but not for the control group receiving informal teaching by the staff. No statistically significant differences in anxiety levels among the three groups were identified.

Researchers in two studies investigated the effects of education before medical procedures. Hjelm-Karlsson (1989) provided structured information describing the procedure of an intravenous pyelography (IVP). The physiologic reactions of cold, sweating, headache, heart rate, and hyperventilation of the control and experimental groups were not significantly different. However the psychological outcomes of calmness, safety, secu-

Table 9.1 – Description of Cognator Intervention Research Studies in Which RAM Was Used (N=10)

Author(s) & Date	Purpose	Sample	Design	Findings
1. Guzzetta (1979)	To determine the relationship between levels of learning, anxiety, and three levels of teaching in adult cardiac patients	Post-acute transmural or subendocardial myocardial infarction adults. (N=45)	Quasi-experimental	The cardiac rehabilitation teaching program was significant in improving patients' knowledge of their illnesses and related health care issues. Learning was greater when teaching was begun at least 1 week after transfer from CCU. There was a significant inverse correlation between learning and psychological anxiety and no correlation between learning and physiologic anxiety.
2. Zonca (1980)	To determine the effects of a formal in-hospital patient education program on anxiety in post-myocardial infarction patients	Adults admitted to the coronary care unit with a diagnosis of acute myocardial infarction (N=60)	Quasi-experimental	Statistically significant differences were found on knowledge tests, and changes in health behavior for the experimental groups.
3. Hjelm-Karlsson (1989)	To determine whether structured information given prior to an IVP for the first time had any effect on the pattern of physiological and psychological responses	Adult patients undergoing IVP (N=60)	Experimental	No differences were found between the groups regarding physiologic reactions such as sweating and heart rate, but there were significant differences in the psychological outcome variables such as calmness and confidence in staff. Less pain and discomfort were experienced in the intervention group.

Author	Purpose	Sample	Design	Results
4. Meeker (1994)	To determine the impact of a preoperative teaching program on the incidence of postoperative atelectasis and patient satisfaction	Adults admitted for either elective general surgery, urological surgery or colorectal surgery (N=144)	Quasi-experimental	There were no significant differences in postoperative complications and patient satisfaction after participating in a preoperative teaching program.
5. Grunstra & Rowe (1992/1993)	To determine the effectiveness of prenatal breast-feeding education on a mother's perceived success at breast-feeding	Primiparous women who had singleton vaginal deliveries (N=20)	Quasi-experimental	Primiparous women who received prenatal breast-feeding education did not report a higher perception of success in breast-feeding than those women who did not receive prenatal breast-feeding education.
6. Vicenzi & Thiel (1992)	To describe college students' AIDS beliefs, condom beliefs, and behaviors, and to determine if a safe sex education workshop would change college students' beliefs and sex practices	College students (N=49)	Quasi-experimental	Pre- and post-test comparisons of safer sex practice scores did not show a significant difference in the number of practice changes. The AIDS education workshop did change several sex beliefs.
7. Gilbert (1990/1991)	To determine the effectiveness of a structured group nursing intervention on adaptation of girls who had been sexually abused	Sexually abused girls (N=47)	Quasi-experimental	There were no significant differences among the three groups over time. All groups achieved scores indicating adaptation in the psychosocial modes.

(continued)

Table 9.1 (continued)

Author(s) & Date	Purpose	Sample	Design	Findings
8. Newman (1991)	To investigate the effect of the arthritis self-help course on self-efficacy, social support, life purpose and arthritis	Adults with arthritis (N=130)	Quasi-experimental	ASHC participants achieved significant increase in arthritis self-efficacy for pain management and other symptoms such as fatigue and frustration. Arthritis self-efficacy for function, perceived social support, purpose and meaning in life, and arthritis impact scores were not affected by participation in the course.
9. Campbell (1992)	To determine the effects of techniques from cognitive therapy for depressed subjects and nurses' ability to identify normal adaptive reactive depression	Geriatric adults with a diagnosis of depression (N=103)	Experimental	The experimental group demonstrated a significant reduction in depressive symptoms. The art and crafts group decreased their depression scores. The control group with no intervention demonstrated no significant change in depression scores.
10. Gaberson (1991)	To determine anxiety levels in preoperative patients who listen to either humorous audiotapes or tranquil music	Preoperative patients (N=15)	Experimental design	No statistically significant differences were found between the experimental and control groups. Subjects in the control group reported the highest levels of preoperative anxiety.

rity, relaxation, control, confidence in staff, and feelings of being cared for by staff were different. The intervention group indicated less pain and discomfort during the IVP than those in the control group indicated.

Meeker (1994) evaluated the effects of a preoperative teaching program on the incidence of postoperative atelectasis and patient satisfaction in 144 adults admitted for either elective general surgery, urologic surgery, or colon-rectal surgery. The control group consisted of 95 patients who received the usual informal patient education. The experimental group consisted of 49 patients who received structured preoperative teaching. No significant differences were observed in either postoperative complications—measured by physiologic outcomes—or patient gratification—measured by psychological outcomes.

Grunstra and Rowe (1992/1993) evaluated the effects of prenatal breast-feeding education on the perception of success in 20 primiparaous women who had singleton vaginal deliveries between 36 and 42 weeks gestation. The experimental group attended a prenatal breast-feeding class; those in the control group did not. Outcomes indicated no significant differences between the experimental group and the control group.

In a study to evaluate the effects of a safer sex education workshop on 49 college students, Vincenzi and Thiel (1992) examined the outcomes of self-esteem, sexual regard, and safe sex practices. Contextual stimuli included subjects' beliefs about AIDS and use of condoms. These beliefs were the focus of the nursing intervention of a safe sex education workshop. The nursing intervention did change several beliefs. For example, after the educational intervention, students reported being more confident about knowing how to use a condom correctly. However increasing safe-sex practices were not reported.

The effects of a structured group nursing intervention on subjects (N=47) who had been sexually abused were evaluated by Gilbert (1990/1991).The experimental group consisted of 17 girls who had been sexually abused and were randomly assigned to the structured group. The control groups consisted of 13 girls who had been sexually abused and received standard agency treatment and 17 community girls who had not been sexually abused. The outcomes investigated included isolation and loneliness, self worth, academic competence, and emotional/behavioral problems. No significant statistical differences were found among the groups over time. All groups achieved scores indicating adaptation in the psychosocial modes.

Newman (1991) evaluated the effects of the Arthritis Self-Help Course (ASHC) in 130 adults with arthritis randomly assigned to experimental and control groups. Arthritis was designated as the focal stimulus. The following outcomes were measured: arthritis self-efficacy, perceived social support, purpose and meaning in life, and arthritis impact. Results indicated that the experimental group achieved significant increases in arthritis self-efficacy for pain management and other symptoms of arthritis such as fatigue and frustration. Arthritis self-efficacy for function, perceived social support, purpose and meaning in life, and arthritis impact scores were not affected by participation in the ASAC.

Cognitive therapy as a nursing intervention was implemented in one study in which focus was on the judgment component of the cognator coping process which encompasses activities such as problem solving and decision making. Campbell (1992) investigated nurses' ability to identify reactive depression and used techniques from cognitive therapy to decrease levels of depression in 103 geriatric adults.

Participants were randomly assigned to three groups: one experimental group who received cognitive therapy, a control group who received no intervention, and another control group who received group art and craft classes. The cognitive therapy was a planned nursing intervention aimed at managing the cognator subsystem and making coping easier through positive input thought patterns. The experimental group had a significant reduction in depressive symptoms. The group receiving craft classes had decreased depression scores, suggesting attention affects depression. The control group with no treatment had no significant change in depression scores. Nurses were able to accurately identify depression in 92% of patients.

The emotion component of the cognator subsystem was the focus of a study conducted by Gaberson (1991). The emotion component of the cognator coping process as described in the RAM encompasses activities in which cognator defenses are used to seek relief from anxiety and to make affective appraisals and attachments. Gaberson investigated anxiety levels in 15 preoperative patients who listened to either humorous audiotapes or tranquil music. Subjects were randomly assigned to one of two treatment groups or to the control group. Each group contained five subjects. One treatment group received the humorous intervention and the other treatment group received the musical intervention. No significant differences in preoperative anxiety levels were found between the two experimental groups. However a moderate effect size (0.496) suggested that the lack of significance may have been because of the small sample size. Subjects who experienced no intervention before surgery reported the highest levels of preoperative anxiety.

Physiologic mode intervention research. In 11 studies, the effects of a physiologic nursing intervention were examined (see Table 9.2). The physiologic mode is associated with the manner in which a person responds physically to environmental stimuli. Behavior in this mode is a manifestation of the physiologic activity of all the cells, tissues, organs, and systems which make up the human body.

In four studies, researchers investigated nursing interventions that provided some form of touch to the subjects involved. Meek (1993) investigated the effects of slow-stroke back massage (SSBM) on blood pressure, heart rate, and skin temperature in 30 adults from two hospice home-care programs. Subjects served as their own controls in this repeated-measures, design. Two preintervention and two postintervention measures of the four dependent variables were completed on the first day and again 24 hours later. The SSBM intervention was considered the focal stimulus. SSBM was associated with decreases in blood pressure and heart rate and with an increase in skin temperature—all indicative of relaxation.

In three studies, researchers investigated the effects of tactile stimulation on either fetal or infant responses. Komara (1991/1992) investigated the effects of music and vibroacoustic stimulation on fetal responses in 30 pregnant women from a private obstetric practice. A modified nonstress test was performed on all subjects. The experimental group ($n=15$) was introduced to music and the control group ($n=15$) was introduced to the vibroacoustic stimulator. The physiologic mode outcomes were heart rate and fetal activity. Results indicated that both music and vibroacoustic stimulation were statistically comparable and provide an effective means for stimulating the fetus during a reactive nonstress test. Music was an effective stimulus for acceleration of fetal movement and heart rate.

Modrcin-McCarthy (1992/1993) examined the physiologic and behavioral effects of a gentle human-touch nursing intervention on 20 medically fragile, preterm infants. Infants were randomly assigned to either a nontouch control group or an experimental touch group receiving 20 minutes of gentle human touch for 10 days from the 7th through 16th days of life. Heart rate, oxygen saturation, state classifications, motor activity, behavioral distress, weight gain, caloric intake, days on oxygen and photo therapy, blood transfusions, discharge weight, and length of stay were recorded. Results indicated that immediate and short-term effects of a gentle human-touch nursing intervention were neither adverse nor stressful to preterm infants. The researcher documented the positive, beneficial effects of the intervention on preterm infants and indicated this type of touching was appropriate for infants in the neonatal intensive care unit.

The effectiveness of an experimental intervention consisting of taste, smell, oral, and tactile stimulation using a lemon glycerin swabstick was examined on preterm infants' respiratory and behavioral state responses during apnea by Garcia and White-Traut (1993). Fourteen preterm infants less than 35 weeks gestation diagnosed with apnea of prematurity were included in the sample. Infants served as their own control. Each infant received four randomly assigned stimulations when they experienced an apneic episode. Physiologic adaptation was measured by the time interval for reinitiation of respiratory effort and changes in behavioral state. The time interval for reinitiation of respiratory effort was significantly shorter

Table 9.2 – Description of Physiologic Intervention Research Studies (*N*=11)

Author(s) & Date	Purpose	Sample	Design	Findings
11. Meek (1993)	To examine the effects of slow stroke back massage (SSBM) on blood pressure, heart rate, and skin temperature	Adults from two ospice home-care programs (*N*=30)	Quasi-experimental	SSBM was shown to produce modest but statistically significant changes in vital signs and skin temperature indicative of relaxation.
12. Komara (1991/1992)	To compare the effects of music and vibroacoustic stimulation on fetal heart rates and fetal movement during nonstress tests	Pregnant women (fetuses in utero) (*N*=30)	Quasi-experimental	Both music and vibroacoustic stimulator were statistically significant in producing a reactive nonstress test. Music was an effective stimulus for provoking fetal heart rate acceleration and fetal movement.
13. Modrcin-McCarthy (1992/1993)	To examine the physiological and behavioral effects of a gentle human touch nursing intervention on medically fragile, preterm infants	Preterm infants 27 to 32 weeks gestational age (*N*=20)	Quasi-experimental	The immediate and short-term effects of a gentle human touch nursing intervention were not adverse or stressful to preterm infants.
14. Garcia & White-Traut (1993)	To compare preterm infants' respiratory and behavioral state responses to traditional tactile and experimental oral tactile stimulation during apnea	Preterm infants with apnea of prematurity (*N*=14)	Quasi-experimental	The time interval for reinitiation of respiratory effort was significantly shorter after infants received the experimental stimulation. Behavior state changed to alertness when the infants received the traditional tactile intervention yet remained unchanged when the experimental stimulation was administered during apnea.

15. Houston (1993)	To evaluate whether elderly subjects exposed to vestibular-proprioceptive stimulation in the form of slow rocking in a rocking chair will manifest a decrease in heart rate, blood pressure and increase in skin temperature	Geriatric adults > 65 years (N=25)	Quasi-experimental	No statistically significant variations in blood pressure occurred. Heart rate showed a statistically significant decline. There was a significant difference in skin temperature.
16. Carson (1991/1992)	To explore the effect of discrete muscle activity on stress response	Healthy adults (N=105)	Quasi-experimental	There was a reduction of subjective stress in the experimental group but no significant differences in physiologic responses to acute stress. Gender, stress perceptions, and fatigue were significant covariate effects.
17. Riegel, Heywood, Jackson, & Kennedy (1988)	To determine effect of place-ment/location of nitroglycerin ointment on patients' reports of headache and flushing	Adults with cardiac disease (N=56)	Quasi-experimental	There were no significant differences in severity of side effects when the three sites were compared.
18. Fahs (1991/1992)	To examine the effects of heparin injectate volume on pain and bruising	Medical surgical patients receiving low-dose heparin (N=50)	Quasi-experimental	The proposed effect of injectate volume on pain of injection, bruise occurrence and size and pain of injection site was not supported.

(continued)

Table 9.2 (continued)

Author(s) & Date	Purpose	Sample	Design	Findings
19. Roberson (1987)	To determine the effect of a small nebulizer inhalation treatment on oral temperatures of adults with chronic and nonchronic conditions requiring varying degrees of supplemental oxygen over specified time intervals	Four groups of 20 adults each: one nonchronic and three chronically ill groups requiring varying degrees of oxygen ($N=80$)	Quasi-experimental	There was no significant difference in oral temperature before or after a small nebulizer inhalation treatment. There was a significant difference in oral temperature by timing of measurement.
20. Smith (1987/ 1989)	To determine the difference in cardiovascular responses during basin bath, tub bath, and shower	Healthy male adults ($N=30$)	Quasi-experimental	There were no significant differences in peak heart rates, presence of cardiac dysrhythmia, and changes in ST segment during basin bath, tub bath, and shower.
21. Jones (1994)	To determine the outcomes of a managed care clinical system in one intensive care nursery	Neonates ($n=260$), parents ($n=105$), professional nurses and health care team members ($n=133$)	Ex post-facto	It is feasible to evaluate the outcomes of a new health care delivery system in a dynamic neonatal setting.

after infants received the experimental stimulation. Behavioral state of the infants changed to alertness when the infants received the traditional tactile intervention. However, level of alertness remained unchanged when the experimental stimulation was administered during apnea thus a sleep state continued.

Investigators in two studies evaluated the effect of bodily movement on stress and relaxation. Houston (1993) evaluated 25 adults over 65 years old who were exposed to vestibular-proprioceptive stimulation in the form of slow rocking in a rocking chair. The effect of slow rocking was evaluated by measuring heart rate, systolic and diastolic blood pressure, and skin temperature. A total of six recordings of the four dependent variables were taken at 5-minute intervals before, during, and after each subject had rocked slowly. No statistically significant variations in blood pressure occurred. A statistically significant decrease in skin temperature and heart rate occurred indicating increased relaxation.

Carson (1991/1992) explored the effect of discrete muscle activity on the stress response in 105 healthy adult subjects. Subjects were exposed to a physically uncomfortable procedure called the cold pressor test. The randomly assigned experimental group was instructed to perform a muscle activity that involved limited movement but required the subject to keep the forearm flat on a table while lifting and dropping a small, wooden barbell. Anxiety, subjective stress, blood cortisol levels, heart rate, and blood pressure were the outcomes measured. Results in the experimental group indicated a reduction of subjectively identified stress but no significant differences in physiologic responses to acute stress. Gender, stress perceptions, and fatigue had significant covariate effects on the subjective response to stress.

In four studies, researchers manipulated some form of treatment as the nursing intervention. Riegel, Heywood, Jackson, and Kennedy (1988) using a repeated-measures design investigated the effect of changing the site of nitroglycerin ointment on 56 adults with cardiac disease who had reported headache and flushing. Results indicated no significant differences in severity of side effects when the three sites were compared.

Fahs (1991/1992) examined the effect of heparin injectate volume on pain and bruising in 50 general medical-surgical patients receiving low-dose heparin therapy. Subjects served as their own controls. Order of treatment and selection of injection site were randomized. Injectate volume was the focal stimulus. Contextual stimuli included dose, technique, syringe, needle, length of injection, depression, age, sex, diagnosis, surgery, adipose tissue, location of site, time of injection, and two classes of medications. Measures of physiologic adaptation following injection included pain at the time of injection, presence and size of bruising, and pain at the site of the injection. Results indicated no significant effect of injectate volume on pain at the site of injection or size of the bruise.

Roberson (1987) examined the effect of a small-nebulizer inhalation treatment on oral temperature in well adults and adults with chronic respiratory disease (N=80). The sample consisted of four groups with 20 subjects in each: nonchronic, chronic requiring no supplemental oxygen, chronic requiring supplemental oxygen at 1 liter per minute continuously, and chronic requiring supplemental oxygen at 2 liters per minute continuously. Oral temperature was assessed before and at various times after a small-nebulizer inhalation treatment. Results indicated no significant differences in oral temperature before or after a small-nebulizer inhalation treatment among the four groups tested. Significant differences occurred in oral temperatures when taken at specified intervals before treatment and at 5, 10, and 15 minutes after completion of treatment.

Smith (1987/1989) investigated the difference in cardiovascular responses in 30 healthy men during basin bath, tub bath, and shower. A nonrandom, convenience sample was used. The bathing activity was labeled the focal stimulus; the cardiovascular system measurements represented physiologic adaptation. Results indicated no significant difference in peak heart rates, presence of cardiac dysrhythmia, and changes in ST segment during basin bath, tub bath, or shower.

Jones (1994) viewed the group as an adaptive system as described by Roy and Anway (1989). The investigator evaluated the effects of a clinical-system change in an investigation in which the outcome variables for a managed-care clinical system were contrasted with those of a conventional system in one intensive care nursery. The sample was composed of neonates, parents, health care team members, and professional nurses. Outcome variables included direct nursing costs per day, costs per Diagnosis-Related Group (DRG) 386 and 387 (physical), job satisfaction of the health team members and the professional nurses (interpersonal), neonatal length of stay, level of neurobehavior, neonates' readmissions, parent satisfaction (role performance), and reimbursement policies (interdependence). Enrolled in the study were 260 neonates and 105 parents. In addition, 133 health care team members, including professional nurses, participated. Physical, interpersonal, role performance, and interdependence systems were evaluated.

The author concluded that the outcomes of a system in a dynamic neonatal setting could be evaluated. Neonates in DRG 386 in the managed-care clinical system had a shorter mean length of stay, increased frequency of complications, and higher mean daily costs than neonates in the conventional system. Neonates in DRG 387 in the managed-care clinical system had a longer mean length of stay and lower mean daily costs than did neonates in the conventional system. Nursing care costs remained constant despite increased neonatal complications. Satisfaction of parents, professional nurses, and health care team members did not differ significantly from the conventional system to the managed-care clinical system.

Interdependence intervention research. In seven studies, the interdependence mode was the focus of the intervention research. Within this mode, which involves interaction with others, each person seeks to have affectional needs met through satisfying relationships (see Table 9.3).

In three studies categorized as interdependence mode interventions, researchers investigated the effects of animal therapy on the elderly. In all three studies animal therapy was the focal stimulus of the subjects; however the researchers evaluated outcomes in different modes. Prelewicz (1993) evaluated the effective pattern of loneliness (interdependence mode) in 10 elderly adults residing in a nursing home using a one-group pre-post-test design. No significant difference in loneliness was found before or after the animal-assisted therapy program. Parlin (1988/1990) evaluated the oxygenation and fluid and electrolyte components of the physiologic mode through the measurement of heart rate and blood pressure in 40 well elderly volunteers petting an unknown dog for 15 minutes. Parlin found that the elderly volunteers experienced a statistically significant reduction in heart rate, but no significant difference in blood pressure when petting an unknown dog.

Francis, Turner, and Johnson (1985) evaluated the functional self-esteem component of the self-concept mode in 40 adult-home residents receiving weekly domestic animal visitation. Subjects from one home comprised the experimental group and subjects from a second home comprised the control group. Multiple instruments were used to measure self-concept including the Affect Balance Scale, Observed Patient Behavior Scale, and Psychosocial Function Scale. The researchers reported significant differences in seven of nine variables measured: social interaction, psychosocial function, life satisfaction, mental functioning, depression, social competence, and psychological well-being.

In two of the seven interdependence intervention studies, effects of family presence were evaluated in two hospital settings: a post-surgery care unit and an operating room. Vogelsang and Ragiel (1987) and Neiterman (1987/1988) examined the presence of family members or significant others within the context of surgical hospital experiences. The focal stimulus for both studies was the presence of family members in presurgical or postsurgical experiences. Vogelsang and Ragiel evaluated the anxiety levels of 60 elective adult surgical patients. The experimental group consisted of patients who had significant others or nurses with them in the immediate postanesthesia period. The control group had no visitation during the immediate postanesthesia period. Vogelsang and Ragiel evaluated coping strategies for threats to self by measuring anxiety levels using the State-Trait Anxiety Inventory the evening before surgery and 20 to 30 hours after discharge from the PACU. They found a statistically sig-

Table 9.3 – Description of Interdependence Intervention Research Studies (N=7)

Author(s) & Date	Purpose	Sample	Design	Findings
22. Prelewicz (1993)	To examine the effect of animal-assisted therapy on loneliness	Elderly adults residing in a nursing home (N=10)	Quasi-experimental	No statistically significant difference in loneliness before or after animal-assisted therapy program.
23. Parlin (1989/1990)	To determine if there were significant changes in blood pressure and heart rate when petting an unknown dog	Well elderly (N=40)	Quasi-experimental	There was a significant reduction in heart rate but not blood pressure.
24. Francis, Turner & Johnson (1985)	To determine the effect of weekly, domestic animal visitation on geriatric adult patients in adult homes on nine psychosocial variables	Geriatric adults residing in adult homes (N=40)	Quasi-experimental	There were significant differences in seven of nine variables–e.g., social interaction, psychosocial function, life satisfaction, and mental function–between the experimental and control groups.
25. Vogelsang & Ragiel (1987)	To evaluate patients' anxiety levels in response to the presence of a significant other or familiar nurse in the immediate postanesthesia period	Elective surgical patients (N=60)	Quasi-experimental	A reduction in mean state anxiety scores was statistically significant for both treatment groups within 30 hours post-PACU.

26. Neiterman (1987/ 1988)	To determine whether parents' presence in the operating room during the induction of anesthesia would increase their child's cooperation and reduce fluctuations in the child's pulse rate	Children undergoing surgery (N=42)	Quasi-experimental	The children who had parents present for anesthesia administration received significantly higher ratings of cooperation, but no significant difference in pulse rates.
27. Shrubsole (1991/1992)	To determine the effects of a mutual aid group on adaptation to the luteal phase of the menstrual cycle	Female adults with premenstrual syndrome (N=51)	Quasi-experimental	There were no statistically significant differences in the number or severity or symptoms during the luteal phase between the two groups.
28. Komelasky (1990)	To determine if home nursing visits would have a significant effect upon parental anxiety levels and CPR learning in families whose infants were on home cardiorespiratory monitors	Families with apnea-monitored infants (N=28)	Experimental	No significant differences were found in anxiety or knowledge over time between the groups. However, the trends of scores showed that families in the treatment group had a greater decrease in anxiety scores and maintained or improved CPR scores.

nificant reduction in state anxiety mean scores for adults who had significant others or familiar nurses present in the postanesthesia care unit.

Neiterman (1987/1988) evaluated the effect of parents' presence in the operating room during the induction of anesthesia on children's cooperation and heart rate in a study of 42 children. One hospital was used for the experimental group and another for the control group. Neiterman evaluated the oxygenation component of the physiologic mode by measuring heart rate and assessed the coping strategies of the self-concept mode by measuring cooperation. Results were that the children who had parents present for anesthesia administration received significantly higher ratings of cooperation but no statistical difference was noted in heart rate.

The effect of a peer support group—as a nursing intervention—on the luteal phase of the menstrual cycle in 51 women with premenstrual syndrome was evaluated by Shrubsole (1991/1992). The women randomly assigned to the experimental group attended six mutual-aid meetings during a 3-month period. The control group received no treatment. The focal stimulus was identified as the luteal phase of the menstrual cycle; the contextual stimulus was identified as the gonadal steroid-induced change in opiate activity; and residual stimuli were identified as family dynamics and social stress. The physical and personal components of the self-concept mode were evaluated by measuring self-esteem, powerlessness, anxiety, helplessness, and shame. The role function mode was evaluated by measuring the inability to cope with activities of daily living. The interdependence mode was evaluated by measuring withdrawal and isolation. The physiologic mode was evaluated by measuring the frequency and severity of headaches, edema, skin problems, increased or decreased appetite, and constipation. Results were that no significant differences existed in the number or severity of symptoms during the luteal phase between the groups. Support-group participants, however, reported more effective coping with their symptoms after attending support meetings.

Komelasky (1990) evaluated the effects of nurses' visits on parental anxiety levels and cardiopulmonary resuscitation (CPR) learning in 28 parents whose infants required cardiorespiratory monitoring for apnea at home. A two-group design was used. Experimental-group families received three visits from the researcher during the 6-week post-discharge period. Komelasky manipulated the variables of learning CPR and monitor use, the environment and timing of instruction, and the opportunity for parents to discuss fears and stresses. The self-concept mode was measured by evaluating parental anxiety levels. The role-function mode was measured by evaluating CPR knowledge. Families in the treatment group had a greater decrease in anxiety scores and either maintained or improved their CPR scores. However these differences were not statistically significant.

Critical Analyses of Reported Research

The 28 intervention research studies were critically analyzed using specific criteria developed by the BBARNS members to assess the quality of the research as described in Chapter 2.

Critical analyses of quantitative research. In approximately 75% of the studies, investigators made at least a partial effort to control for threats to internal or external validity (see Table 9.4). Instrument reliability and validity data were reported completely in 70% of the studies. Investigators for approximately 73% of studies appropriately analyzed data, and 90% reported results accurately. Consistency between the findings and conclusions was present in most of the studies. In most studies, convenience samples were used and most investigators discussed the effects of the homogeneity of the samples on the generalizability of the findings.

In approximately half of the studies, researchers took adequate measures to control for threats to internal validity. For example, Carson (1991/1992) controlled for internal validity by randomly assigning subjects to control and experimental groups. Additionally, the study data were collected in two humidity- and temperature-controlled, sound-attenuated rooms connected via wires to an adjoining control room where the experimental apparatus was located. In this laboratory setting, the subjects were exposed to a physically uncomfortable procedure called the cold pressor test. Subjective and physiologic measures were obtained at points before, during, and after the testing. Variables such as gender, fatigue, and present level of stress were tested for possible covariate effects by using standardized instruments with known reliability.

Shrubsole (1991/1992) made efforts to control for internal validity by using a post-test only control-group design and a convenience sample with random assignment of subjects. The exclusion criteria for the sample made controlling for internal validity easier. For example, the sample criteria included the following: age range in the reproductive years; not taking nutritional supplements, diuretics, oral contraceptives, or other regular medication; not planning to become pregnant or move; having regular menses; absence of significant gynecologic conditions; and presence of moderate to severe premenstrual symptoms that interfered with adaptation.

In one-fourth of the studies, researchers only partially met the criteria for controlling for internal validity. For example, Jones (1994) evaluated the outcome measures of a managed-care clinical system compared to a conventional system in one intensive care nursery. Threats to internal validity included effects of history such as the opening of a maternal-fetal diagnostic and treatment center and an institution-wide, cost-effectiveness study during the period when implementation of the managed-care system was taking place. These environmental changes could have influ-

Table 9.4 – Critical Analysis of Intervention Research (N=28)

Criteria	Evaluation		
	Yes	*Partially*	*No*
Design			
Efforts to control for threats to internal validity	3, 7, 8, 9, 10, 11, 12, 13, 14, 16, 18, 19, 27	1, 15, 17, 21, 22, 23, 24, 28	2, 4, 5, 6, 20, 25, 26
Efforts to control for threats to external validity	3, 7, 8, 9, 10, 11, 12, 13, 14, 16, 17, 18, 19, 27	1, 6, 15, 20, 21, 22, 23, 24, 25, 28	2, 4, 5, 26
Measurement			
Reliability of instruments addressed	2, 4, 6, 7, 8, 10, 13, 14, 15, 16, 17, 18, 19, 22, 23, 24, 25, 27, 28	1, 3, 5, 9, 11, 12, 21, 26	20
Validity of instruments addressed	2, 4, 6, 7, 8, 10, 11, 12, 13, 14, 16, 17, 18, 19, 20, 21, 22, 23, 25, 27, 28	1, 3, 5, 9, 12, 15, 24	26
Data analysis			
Appropriate	1, 3, 4, 5, 6, 7, 8, 10, 12, 13, 14, 15, 16, 17, 18, 19, 20, 21, 22, 23, 25, 27	2, 9, 11, 24, 26, 28	
Interpretation of results			
Consistency of findings with conclusions	1, 3, 4, 5, 6, 7, 8, 9, 10, 11, 12, 13, 14, 16, 17, 18, 19, 20, 21, 22, 23, 24, 27	2, 15, 25, 26, 28	

Key: 1=Guzzetta, 1979; 2=Zonca, 1980; 3=Hjelm-Karlsson, 1989; 4=Meeker, 1994; 5=Grunstra & Rowe, 1992/1993; 6=Vincenzi & Thiel, 1992; 7=Gilbert, 1991/1992; 8=Newman, 1991; 9=Campbell, 1992; 10=Gaberson, 1991; 11=Meek, 1993; 12=Komara, 1991/1992; 13=Modrcin-McCarthy, 1992/1993; 14=Garcia & White-Traut, 1993; 15=Houston, 1993; 16=Carson, 1991/1992; 17=Riegel, Heywood, Jackson, & Kennedy 1988; 18=Fahs, 1991/1992; 19=Roberson, 1987; 20=Smith, 1989; 21=Jones, 1994; 22=Prelewicz, 1993; 23=Parlin, 1988/1990; 24=Francis, Turner, & Johnson, 1985; 25=Vogelsang & Ragiel, 1987; 26=Neiterman, 1987/1988; 27=Shrubsole, 1991/1992; 28=Komelasky, 1990.

enced the outcome measures including the complexity of behavioral responses of the neonates. The fact that the study included only one facility was a threat to external generalizability.

In approximately half of the studies, investigators took adequate measures to control for threats to external validity. Gilbert (1990/1991) controlled for threats to external validity by randomly assigning girls who had been sexually abused to a structured-group nursing intervention. The control groups consisted of 13 girls who had been sexually abused and received standard treatment and a group of 17 girls from the community who were not sexually abused and did not receive treatment. Repeated-measures methodology was used and means derived from the same subjects were measured over time, thus reducing the required sample size. Preparing for attrition, Gilbert set a goal of 45 for sample size and, therefore, had an adequate sample size.

In one-fourth of the studies, investigators made at least partial efforts to control for threats to external validity. For example, in studying the effect of weekly domestic-animal visits on geriatric patients, Francis and colleagues (1985) used a pre- post-test, control-group design. Participants were not randomly selected but were assigned according to their residence.

Gaberson (1990) provided an example of efforts to address appropriately both internal and external validity. This investigator evaluated the effect of humorous distraction on preoperative anxiety, using an experimental post-test design with clear sample-exclusion criteria. Preoperative anxiety was measured using a visual analog scale, which had been tested and highly correlated in a previous study with the Spielberger State Anxiety Inventory. However, in this pilot study, the small sample size ($N=15$) might not have met basic statistical assumptions.

In two-thirds of the studies, researchers adequately described the reliability and validity of the instruments. For example, in exploring the effect of discrete muscle activity on stress response, Carson (1991/1992) used plasma specimens to measure blood cortisol levels. Reliability of the testing procedures was described as follows: (a) a known-value control substance provided by Travenol-Genentech Diagnostics was included in every batch of cortisol testing—and in order to be accepted, results had to be within two standard deviations; and (b) laboratory personnel had participated in periodic testing surveys by the College of American Pathologists. The author also used the Hassles and Uplifts Scale and the State-Trait Anxiety Inventory.

In over three-fourths of the studies, investigators used appropriate data analysis and reported conclusions consistent with the findings. Riegel and colleagues (1988) used multivariate analysis of variance with repeated measures and analysis of variance (ANOVA) to analyze data comparing topical placement of nitroglycerin ointment and patients' reports of headache and flushing. Data on headache and flushing were obtained from patients by using a visual analog scale for pain that had been tested previously for reliability and validity. Riegel and colleagues (1988) concluded that the common nursing intervention of teaching patients that side effects of NTG can be decreased by placing the drug at one of these alternate sites may not be effective. The conclusion was based on data from a study of 56 patients with cardiac disease in which researchers found that severity of headache and flushing was not significantly different whether NTG ointment was placed on the upper arm, chest, or pelvis.

Evaluation of Relationships to the Roy Adaptation Model

The 21 intervention studies that were judged to meet the criteria set for empiric adequacy were evaluated for relationships to the RAM. The studies that met criteria for adequacy of the research in the critical analysis and that showed linkages with the model were then used to test propositions from the RAM.

Evaluation of Linkages to the RAM

Evaluation of the linkages of variables in 21 intervention studies and the RAM is summarized in Table 9.5. Two-thirds of the authors explicitly identified the model and linked the research variables with the concepts of the RAM. One-third of the authors discussed the RAM as the conceptual framework for the study and implied linkage to the research variables. Likewise, all authors either explicitly or implicitly linked the research variables with the empiric measures. However, in one third of the studies, the authors did not describe the findings as related to the model. About half that many authors implied the linkage between the model and findings.

Gilbert (1990/1991) and Newman (1991) explicitly discussed the links among the research variables, empiric measures, and findings with the RAM. For example, Newman designated the focal stimulus as arthritis. Demographic and background data such as arthritis education and type of arthritis were designated the contextual stimuli. The physiologic mode was represented by the variable arthritis self-efficacy; the interdependence mode, by perceived social support; the self-concept mode, by purpose and meaning in life; and the mastery aspect of the role function mode, by arthritis impact. Instruments were selected to measure each variable based on an adaptive mode.

The physiologic intervention studies generally explicitly or implicitly indicated the linkages between the research variables and the RAM. The four studies with a nursing intervention providing some form of touch to the subjects explicitly indicated the linkage between the research variables and the RAM (Garcia & White-Traut, 1993; Komara, 1991/1992; Meek, 1993; Modrcin-McCarthy, 1992/1993). All studies indicated tactile stimulation as stimuli and measured some type of physiologic response such as heart rate, blood pressure, or skin temperature.

Table 9.5 – Evaluation of Linkages to the RAM (N=21)

Linkages	Evaluation		
	Explicit	*Implicit*	*Absent*
Research variables	1, 7, 8, 11, 12, 13, 14, 17, 18, 21, 22, 23, 24, 28	3, 9, 10, 15, 16, 19, 27	
Empiric measures	7, 8, 11, 12, 13, 17, 21, 22, 23, 24	1, 3, 9, 10, 14, 15, 16, 18, 19, 27, 28	
Findings	3, 7, 8, 13, 14, 16, 17, 18, 21, 22, 23	1, 15, 27	9, 10, 11, 12, 19, 24, 28

Key: 1=Guzzetta, 1979; 3=Hjelm-Karlsson, 1989; 7=Gilbert, 1991/1992; 8=Newman, 1991; 9=Campbell, 1992; 10=Gaberson, 1991; 11=Meek, 1993; 12 =Komara, 1991/1992; 13=Modrcin-McCarthy, 1992/1993; 14=Garcia & White-Traut, 1993; 15=Houston, 1993; 16=Carson, 1991/1992; 17=Riegel et al., 1988; 18=Fahs, 1991/1992; 19=Roberson, 1987; 21=Jones, 1994; 22=Prelewicz, 1993; 23=Parlin, 1990; 24=Francis et al., 1985; 27=Shrubsole, 1991/1992; 28=Komelasky, 1990.

Riegel and colleagues (1988), and Fahs (1991/1992) explicitly defined the relationship between the research variables and linkage to the RAM. Fahs included a diagram that specifically designated the conceptualization of each variable in the study within the framework of the RAM. In both studies, investigators either explicitly or implicitly related the findings to the model.

Four interdependence intervention studies explicitly indicated research variables linked to the RAM by identifying the intervention as the focal or contextual stimulus (Francis et al., 1985; Komelasky, 1990; Parlin, 1988/1990; Prelewicz, 1993). For example, in the three studies that investigated the effects of animal therapy on the elderly, Francis and colleagues as well as Prelewicz labeled the animal therapy as the focal stimulus. Each study evaluated a different adaptive mode in relation to the outcome of animal therapy.

Approximately half of the authors explicitly identified the model and linked findings to concepts of the RAM. Hjelm-Karlsson (1989) stated the information provided was "accepted" by the cognator subsystem then processed and stored through two cognitive-emotive channels labeled as information processing and learning. During the medical procedure, numerous internal and external stimuli come into focus and are processed by in the regulator and cognator subsystems. Responses to the stimuli were produced and manifested within the four behavioral modes. Houston (1993) investigated rocking as a relaxation technique for the elderly and addressed the interpretation of the findings of the study by discussing components of the RAM.

Evaluation of linkages between the intervention studies and the RAM supported effectiveness of the model in guiding nursing research. All the studies explicitly or implicitly indicated linkage of the research variables and empiric measures to the model—showing support for use of the RAM for experimental and quasi-experimental studies. Gaps in linkages between the findings and the model were present more frequently in articles than in dissertations or theses. Perhaps the space limitations of journals was an issue.

Testing of Propositions from the RAM

All 12 RAM propositions were tested by findings from the 21 studies (See Table 9.6). Regulator and cognator processes affecting innate and acquired ways of adapting at the individual level was illustrated by Campbell (1992) and Hjelm-Karlsson (1989) and at the same time not supported by Hjelm-Karlsson. One study could possibly have multiple results and therefore, findings could support and at the same time not support the same proposition. Campbell (1992) demonstrated the use of techniques from cognitive therapy, which decreased depression in the elderly. Hjelm-Karlsson (1989) reported that people given structured information before undergoing IVP were better able to form mental images of the event than those not given the structured information. However, structured information given to patients did not affect physiologic reactions or adaptation to IVP.

Two authors addressed stabilizer and innovator processes that affected adaptation at the group level. In evaluating nurses' ability to identify reactive depression, Campbell (1992) determined that 92% of the time, nurses were able to accurately identify people who were depressed. In contrast, Fahs (1991/1992) examined the effect of nurses regulating heparin injectate volume on pain and bruising then concluded that volume did not affect either cost of preparation or adaptation to subcutaneous heparin injection.

Three studies showed that characteristics of the internal and external stimuli influence adaptive responses (Garcia & White-Traut, 1993, Houston, 1993; Modrcin-McCarthy, 1992/1993). The following six studies did not show support for the proposition: Houston (1993); Komelasky (1990); Guzzetta (1979); Riegel and colleagues (1988); Gilbert (1990/1991); and Fahs (1991/1992). Garcia and White-Traut (1993) compared preterm infants' respiratory and behavioral state adaptive responses to varied external stimuli during apnea. There were significant differences between tactile stimulation and experimental taste and smell stimulation on length of time required to reinitiate respiratory efforts in infants. The results of this study showed clear support for the proposition.

Modrcin-McCarthy (1992/1993) suggested that external stimuli such as receiving gentle human touching influenced adaptation of infants by increasing time awake over the 10-day study period compared to those in the control group. Infants in the experimental group appeared more relaxed. In contrast, Houston (1993) concluded that elderly adults exposed to the external stimulus of rocking had decreases in heart rate, yet showed no significant variation in either systolic or diastolic blood pressure.

Komelasky (1990) reported that the external stimulus of home nursing visits did not have a significant effect upon parental anxiety levels and learning of CPR. Gilbert (1990/1991) found no significant difference between the experimental and control groups when evaluating the effectiveness of a structured group nursing intervention in promoting adaptation of girls who had been sexually abused.

Riegel and colleagues (1988) reported no significant differences in the severity of headache or flushing among three nitroglycerin placement sites. Fahs (1991/1992) examined the effect of heparin injectate volume on pain and bruising and found that volume did not affect bruise formation, size, or pain.

The effects of internal and external stimuli on the adequacy of cognitive and emotional processes was supported by Guzzetta (1979), Gaberson (1991), and Carson (1991/1992). Guzzetta found that the mean level of anxiety varied with the timing of teaching. Gaberson concluded that subjects who experienced no intervention during their wait before surgery reported the highest levels of preoperative anxiety. Gaberson also reported that anxiety levels did not significantly differ in preoperative patients who listened to either humorous audiotapes or tranquil music as external stimuli. Carson concluded that the external stimulus of discrete muscle activity appeared to have a positive effect on stress response as indicated in subjective reports.

The adequacy of cognator and regulator processes affecting adaptive responses was tested and supported by Roberson (1987). No significant differences in oral temperature before and after small-nebulizer inhalation treatment were found among the four groups of subjects.

Adaptation in one mode being affected by adaptation in other modes through cognator and regulator connectives was demonstrated by Francis and colleagues (1985), Newman (1991), and Guzzetta (1979). Those who did not support that finding included Fahs (1991/1992), Carson (1991/1992), Newman (1991), Guzzetta (1979), and Hjelm-Karlsson (1988). Francis and colleagues (1985) found that subjects receiving animal visitation showed significant differences in social interaction, psychosocial function, life satisfaction, mental function, depression, social competence, and

Table 9.6 – Testing of Propositions from the RAM (*N*=21)

Propositions from the RAM	Ancillary and practice propositions	Supported by results	Not Supported by results
1. At the individual level, regulator and cognator processes affect innate and acquired ways of adapting.	a. Cognitive therapy decreases depression.	Campbell (1992)	
	b. Education assists in forming mental images of the event.	Hjelm-Karlsson (1989)	
	c. Education affects physiologic reactions.		Hjelm-Karlsson (1989)
2. At the group level, stabilizer and innovator processes affect adaptation.	a. Nurses are able to accurately identify individuals who are depressed.	Campbell (1992)	
	b. Nurses can affect preparation costs of injections by decreasing dose injectate volume.		Fahs (1991/1992)
3. The characteristics of the internal and external stimuli influence adaptive responses.	a. Taste/smell stimulation shortens time required to reinitiate respiratory effort in infants.	Garcia & White-Traut (1993)	
	b. Taste/smell stimulation requires a shorter period of intervention for infants.	Garcia & White-Traut (1993)	
	c. Infants receiving taste/smell stimulation maintain baseline sleep state after intervention.	Garcia & White-Traut (1993)	
	d. Tactile stimulation changed sleep state from sleep to alert in infants.	Garcia & White-Traut (1993)	

e. Gentle human touching stimulation decreases active sleep of infants.	Modrcin-McCarthy (1992/1993)
f. Gentle human touching decreases motor activity in infants.	Modrcin-McCarthy (1992/1993)
g. Gentle human touching decreases motor activity, movement, behavioral distress cues, drowsiness; and increases quiet sleep.	Modrcin-McCarthy (1992/1993)
h. Vestibular-proprioceptive stimulation (rocking) facilitates a decrease in heart rate.	Houston (1993)
i. Rocking affects blood pressure.	Houston (1993)
j. Home nursing visits affect parental anxiety or learning.	Komelasky (1990)
k. Time of learning and physiologic anxiety is correlated in patients.	Guzzetta (1979)
l. Placement site of topical medication effects severity of headache or flushing.	Riegel et al., 1988
m. Subsequent doses of topical medication affect headache and flushing when placed at different sites compared with severity of such side effects when placed at previous sites.	Riegel et al., 1988
n. Education and support effects adaptation.	Gilbert (1990/1991)

(continued)

Table 9.6 (continued)

Propositions from the RAM	Ancillary and practice propositions	Supported by results	Not Supported by results
	o. Injectrate volume affects size of bruise formation and pain.		Fahs (1991/1992)
4. The characteristics of the internal and external stimuli influence the adequacy of cognitive and emotional processes.	a. Timing of teaching affects psychological anxiety.	Guzzetta (1979)	
	b. Music and humor reduce anxiety.	Gaberson (1991)	
	c. Discrete muscle activity has a positive psychological effect on stress response.	Carson (1991/1992)	
5. The adequacy of cognator and regulator processes will affect adaptive responses.	Respiratory treatment does not affect oral temperature.	Roberson (1987)	
6. Adaptation in one mode is affected by adaptation in other modes through cognator and regulator connectives.	a. Animal visitation positively affects social interaction, psychosocial function, life satisfaction, mental function, depression, social competence, and psychologic well being.	Francis et al. (1985)	
	b. Self-help group facilitates self-efficacy for pain management.	Newman (1991)	
	c. Psychological anxiety and learning are inversely correlated.	Guzzetta (1979)	

d. Animal visitation affects health self concept despite changes in social interaction, psycho-social function, life satisfaction, mental function, depression, social competence and psychologic well being. — Francis et al. (1985)

e. There is an association between size of bruise formation and pain response. — Fahs (1991/1992)

f. Discrete muscle activity has an effect on physiologic stress response. — Carson (1992)

g. Self-help group affects self-efficacy for function, perceived social support, arthritis impact scores, and total life purpose. — Newman (1991)

h. There is a correlation between levels of urinary cortisol and psychological anxiety. — Guzetta (1979)

7. The pooled effect of focal, contextual, and residual stimuli determines the adaptation level.

a. Vestibular-proprioceptive stimulation (rocking) facilitates a decrease in heart rate. — Houston (1993)

b. There are gender differences in heart rate and systolic blood pressure and subjective stress response. — Carson (1991/1992)

c. Rocking affects blood pressure. — Houston (1993)

8. Adaptation is influenced by the integration of the person with the environment.

Activity and heart rate are increased when exposed to music or vibroacoustic stimulation. — Komara (1991/1992)

(continued)

Table 9.6 (continued)

Propositions from the RAM	Ancillary and practice propositions	Supported by results	Not Supported by results
9. The variable of time influences the process of adaptation.	a. Learning is affected by timing of teaching during recovery.	Guzzetta (1979)	
	b. Oral temperature is affected by timing of measurement after respiratory treatments.	Roberson (1987)	
10. The variable of perception influences the process of adaptation.	Satisfaction changes under a managed care system versus a conventional care system.		Jones (1994)
11. Perception influences adaptation through linking the regulator and cognator subsystems.	a. Education prior to medical procedure reduces pain and discomfort.	Hjelm-Karlsson (1989)	
	b. Level of stress and fatigue affect psychologic perception of a stressful event.	Carson (1991/1992)	
12. The goal of nursing interventions is to enhance adaptation by managing input to adaptive systems.	a. Teaching increases learning.	Guzzetta (1979)	
	b. Massage promotes relaxation.	Meek (1993)	
	c. Petting a dog reduces blood pressure but not heart rate.	Parlin (1988/1990)	
	d. Animal-assisted therapy decreases loneliness.		Prelewicz (1993)
	e. Education and support groups affect severity of symptoms.		Shrubsole (1991/1992)

psychological well being. Newman (1991) reported that arthritis self-efficacy for pain-management scores were significantly higher for those in a self-help course than for those of nonparticipants. However Newman found no significant differences in scores in arthritis self-efficacy for function, perceived social support, arthritis impact scores, and purpose in life between groups; and thus did not support the proposition.

Guzzetta (1979) found that psychological anxiety and learning are inversely correlated when exploring the relationship among learning, anxiety, and timing of a teaching intervention in adult cardiac patients, which supported the proposition. Guzzetta also found no correlation between levels of urinary cortisol and psychological anxiety, which did not support the proposition.

The pooled effect of focal, contextual, and residual stimuli on determining adaptation level was illustrated by Carson (1991/1992). The effect of discrete muscle activity on stress response revealed significant gender differences in regard to heart rate, systolic blood pressure, and subjective stress response.

Komara (1991/1992) investigated the effects of music and vibroacoustic stimulation on fetal heart rate and fetal movement during nonstress tests and observed that both increased when either music or the vibroacoustic stimulator was introduced. Adaptation was influenced by the integration of the person with the environment.

The effects of time on adaptation was supported by Guzzetta (1979) and Roberson (1987). Guzzetta (1979) found that learning was significantly increased when begun at least 1 week after transfer from the CCU. Roberson (1987) reported oral temperatures were affected by the timing of measurement when patients were using small-nebulizer inhalation treatments.

The variable of perception influencing adaptation through cognator and regulator processes was not supported by Jones (1994). Reports of satisfaction of parents, professional nurses, and health care team members did not change under the managed-care system when compared with the conventional system in a neonatal intensive care unit (ICU). However, this proposition was supported by Hjelm-Karlsson (1988) and Carson (1991/1992). Hjelm-Karlsson (1988) found less pain and discomfort during IVP in the group which had received the preteaching. When exploring the effect of discrete muscle activity on stress response, Carson reported that stress level and fatigue appeared to have significant covariate effects on perception of a stressful event.

Three studies showed that the goal of nursing intervention is to enhance adaptation by managing input to adaptive systems. Guzzetta (1979) concluded that learning was significantly greater after cardiac rehabilitation teaching. Meek (1993) reported that SSBM produced statistically significant decreases in blood pressure, heart rate, and increases in skin temperature, thereby enhancing adaptation in hospice patients. Parlin (1988/1990), who evaluated physiologic changes in the elderly when petting an unknown dog, reported a statistically significant reduction in blood pressure but not heart rate. Interventions reported by Prelewicz (1993) and Shrubsole (1992) did not decrease loneliness or severity of symptoms, respectively, and therefore did not support the proposition.

Synthesis of Intervention Research: Contributions to Nursing Science

Included in this section is information about the 21 studies that met the guidelines for adequate critical analysis and linkages to the RAM. Intervention research is discussed relative to implications for nursing practice, research, and further theory development.

Applications to Nursing Practice

The findings from six studies conducted by Campbell (1992), Carson (1991/1992), Hjelm-Karlsson (1988), Gaberson (1991), Guzzetta (1979), and Newman (1991) have good potential for being implemented in nursing practice (Table 9.7). Based on the fact that these researchers introduced interventions that exposed the patient to minimal risk and significant benefits, their studies were rated as having a high potential for implementation. The BBARNS investigators encourage replication of intervention studies in other settings and with other populations to ensure the well being of clients and to promote nursing practice based on a solid foundation of nursing research.

Campbell (1992) used techniques from cognitive therapy to care for depressed elderly patients. Cognitive therapy, used often in the practice of behavioral medicine, is based on a body of research that has substantiated its effectiveness. Nurses are in a particularly good position to use cognitive therapy with a variety of patient groups and settings.

The intervention of using discrete muscle activity to lift a small barbell is risk free and showed a positive effect on psychological adaptation to stress (Carson, 1991/1992). The intervention might be appropriate as a distraction for a burned patient when a nurse is implementing a painful treatment such as changing a dressing.

Structured information is an appropriate intervention before any potentially painful medical procedure (Hjelm-Karlsson, 1988). The cost of the intervention reviewed was minimal and the benefits were significant for patients.

The nursing intervention used by Gaberson (1991) required little time, yet provided worthwhile outcomes. Offering music and humor audiotapes to subjects having medical procedures or surgery may be an appropriate nursing action in many situations. Patients about to participate in a painful stretching session during rehabilitation may benefit from such an intervention.

Guzzetta (1979) evaluated the relationship among learning levels, anxiety, and teaching levels in adult cardiac patients and found that anxiety and learning are inversely correlated. The timing of teaching affected reported anxiety levels for post-MI patients but did not alter physiologic effects of anxiety. Whether nurses practice in an ICU or in a rehabilitation hospital, selecting the best time for patient teaching can enhance patient learning. This becomes possible when nurses understand the relationship between anxiety and learning.

Newman (1991) reported that the arthritis self-help group facilitated arthritis self-efficacy for pain management and other symptoms. Nurses are in a position to provide these courses to reduce the symptoms of this chronic illness.

It was concluded that the following studies need clinical further evaluation before implementation. The intervention described by Fahs (1991/1992) is noteworthy and significant to nurses concerned about pain or discomfort associated with frequent injections. However further clinical evaluation is necessary to determine the applicability of the finding to nurses giving other injections, such as insulin. Likewise, nurses in home care and other settings could continue to evaluate the effectiveness of animal visitation in promoting adaptation in multiple modes.

Garcia and White-Traut (1993) found that the length of time required to reinitiate respiratory effort using the swabstick was shorter than traditional tactile stimulation. The intervention appeared to meet the goal of reinitiating respiration while promoting physiologic adaptation and decreasing energy expenditure. Clinical nurse experts can evaluate the intervention in this population for its effectiveness in comparison with other interventions. Other examples of nursing interventions which are cost effective, clinically relevant, and feasible to implement with minimal resources include those used by Houston (1993) and Meek (1993). Clinical nurse experts should continue evaluating effects of vibroacoustic stimulation (Komara, 1991/1992) and gentle touching (Modrcin-McCarthy, 1992/1993) to identify and manage focal and contextual stimuli for this vulnerable population.

Nurses often teach patients that nitroglycerin side effects can be decreased by alternating sites, but Riegel and colleagues (1988) did not find support for this intervention. Because the knowledge is important for nurses working with patients who may have limited placement sites, such research should be replicated and expanded. Nurses should also be aware that respiratory treatments can have an effect on oral temperatures (Roberson, 1987).

<u>Table 9.7 – Potential for Implementation from Intervention Research</u>
<u>(N=21)</u>

Category One: High potential for implementation
Campbell (1992)
Carson (1991/1992)
Hjelm-Karlsson (1989)
Gaberson (1991)
Guzzetta (1979)
Newman (1991)

Category Two: Needs further clinical evaluation before implementation
Fahs (1991/1992)
Francis et al. (1985)
Garcia & White-Traut (1993)
Houston (1993)
Komara (1991/1992)
Meek (1993)
Modrcin-McCarthy (1992/1993)
Parlin (1988/1990)
Riegel et al. (1988)
Roberson (1987)

Category Three: Further research indicated before implementation
Jones (1994)
Gilbert (1990/1991)
Komelasky (1990)
Shrubsole (1991/1992)
Prelewicz (1993)

The following studies should be tested further before findings are implemented in practice. Jones (1994) evaluated the outcomes of a managed-care system versus a conventional system in one intensive care nursery. However the study should be replicated because the results contradict findings from other research. Investigators of three studies (Komelasky, 1990; Gilbert, 1990/1991; Shrubsole, 1991/1992) reported education or support groups were not effective in promoting adaptation. These studies should be replicated because some evidence indicates that such intervention might be effective in certain circumstances. Education and support-group interventions vary and thus must be clearly described in reports of research so that they may be evaluated and replicated.

Prelewicz (1993) reported that elderly residents of long-term care who participated in animal-assisted therapy did not experience decreased loneliness. This study could be replicated in combination with the studies by

Francis and colleagues (1985) and Parlin (1988/1990) to determine effectiveness of this intervention over time and reevaluate its effects on physiologic, self concept, and interdependence modes.

Recommendations for Model-Based Research

Recommendations for future research using the RAM are derived from the critical analysis and also relate to sample selection and size. A full research report includes evidence that investigators considered requirements of sample size needed to test the hypotheses using techniques such as power analysis. Such considerations can add to the advancement of nursing science. While studies considered in this monograph generally indicated exclusion criteria for subjects, randomization of subject treatment was not often addressed.

Conflicting results among studies can occur and such studies will be evaluated and replicated. For example, Francis and colleagues (1985) reported that animal visitation positively affected social interaction, psychosocial function, life satisfaction, mental function, depression, social comptentence, and psychological well-being. Parlin (1988/1990) reported a decrease in blood pressure when elderly clients petted an unknown dog. Prelewicz (1993) reported that animal therapy did not decrease loneliness. If such studies were repeated in different settings or with different populations, generalizability could increase.

Replication of studies was uncommon among those included in this chapter. However replication is crucial for developing a body of knowledge on which to base nursing practice. Description of intervention protocols is important and should be detailed so that studies can be replicated to help ensure generalizability.

Results from Komelasky (1990), Gilbert (1990/1991) and Shrubsole (1991/1992) indicated that education and support groups were not effective in promoting adaptation while results reported by Newman (1991) and Hjelm-Karlsson (1988) supported that such groups were effective. Further investigation into the elements of education and support group interventions that are effective will be helpful in designing and testing future interventions for practice.

Investigations of interventions that facilitate relaxation are particularly pertinent to nursing practice. Meek (1993) and Houston (1993) examined methods to promote relaxation laying the groundwork for future research to promote effective relaxation for many patient populations in many age groups and settings.

Directions for Theory and RAM Development

Nursing intervention research based on the RAM was used to derive directions for further development of theory and the nursing model. From the seven propositions not supported by the research, three specific areas were identified for future model development. Characteristics of the internal and external stimuli that influence adaptation should be further developed and clarified. While specific stimuli were evaluated, results indicated that they did not influence adaptation. For example, Guzzetta (1979) reported that time of learning and physiologic anxiety were not correlated. Riegel and colleagues (1988) concluded that placement site of nitroglycerin does not affect severity of headache or flushing. The proposition that adaptation in one mode is affected by adaptation in other modes through cognator and regulator connectives was not supported in four studies. Indications were that adaptation in one mode might not influence adaptation in other modes through cognator and regulator subsysems, which necessitates further clarification of the propositions.

The goal of enhancing adaptation through interventions that manage input to adaptive systems was not supported in two studies. The interventions tested did not enhance adaptation, despite management of input. Possible reasons for negative findings include the inherent difficulty of designing intervention studies and selecting adequate methods for measuring outcomes. Further clarification of this proposition is necessary to provide direction for definitive research on such interventions as managing stimuli.

Summary

Studies that were focused on nursing interventions as derived from the RAM were reviewed in this chapter. Of the 163 studies included in this monograph, 28 were identified as intervention research. The research studies were critically analyzed, relationships of the studies to the RAM were evaluated, and contributions of the studies to nursing science were synthesized.

Study results indicate support for the use of the RAM in guiding intervention research and nursing practice. In addition, the use of the RAM facilitates further knowledge development for understanding interrelationships among theory, research, and practice.

References

Campbell, J.M. (1992). Treating depression in well older adults: Use of diaries in cognitive therapy. *Issues in Mental Health Nursing, 13*, 19-29.

Carson, M.A. (1992). The effect of discrete muscle activity on stress response (Doctoral dissertation, Boston College, 1991). *Dissertation Abstracts International, 52*, 5757-B.

Fahs, P.S. (1992). Effect of heparin injectate volume on pain and bruising using the Roy Model (Doctoral dissertation, University of Alabama, 1991). *Dissertation Abstracts International, 52*, 5195-B.

Francis, G., Turner, J.T., & Johnson, S.B. (1985). Domestic animal visitation as therapy with adult home residents. *International Journal of Nursing Studies, 22,* 201-206.

Gaberson. K.B. (1991). The effect of humorous distraction on preoperative anxiety. *AORN Journal, 54,* 1258-1264.

Garcia, A.P., & White-Traut, R. (1993). Preterm infants' responses to taste/smell and tactile stimulation during an apneic episode. *Journal of Pediatric Nursing, 8,* 145-52.

Gilbert, C.M. (1991). A structured group nursing intervention for girls who have been sexually abused utilizing Roy's theory of the person as an adaptive system (Doctoral dissertation, University of South Carolina, 1990). *Dissertation Abstracts International, 52,* 1350-B.

Grunstra, E.A., & Rowe, S. (1993). The effects of a prenatal breast-feeding class on breast-feeding success and maternal perception of the infant: A replication (Master's thesis, Grand Valley State University, 1992). *Masters Abstracts International, 31,* 1736.

Guzzetta, C.E. (1979). Relationship between stress and learning. *Advances in Nursing Science, 1*(4), 35-39.

Hjelm-Karlsson, K. (1989). Effects of information to patients undergoing intravenous pyelography: An intervention study. *Journal of Advanced Nursing, 14,* 853-62.

Houston, K. A. (1993). An investigation of rocking as relaxation for the elderly. *Geriatric Nursing, 14,* 186-89.

Jones, M.L.H. (1994). Outcome measures of managed care in an intensive care nursery. Unpublished doctoral dissertation, University of Florida, Gainesville.

Komara, C.A. (1992). Effects of music on fetal response (Master's thesis, Bellarmine College, 1991). *Masters Abstracts International, 30,* 300.

Komelasky, A.L. (1990). The effect of home nursing visits on parental anxiety and CPR knowledge retention of parents of apnea-monitored infants. *Journal of Pediatric Nursing, 5,* 387-92.

Meek, Sr. S. (1993). Effects of slow stroke back massage on relaxation in hospice clients. *Image: Journal of Nursing Scholarship, 25,* 17-21.

Meeker, B.J. (1994). Preoperative patient education: Evaluating postoperative patient outcomes. *Patient Education and Counseling, 23,* 41-47.

Modrcin-McCarthy, M.A.J. (1993). The physiological and behavioral effects of a gentle human touch nursing intervention on preterm infants (Doctoral dissertation, The University of Tennessee, 1992). *Dissertation Abstracts International, 54,* 1336-B.

Neiterman, E. W. (1988). Assessment of parents' presence during anesthesia induction of children (Master's thesis, University of Lowell, 1987). *Masters Abstracts International, 26,* 109.

Newman, A.M. (1991). The effect of the arthritis self-help course on arthritis self-efficacy, perceived social support, purpose and meaning in life, and arthritis impact in people with arthritis (Doctoral dissertation, University of Alabama at Birmingham, 1991). *Dissertation Abstracts International, 52,* 2995-B.

Parlin, C.A. (1990). Physiological manifestations of human/animal interaction in the adult population over fifty-five (Master's thesis, University of Nevada, Reno, 1988). *Masters Abstracts International, 28,* 113.

Prelewicz, T.N. (1993). The effects of animal-assisted therapy on loneliness in elderly residents of a long-term care facility utilizing Roy's adaptation model (Master's thesis, D'Youville College, 1993). *Masters Abstracts International, 31,* 1749.

Riegel, B., Heywood, G., Jackson, W., & Kennedy, A. (1988). Effect of nitroglycerin ointment placement on the severity of headache and flushing in patients with cardiac disease. *Heart & Lung, 17,* 426-431.

Roberson, E.L.M. (1987). Changes in oral temperature after small nebulizer inhalation treatment in adult clients. Unpublished master's thesis, Northwestern State University, Shreveport.

Roy, C., & Andrews, H. (1991). *The Roy Adaptation Model: The Definitive Statement.* East Norwalk, CT: Appleton & Lange.

Roy, C., & Andrews, H. (1999), *The Roy adaptation model.* Stamford, CT: Appleton & Lange.

Roy, C., & Anway, J. (1989). *Roy's Adaptation Model: Theories for nursing administration.* In B. Henry, M. DiVincenti, G. Marriner-Tooney (Eds.) Dimensions of nursing administration: Theory, research, education and practice (pp. 75-88). St. Louis, MO: Mosby.

Shrubsole, J.L. (1992). Mutual aid: Promoting adaptation in women with premenstrual syndrome (Master's thesis, D'Youville College, 1991). *Masters Abstracts International, 30,* 1301.

Smith, C.J. (1989). Cardiovascular responses in healthy males during basin bath, tub bath and shower (Master's thesis, Texas Woman's University, 1987). *Masters Abstracts International, 27,* 103.

Vincenzi, A.E., & Thiel, R. (1992). AIDS education on college campus: Roy's adaptation model directs inquiry. *Public Health Nursing, 9,* 270-76.

Vogelsang, J., & Ragiel, C. (1987). Anxiety levels in female surgical patients. *Journal of Post Anesthesia Nursing, 11,* 230-36.

Zonca, B.J. (1980). The effects of a formal in-hospital patient education program on anxiety in postmyocardial infarction patients (Doctoral dissertation, Wayne State University, 1980). *Dissertation Abstracts International, 41,* 1418-A.

Bibliography

Beck, S. (1991). *Designing a study.* In M. Mateo & K. Kirchoff (Eds.) *Conducting and using nursing research in the clinical setting* (pp. 167-174). Baltimore, MD: Williams & Wilkins.

Mateo, M. & Schira, M. (1991). *Exploring innovative ways in giving nursing care.* In M. Mateo & K. Kirchoff (Eds). Conducting and using nursing research in the clinical setting (pp. 81-91). Baltimore, MD: Williams & Wilkins.

Chapter 10

Measurement of the Model Concepts

Measurement of the concepts from the Roy Adaptation Model (RAM) was an important dimension in all phases of the research project. Evaluation of measurement strategies used in the research based on RAM consisted of analysis of instruments used in the 163 studies—both existing instruments and those developed specifically for the research. The purposes of this chapter are to (a) evaluate the appropriateness of instruments used to measure major concepts of the RAM; (b) identify contributions to nursing science from instrument-development studies for measurement of model concepts; and (c) derive directions for future work on measurement of the RAM concepts.

Each of the instruments identified in the analysis of research in Chapters 3 through 9, was classified according to the major concepts of the model. Reliability and validity of the measures and tools were reported as part of the critical analyses in the content chapters. Studies that were focused on instrument development were analyzed for contributions to measurement of the RAM concepts. Instruments that met a given standard related to criteria for critical analysis were considered appropriate for research using the RAM and were therefore included in the chapter. The standard of criteria analysis for instruments consisted of two basic assumptions for model-based research: first, consistency of research variables with model concepts, and second, consistency of empiric measures with concepts. Contributions to nursing science included identification of available instruments appropriate for measuring model concepts and areas where further work on measurement of the RAM is needed.

Instrument Evaluation

Instruments were categorized as measuring one of the seven major concepts of the RAM. These were the same concepts that served as the basis for organization of the model-based research (see Chapter 2); the four adaptive modes, stimuli, intervention, and adaptive processes. Theoretic definitions of the concepts (see Table 10.1) were derived from published works of the theorist, primarily Roy and Andrews (1991).

Classification of Instruments

The first classification of instruments was according to the major design categories of quantitative, qualitative, and methodologic or instrument-development studies. Of the studies, 137 were classified as quantitative, 16 as qualitative, and 9 as instrument development. For a study to be classified as an instrument-development study, the major aim of the study was to develop an instrument to specifically test one of the concepts of the RAM. In some cases, instrument design was part of a study classified as qualitative or quantitative. Furthermore, in many of the quantitative studies the researchers used strategies such as interview schedules or open-ended questionnaires to obtain qualitative data about RAM concepts.

Critical analysis for each measurement strategy was accomplished through several steps. Members of BBARNS, using the seven content areas based on the major concepts of the model, completed a critical appraisal form for all measures used in each study. The form included identification of the concept and empiric measurement, description of the measurement, and an evaluation of the relationships of the research variable and the empiric indicators to the model concepts (see Table 10.2). Measurement strategies were analyzed based on the primary focus of the content chapter and other major concepts that were reported in the study. For example, in Chapter 4, Physiologic Adaptation, if the author stated that responses were measured in adaptive modes in addition to the physiologic mode, then those instruments were also included.

Critical appraisal forms were then used to categorize all instruments by concept area. This step facilitated analyzing similarities and differences among researchers in measuring the same concept.

Criteria for Critical Analysis

Critical analyses of measurement strategies consisted of two basic assumptions for model-based research. The first was that the empiric indicator was clearly related to the model concept. The second required consistency between the operational and theoretic definitions. Instruments and tools that met these criteria were considered appropriate for research using the RAM and were therefore included in the evaluation.

Three areas were considered in appraising the relationship of each operational indicator to the model: (a) the model concept the researcher purported to measure, (b) identification of the research variable, and (c) the name of the instrument or the specific strategy used to collect the relevant data. Further, both the relationships of the research variable and the empiric indicator to the RAM concept were required to be either explicitly or implicitly identified. Relationships of the research variable and the empiric indicator to the RAM concept were verified by at least two members of the research team for the measure to be included.

Appropriateness of the measure was also determined by comparing the description of the instrument with the theoretic definition. The intent was not an in-depth analysis of the instruments, but that the relationship

Table 10.1 – Theoretic Definitions of Major Concepts from the RAM

Major concept	Theoretic definitions
1. Physiologic adaptive mode	The needs and processes whereby an individual maintains physiologic integrity. Includes structures that promote physiologic adaptation related to needs for oxygenation, nutrition, elimination, rest and activity, and protection, and the complex process of fluid and electrolytes, endocrine, and neurologic balance.
2. Self-concept adaptive mode	The composite of beliefs and feelings one holds about oneself aimed at maintaining psychic integrity. It includes perceptions of the physical self (body sensation and body image), and the personal self (self-consistency, self-ideal, and the moral-ethical, spiritual self).
3. Role function adaptive mode	Behavior related to interactive positions in a society that strives for social integrity. Roles involve sets of expectations about how a person occupying a given position in society behaves toward a person occupying another position.
4. Interdependence adaptive mode	Interactions in close relationships that maintain "affectional adequacy." The mode emphasizes the willingness and ability to give and receive love, respect, and value in relations with others.
5. Stimuli	Three types of stimuli make up the adaptation level. (a) Focal- The factor most immediately confronting the person that calls for an adaptive response. (b) Contextual - Other factors present that contribute to the behavior initiated by the focal stimulus. (c) Residual - Background factors that affect the situation but cannot be validated or measured directly.
6. Interventions	Nursing interventions that are based on the model and identify the stimuli that are managed in the intervention. The goal of nursing interventions is to facilitate adaptation by managing internal and external stimuli.
7. Adaptive processes	All the innate and acquired ways of responding to the changing environment. The primary adaptive processes for the individual are inherent in the regulator subsystem that includes neural, chemical, and endocrine processes; and the cognator subsystem that includes perceptual and information processing, learning, judgment, and emotion to cope with a changing environment. For group adaptive processes, the comparable subsystems are the stabilizer and the innovator

Table 10.2 – Critical Appraisal of Measurement Used with RAM Research

Chapter: _____

BBARNS Member: _____

Research: Author(s) name, year, & title

Concept according to RAM	Linkage of research variable with RAM concept: (Explicit, Implicit, Absent)	Linkage of empirical measurement with RAM Concept: (Explicit, Implicit, Absent)	Description of measurement used
1.			
2.			
3.			
4.			
5.			

between the theoretic and operational definitions was consistent. Relationships between the two definitions were validated by at least two members of the research team. When there was lack of agreement between the two experts, a third member was involved until a consensus was reached.

Evaluation of the measurement strategies is first presented under the larger categorics, use of existing instruments and newly developed instruments. Within each of the categories, the measures are categorized according to major concepts of the RAM.

Use of Existing Instruments

Because of the small number of instrument-development studies, the majority of researchers used existing instruments in their studies. Although studies were assigned to one of seven content chapters, all researchers reported measuring at least two of the model concepts, with the average number of concepts measured being 3.5 per study. In studies assigned to the stimuli category (Chapter 8), the highest number of measured concepts was reported—an average of 5.2 concepts per study. Research that was focused on either self-concept (Chapter 4) or role function (Chapter 5) had an average of 2.3 concepts measured per study.

Physiologic adaptive mode. Numerous biologic measures were used to collect data for measuring responses in the physiologic mode (see Table 10.3). Consistency was present between the theoretic and operational definitions for physiologic adaptation in most studies. In general, many of the instruments were specifically related to the focus of the research and were appropriate measures for the selected physiologic needs and processes. For example, in studies focusing on oxygenation, the measure for change in infants was frequently arterial oxygen saturation levels, while heart rate and blood pressure were used to record changes in adults. Likewise, studies that focused on temperature and the sensory system used standard devices that were accurate and appropriate for recording either temperatures or visual and hearing acuity.

Other instruments used to measure physiologic responses were pain inventories, physiologically based classifications such as the APACHE, and behavioral assessments. Pollock (1986, 1989) developed physiologic measures which had been validated and weighted by experts for each chronic illness studied. Advantages of using weighted values included availability of a total physiologic adaptation score and comparison of physiologic adaptations among groups with different chronic illnesses.

The large number of model-based studies that included a physiologic measure reflects recognition that the outcomes of nursing care should include a physiologic dimension. It is also indicative of the holistic nature of the RAM, in that researchers are motivated to look at physiologic as well as psychosocial outcomes.

Self-concept adaptive mode. Researchers used paper and pencil instruments exclusively to collect data about the self-concept adaptive mode. Researchers were consistent in identification of similar instruments to measure concepts of the mode, and they clearly specified the relationship of the empiric indicator to the self-concept adaptive mode.

Instruments used for the identified concepts of this mode were primarily measures of self concept, self-esteem, anxiety, depression, powerlessness, and hope (See Table 10.4). The measures were consistent with theoretic definitions and had been identified as key concepts of the personal self component of the mode (Roy & Andrews, 1991). However, the other components of the self-concept adaptive mode were not identified for use in the research reviewed, and therefore were not measured.

Role-function adaptive mode. Relatively few instruments were used to measure concepts of the role function adaptive mode (see Table 10.5). However a program of research focused on instruments of functional status was reviewed. The focus of the instruments was either on adjustment to a role such as the maternal role, or effects of being in such roles as nurse or caregiver. Effects were measured by burnout or burden. Contin-

Table 10.3 – Measures for Concepts in the Physiologic Adaptive Mode

Measurement	References	Studies using measurement
Brief symptom inventory	Derogatis & Spencer (1982)	7-9 Smith (1987/1989)
Physical distress scale	Johnson (1984), Zeimer (1983)	6-16 Fawcett, Pollio, Tully, Baron, Henklein, & Jones (1993)
Functional independence; FONE FIM Modified	Smith, Hamilton, & Granger (1990)	3-13 Barone (1993/1994)
McGill Pain Questionnaire	Melzack (1975, 1983)	4-14 Calvillo (1991/1992) 4-15 Calvillo & Flaskerud (1993)/ 9-18 Fahs (1991/1992)
Pain intensity scale	Johnson (1984), Zeimer (1983)	6-16 Fawcett, Pollio, et al. (1993)
Acute Physiology & Chronic Health Evaluation Scale (APACHE)	Knaus, Zimmerman, Wagner, Draper, & Lawrence (1983)	3-28 Jackson, Strauman, Frederickson, & Strauman (1991)
Therapeutic Intervention Scoring System (TISS)	Keene & Cullen (1983)	3-28 Jackson, et al. (1991)
Physiological Adaptation to Chronic Illnesses: PAD, PAR, PAH	Pollock (1984)	3-11 Pollock (1986) 3-12 Pollock (1989)
24-Hour Behavioral Assessment Log	O'Leary, Haley, & Paul (1993)	4-12 O'Leary, Haley, & Paul (1993)
Neonatal Assessment Coding Sheet (NACS)	Harrison & Woods (1991)	9-13 Modrcin-McCarthy (1993)

Brazelton Scale	Brazelton (1984)	9-14 Garcia & White-Traut (1993)
Sleep characteristics	Verran & Snyder (1988)	4-13 Cheng (1990/1991)
Sequelae of Spinal Cord Injury	Cyr (1989)	3-13 Barone (1993/1994)
Couvade syndrome		4-5 Khanodbee, Sukratanachaiyakil, & Gay (1993)
Visual analog; Headache and flushing		9-17 Riegel, Heywood, Jackson, & Kennedy (1988)
Visual analog: Pain at time of injection		9-18 Fahs (1991/1992)
Visual analogs: Fatigue, Stress, Control, and Discomfort		9-22 Carson (1991/1992)
Lighthouse Near & Distance Visual Acuity Tests		4-17 Kelly (1993/1994)
Ventilator status		4-16 Gujol (1994)
Holter cardiac monitor		9-20 Smith (1987/1989)
Bruise measurement		9-18 Fahs (1991/1992)
Hemoglobin A1C		3-14 Grey, Cameron, & Thurber (1991)
24 hour urinary cortisol		9-1 Guzetta (1979)

(continued)

Table 10.3 *(continued)*

Measurement	References	Studies using measurement
Blood cortisol level		9-1 Guzetta (1979)
Eosinophil count		9-2 Zonca (1980)
Plasma non-esterified fatty acids		9-2 Zonca (1980)
Fraction of inspired transcutaneous oxygen pressure ($TcPO_2$)		4-1 Cheng & Williams (1989) 4-3 Norris, Campbell, & Brenhert (1982)
Arterial oxygen saturation levels		4-2 Harrison, Leeper, & Yoon (1990) 4-4 Shogan & Schumann (1993) 9-13 Modrcin-McCarthy (1992/1993)
Compressed respiratory wave graph (CRG)		9-14 Garcia & White-Traut (1993)
Fetal heart rate, Fetal uterine movement		9-12 Komara (1991/1992)
Blood pressure		9-11 Meek (1993) 9-15 Houston (1993) 9-16 Carson (1991/1992) 9-23 Parlin (1988/1990)
Pulse rate		9-26 Neiterman (1987/1988)

Heart rate

4-2 Harrison, Leeper, & Yoon (1990)
9-11 Meek (1993)
9-13 Modrcin-McCarthy (1992/1993)
9-15 Houston (1993)
9-16 Carson (1991/1992)
9-20 Smith (1987/1989)
9-23 Parlin (1988/1990)

Body temperature

4-19 Hunter (1991)
4-20 Pontious, Kennedy, Shelly, &
Mitttracker (1994)
9-19 Roberson (1987)

Skin temperature

9-11 Meek (1993)
9-15 Houston (1993)
9-16 Carson (1991/1992)

Key: Numbers indicate chapter number followed by study number.

Table 10.4 – Measures for Concepts in the Self Concept Adaptive Mode

Measurement	References	Studies using measurement
Management of Emotional Concerns in Daily Life	Varvaro (1986)	3-3 Varvaro (1991)
Health Self Concept Index	Jacox & Stewart (1973)	9-24 Francis, Turner, & Johnson (1985)
Coopersmith Self-Esteem Scale	Coopersmith (1967,	5-1 Holcombe (1986); Self-Esteem Scale 1981, 1987); 5-4 Foster (1990); 5-5 Stein (1992); 5-6 Robinson (1991); 5-7 Robinson & Frank (1994)
Rosenberg Self-Esteem Scale	Rosenberg (1965, 1979)	3-36 Rich (1992); 5-3 McRae (1991); 5-8 Edwards (1992); 5-9 Christian (1993); 5-10 Chen (1994); 7-9 Smith (1989/1990); 7-18 Limandri (1986)
Beck Depression Inventory	Beck (1978); Beck & Beanersderfer (1974); Beck, Ward, Mendelson, Mock, & Erbaugh (1987)	5-11 Bergin (1986) 9-24 Francis, Turner, & Johnson (1985)
Center for Epidemiologic Studies Depression Scale (CES-D)	Radloff (1977)	9-18 Fahs (1991/1992)
Self-Rating Depression Scale (SDS)	Zung (1965)	9-9 Campbell (1992)
Tennessee Self-Concept Scale	Fitts (1965)	3-24 Scherubel (1985/1986) 5-13 Lamb (1991)

Instrument	Source	Studies
Spielberger State-Trait Anxiety Inventory (STAI)	Spielberger, Gorsuch, Lushene, Vagy, & Jacobs (1970, 1983)	4-14 Calvillo (1991/1992) 4-15 Calvillo & Flaskerud (1993) 6-21 Kiker (1983); 8-15 Cornell (1990); 9-2 Zonca (1980) ; 9-16 Carson (1991/1992); 9-28 Komelasky (1990)
Anxiety Affect Adjective List	Zuckerman & Lubin (1965)	3-16 Roy (1977)
Miller Hope Scale	Miller (1988)	5-15 McGill (1991/1992); 5-16 McGill & Paul (1993)
Heath Illness Powerlessness Scale	Roy (1977)	3-16 Roy (1977)
Purpose in Life Test (PIL)	Crumbaugh (1968)	9-8 Newman (1991)
Post-Partum Self-Evaluation Questionnaire (PSQ)	Lederman et al. (1981)	6-6 Tulman, Fawcett, Groblewski, & Silverman (1990)
Child Mental Health Self-Care Inventory	Gast (1988)	6-7 Tulman & Fawcett (1990)
Visual Analog: Body Image	Mock (1987)	9-7 Gilbert (1990/1991)
Visual Analog: Self-Esteem		5-13 Lamb (1991)
Visual Analog: Body Image		5-13 Lamb (1991)
Visual Analog: Preoperative Anxiety		9-10 Gaberson (1991)

Key: Numbers indicate chapter number followed by study number.

Table 10.5 - Measures for Concepts of Role Function Adaptive Mode

Measurement	References	Studies using measurement
Alienation from Work Scale	Maddi, Kobasa, & Hoover (1979)	3-36 Rich (1991/1992)
Jones Burnout Scale	Jones (1980)	3-36 Rich (1991/1992)
Nursing Stress Scale	Cronin-Stubbs & Rooks (1985)	3-36 Rich (1991/1992)
Role Strain Scale	Katz & Peotrkowski (1983)	7-1 Artinian (1989); 7-2 Artinian (1991); 7-3 Artinian (1992)
Inventory of Functional Status after Childbirth (IFSAC)	Fawcett, Tulman, & Myers (1988)	6-1 Fawcett, Tulman, & Myers (1988) 6-6 Tulman, Fawcett, Groblewski, & Silverman (1990); 6-7 Tulman & Fawcett (1990) ; 6-16 Fawcett, Pollio, et al. (1993)
Inventory of Functional Status-Antepartum Period	Tulman, Higgins, et al. (1991)	6-2 Tulman, Higgins, et al. (1991)
Inventory of Functional Status-Fathers	Tulman, Fawcett, & Weiss (1993)	6-3 Tulman, Fawcett, & Weiss (1993)
Inventory of Functional Status-Cancer	Tulman, Fawcett, & McEvoy (1991)	6-4 Tulman, Fawcett, & McEvoy (1991)
Inventory of Functional Status in the Elderly	Paier (1994)	6-5 Paier (1994)
Post-Partum Self-Evaluation Questionnaire (PSQ)	Lederman et al. (1981)	6-20 Weiss (1990/1991)

Key: Numbers indicate chapter number followed by study number.

Table 10.6 – Measures for Concepts in the Interdependence Adaptive Mode

Measurement	References	Studies using measurement
Dyadic Adjustment Scale	Spanier (1976)	7-1 Artinian (1988/1989); 7-2 Artinian (1991); 7-3 Artinian (1992); 7-20 Pruden (1991)
Feelings about Baby Scale	Leiffer (1977)	6-16 Fawcett, Pollio, Tully, Baron, Henklein, & Jones (1993)
Relationship Change Scale	Guerney (1977)	6-16 Fawcett, Pollio, et al. (1993)
Empathetic Tendency Questionnaire	Mehrabian & Epstein (1972)	7-9 Smith (1987/1989)
Affection-Obligation Scale	Montgomery & Borgatta (1985)	7-10 Perkins (1988)
Burden Scale	Montgomery & Borgatta (1985)	7-10 Perkins (1988)
Caregiver Burden Interview	Zarit, Reever, & Bach-Peterson (1980)	7-9 Smith (1989)
UCLA Loneliness Scale	Russell (1982)	5-10 Chen (1994); 7-19 Calvert (1989); 7-20 Pruden (1991); 9-7 Gilbert (1991); 9-22 Prelewicz (1993);
Family Environment Scale	Moos (1974)	3-23 Wright (1993)
Family APGAR	Hillard, Gjerde, & Porker (1986)	7-11 Smith, Mayer, Parkhurst, Perkins, & Pringleton (1991)

(continued)

Table 10.6 *(continued)*

Measurement	References	Studies using measurement
House & Wells Social Support	House (1978/1981);	3-36 Rich (1991/1992)
Social Support Scale	Zich & Temoshok (1987)	4-14 Calvillo (1991/1992); 4-15 Calvillo & Flaskerud (1993)
Norbeck Social Support Questionnaire	Norbeck (1981, 1984)	7-1 Artinian (1988/1989); 7-2 Artinian (1991); 7-3 Artinian (1992); 7-15 Eves (1992/1993); 7-18 Limandri (1986)
Personal Resources Questionnaire	Brandt & Weinert (1981)	7-20 Pruden (1991/1992); 9-8 Newman (1991)
Self-Perception Profile for Children	Harter (1985)	9-7 Gilbert (1990/1991)
Visual Analog: Sexual functioning		5-13 Lamb (1991)
Visual Analog: Caregiver burden	Aitken (1969)	7-10 Perkins (1987/1988)

Key: Numbers indicates chapter number followed by study number.

Table 10.7 – Measures for the Concept of Adaptation (Global Adaptation)

Measurement	References	Studies using measurement
Adolescent Life-Change Event Scale	Yeaworth, York, Hussey, Ingle, & Goodwin (1980)	3-6 Thomas, Shoffner, & Groer (1988)
Instrumental Activities of Daily Living	Lawton & Brody (1969)	3- 31 Collins (1993)
Activities of Daily Living	Katz & Peotrkowski (1983)	4-12 Cheng (1990/1991)
Inventory of Functional Status (IVS)	Kelly (1993/1994)	4-17 Kelly (1993/1994)
Functional Assessment Inventory	Pfeiffer (1985)	7-10 Perkins (1987/1988)
Functional Adaptation Index	Fortinsky, Granger, & Seltzer (1981)	3-29 Strohmyer, Noroian, Patterson, & Carlin (1993)
Philadelphia Geriatric Center Multilevel Assessment	Lawton, Moss, Fulcomer, & Kleban (1982)	5-15 McGill (1992) 5-16 McGill & Paul (1993)
Adaptation Index	Tasto, Colligan, Skjel, & Polly (1978)	3-18 Phillips (1991) 3-27 Phillips & Brown (1992)
Sickness Impact Profile (SIP)	Bergner, Bobbitt, Pollard, Martin, & Gibson (1976) Bergner et al. (1981)	3-22 Frederickson, Jackson, Strauman, & Strauman (1991)
Symptom Distress Scale	McCorkle & Quint-Benoliel (1983)	3-22 Frederickson, Jackson, Strauman, & Strauman (1991) 3-29 Jackson, Strauman, Frederickson, & Strauman (1991) *(continued)*

Table 10.7 *(continued)*

Measurement	References	Studies using measurement
Menstrual Distress Questionnaire	Moos et al. (1986)	9-27 Shrubsole (1992)
Premenstrual Assessment Form	Halbreich, Endicott, & Schacht (1982)	9-27 Shrubsole (1992)
Parenting & Stress Index	Abidin (1983)	3-17 Dow (1992/1993)
Impact of Arthritis Scale	Meenan, Geetman, & Mason (1980)	3-33 Selman (1989)
Arthritis Impact Scale	Wallston et al. (1989)	9-8 Newman (1991)
Prosthetic Problem Inventory Scale	Huber, Medhat, & Carter (1988)	4-9 Huber, Medhat, & Carter 1988 4-10 Medhat, Huber, & Medhat (1990)
Severity Body Cathexis Survey	Secord & Jourad (1953)	8-14 Leech (1982)
Perception of Birth Scale	Marut & Mercer (1979)	6-16 Fawcett, Pollio, Tully, Baron, Henklein & Jones (1993); 6-17 Fawcett & Weiss (1993); 6-18 Fawcett, Tulman, & Spedden (1994)

Key: Numbers indicate chapter number followed by study number

Table 10.8 – Measures for the Concepts of Psychosocial Adaptation (Self Concept, Role Function, and Interdependence)

Measurement	References	Studies using measurement
Psychosocial Adaptation to Illness Survey (PAIS)	Derogatis (1986)	3-11 Pollock (1986); 3-12 Pollock (1989); 3-13 Barone (1993/1994); 7-4 Gardner (1994)
Psychosocial Function Scale	Putnam (1973)	9-24 Francis, Turner, & Johnson (1985)
Inventory of Current Concerns	Weisman & Worden (1977)	3-28 Jackson, Strauman, Frederickson, & Strauman (1991)
Strain Questionnaire	Lefebvre & Sandford (1985)	7-1 Artinian (1989); 7-2 Artinian (1991) 7-3 Artinian (1992)
Affects Balance Scale	Bradburn (1969) Derogatis (1975)	3-25 Dobratz (1993) ; 6-9 Razmus (1994) 9-24 Francis, Turner, & Johnson (1985)
Profile of Mood State	McNair, Lorr, & Droppleman (1971)	3-27 Phillips & Brown (1992)
Grief Experience Inventory	Sanders, Mauger, & Strong (1985)	7-15 Robinson (1991)
Philadelphia Geriatric Center Morale Scale	Lawton (1975)	3-31 Collins (1994/1993) ; 8-1 Armer (1988/ 1989)
Observed Patient Behavior	Barjas (1971)	9-24 Francis, Turner, & Johnson (1985)
Satisfaction with Life	Converse & Robinson (1973)	9-24 Francis, Turner, & Johnson (1985)
Quality of Life Index	Ferrans & Powers (1985)	3-17 Dow (1992/1993) *(continued)*

Table 10.8 (continued)

Measurement	References	Studies using measurement
Quality of Life Scale	Olson et al. (1982)	3-3 Varvaro (1991)
Youth Self Report	Achenbach (1988)	9-7 Gilbert (1991)
Visual Analog: Quality of life		4-14 Morris (1992)

Key: Numbers indicate chapter numbers followed by study numbers

Table 10.9 – Measures for Concepts of Adaptive Processes of the RAM

Measurement	References	Studies using measurement
Ways of Coping Checklist	Folkman, Lazarus, Dunelk, Schetter, DeLongis, & Green (1986)	3-11 Pollock (1986) 3-13 Barone (1993/1994)
Cognitive Appraisal Index	Folkman, Lazarus et al. (1986)	8-1 Armer (1988/1989)
Hassles and Uplift Scales	Lazarus & Folkman (1989)	9-16 Carson (1991/1992)
Revised Jalowiec Coping Scale	Jalowiec (1987)	3-18 Phillips (1991); 3-27 Phillips & Brown (1992); 7-15 Robinson (1992)
Coping Skills Index	Billings & Moos (1981)	8-1 Armer (1988/1989)
Indices of Coping Responses	Moos, Cronkite,. et al. (1986)	7-1 Atinian (1989); 7-2 Artinian (1991)

Instrument	Source	Study
Coping Health Inventory for Parents (CHIPS)	McCubbin, McCubbin et al. (1983)	7-16 Eves (1993)
Family Coping Scale	McCubbin & Thomas (1986)	7-11 Smith, Mayer, Parkhurst, Perkins & Pingleton (1991)
Chronic Impact and Coping Instrument: Parent Questionnaire	Hymovich (1984)	7-16 Eves (1993)
Health Related Hardiness Scale (HRHS)	Pollock (1984)	3-11 Pollock (1986); 3-12 Pollock (1989) 3-13 Barone (1993/1994)
Adaptation after Surviving Cancer Profile	Dow (1992/1993)	3-17 Dow (1992/1993)
Multidimensional Measure of Control	Levenson (1974)	9-16 Carson (1991/1992)
Arthritis Self-Efficacy Scale	Lorig et al. (1989)	9-8 Newman (1991)
Decision Making Styles Inventory	Janis & Mann (1977)	3-24 Scherubel (1986)
Circadian Type Indicator	Folkard, Monk, & Lobban (1979)	3-18 Philips (1991); 3-27 Philips & Brown (1992)
Adaptation to Hospital Stress Scale	Roy (1977)	3-16 Roy (1977)
Mini-Mental State Exam (MMSE)	Folstein, Folstein, & McHugh (1975)	4-12 O'Leary (1991)

Key: Numbers inidcate chapter number followed by study number.

ued work in the area of functional-status instruments can contribute to measurement of the role-function adaptive mode.

Reported instruments that measured concepts of the role function mode were clearly linked with the model, and descriptions of the empiric indicators were consistent with the theoretic definitions. Many researchers used structured interview or open-ended questions to obtain data about role function or performance.

Interdependence adaptive mode. The interdependence adaptive mode is focused on interactions with others and with support systems. Researchers frequently used social support measures, dyadic and family adjustment scales, and loneliness measures to collect data about concepts of interest from this mode (see Table 10.6). The measures are consistent with the key concepts identified by Roy and Andrews (1991) and with the theoretic definitions. Researchers often used demographic data such as marital status or size of family for comparison of outcomes that reflected the effects of significant others and support systems. Identification of appropriate instruments that measure family functioning and adjustment is needed to promote family research using the RAM.

Adaptation. The term adaptation refers to responses in all four modes. While the terms global or total adaptation were not frequently used in the research, authors identified specific instruments that were used to measure responses in all four modes (see Table 10.7). Instruments frequently used included items or subscales related to functioning, activities, or losses in all four modes. Although the term total or global adaptation was not theoretically defined, there was consistency among the researchers in describing how the instrument measured responses in all four modes. The empiric indicators were clearly related to the appropriate concepts of the RAM. Efforts to measure all four adaptive modes emphasizes the need for further attention to global or total adaptation. The construct should be theoretically defined and instruments that measure the construct should be evaluated based on their relationship to the RAM and the consistency between the theoretic and operational definitions. Global or total adaptation is a promising area for development of new instruments based on the model.

Psychosocial adaptation. Similarly, the category of psychosocial adaptation was created based on the review of research included in the monograph. Frequently the researchers reported using instruments that measured the construct of psychosocial adaptation (see Table 10.8). While the term psychosocial adaptation was not theoretically defined, some authors identified and described questions used to elicit responses for the three psychosocial modes. For example, Pollock (1986, 1989) used the psychosocial adjustment to illness scale (Derogatis & Spencer,1982) to determine psychosocial adaptation and described specific subscales that measured self concept, role function, and interdependence adaptation. Other frequently used measures were mood and affect scales, life satisfaction indices, and quality of life instruments.

Quality of life measures were categorized as measurements of psychosocial adaptation based on descriptions of the items included. If quality of life instruments included items or subscales that focused on physiologic adaptation, they could be categorized as measuring global adaptation. Support for the use of quality of life measures was provided by Frederickson and Pollock (1994). The authors hypothesized that the adaptation outcome or degree to which a person's psychosocial (and physiologic) integrity are promoted can be represented by quality of life.

Further theoretic clarification of responses in the three psychosocial modes is indicated and identification of appropriate operational indicators is needed. Numerous valid and reliable instruments are available to measure relevant psychological and sociologic concepts. The problem lies with determining their applicability to research based on the RAM.

Measurement of Stimuli. Focal and contextual stimuli were identified in the majority of studies included in the monograph. The naming and description of the stimuli has contributed to clarifying the internal and external events that confront the individual and their effect on adaptation. Most stimuli identified as variables required reporting factors as present rather than using tools or tests to measure them.

The focal stimulus was identified as the most immediate challenge confronting the individual. In many studies the immediate threat was an illness or injury to self that the person was facing or a health problem of a child or significant other. Commonly identified health problems for the individual were a coronary event, surgery, cancer or treatment such as chemotherapy, chronic illnesses such as insulin dependent diabetes mellitus, disabilities such as incontinence and impaired vision, pain from surgery or illness, fever in children and adults, apneic episodes in infants, and effects of medications or treatments. An interesting threat identified by Campbell-Heider (1988; 1993) was adaptation of adults to invasive and noninvasive technological stimuli.

Adaptation to events of a more psychosocial nature were the second most frequently identified category of focal stimuli. Examples included adaptation to new roles such as pregnancy, childbirth, and parenthood, and relocation to a new residence or type of living situation. Other threats that involved the self concept and interdependence adaptive modes were stressors related to work environment, grief responses of widows, living alone in a rural environment, and—especially in the elderly—loneliness.

The third most frequently identified category of focal stimuli included those related to interdependence mode functioning such as parents coping with health problems of their children, spouses adjusting to changes or illnesses in their partners, and caring for a family member in the home. Several studies focused on the adjustment of parents to specific stimuli impinging on their children: the diagnosis of cancer in a child (Smith, Garvis, & Martinson, 1983), caring for a chronically ill child in the home (Eves, 1992/1993; Gibson, 1993/1994), or adjusting to infants on home cardio-respiratory monitors (Komelasky, 1990). The immediate threat for spouses in several studies was their partner's experiencing and adjusting to events such as cardiac surgery, stroke, and head injury. Specific stressors of caregiving included caring for ventilator-dependent adults at home (Smith et al., 1991) and caring for relatives dependent on total parenteral nutrition (Smith et al., 1993).

Contextual stimuli have been defined as the internal and external factors that influence how the person deals with the focal stimulus. The difference between contextual and residual stimuli is that the effects of the latter are unknown or unclear in the current situation. Therefore, residual stimuli generally were not the focus of measurement research based on the RAM. The major consistency among the studies related to contextual stimuli was inclusion of demographic variables.

Other data researchers designated as contextual stimuli included strategies that had facilitated coping with the focal stimulus and previous experience with similar stressful situations. Another important variable was the length of time involved such as how long people had been living with a chronic illness or in a caregiver role. However, demographic characteristics and other variables that influenced the effect of the focal stimulus often were not explicitly identified by the researchers as contextual stimuli.

According to the RAM, the goal of nursing interventions is to facilitate adaptation by managing stimuli from the internal and external environment including cognator-regulator effectiveness. Nurses intervene to modify the effect of the focal stimulus and such interventions can be viewed as a contextual stimulus. The measured effectiveness of the intervention is determined by the adaptive behavior of the individual. While reports of studies that involved interventions provided descriptions of the nursing action and the expected outcomes, many researchers did not identify interventions as contextual stimuli according to the model.

Adaptive processes. Individual and family coping scales were frequently used for measuring adaptive processes (see Table 10.9). Specifically the instruments were used to measure concepts related to cognitive processes such as appraisal, coping, control, and hardiness. None of the measurement strategies used were focused specifically on the regulator processes of the RAM.

Several explanations exist for the lack of instruments for use in measuring adaptive processes. Many of the measures reported to record physiologic responses also involve the regulator subsystem. Concepts of adaptive processes were explored and described in many of the qualitative studies. While the theoretic relationships between the cognator and regulator subsystems and the four adaptive modes emphasize the holistic nature of the model, the complexities of the interactions are difficult to measure. Therefore, further theoretic work is indicated to clarify these interactions to provide better direction for measurement of the adaptive processes.

Contributions from Instrument-Development Studies

While only 9 of the 163 studies in the monograph were classified as instrument-development studies, many researchers used visual analog scales or structured interview questions to elicit information about concepts of interest. The major area of concentrated effort to measure concepts of the model was from the development of functional-status instruments. The work done by Fawcett, Tulman, and colleagues (1988, 1991, 1993) measured functional status related to maternal and parental roles during such times as the antepartum and postpartum period. Two other inventories of functional status were developed—one for cancer patients (Tulman, Fawcett, & McEvoy, 1991) and the other for elderly patients (Paier, 1994).

Three instruments using elements of the RAM were developed to measure various aspects of physiologic adaptation. The Joseph Continence Assessment Tool focused on a holistic assessment of men following prostatectomies before implementing bladder interventions (Joseph, 1994). O'Leary (1993) developed a behavioral assessment for users to provide descriptions of adaptive and ineffective behaviors of people with Alzheimer's Disease.

The Prosthetic Problem Inventory Scale (Huber et al., 1988) was developed to identify problem areas in the use of prostheses. An instrument to measure the interdependence functioning of mothers after childbirth was developed by Short (1994). Based upon findings from a qualitative inquiry of women surviving cancer, Dow (1992/1993) developed the instrument, Adaptation After Surviving Cancer. The nine instrument studies have made a beginning contribution to clarify and refine several major concepts of the RAM.

Contributions to Measurement of RAM Concepts

Most investigators used existing instruments to measure the major concepts of the RAM. Approximately 120 instruments, including those described in the section on instrument-development studies, and more than 20 physiologic and biologic indicators were used in the model-based research reviewed for this monograph. The measures were classified according to the major concepts of the model. The identified measures have support for reliability and validity, are theoretically related to the model, and have been identified as appropriate for use with research based on the RAM. Many instruments are available for measuring various concepts of the physiologic and self-concept modes, functional status of the role function adaptive mode, and social support of the interdependence adaptive mode. Additionally, several instruments are available that are appropriate for measuring the coping processes of adaptation.

Many researchers included physiologic measures, a fact which supports the strength of the model for allowing users to view the adapting person holistically. Continued examination of biologic processes along with psychosocial outcomes is warranted. Indicators from the field of psychoneuroimmunology may provide a promising avenue for incorporating several of the major concepts from the model in future research.

Stimuli were accurately identified in the majority of studies. Quantification of the quality and strength of the stimulus, as well as the relationships among stimuli, as described by Pollock (1981/1982), could be used as directions for continued theoretic work on measurement of the concepts of the model. Complexities of the interactions between the regulator and congator subsystems, and the adaptive processes used by groups such as families and communities, should to be further clarified to facilitate RAM research in these areas.

Many researchers used a specific instrument to measure psychosocial adaptation or global adaptation. Researchers accurately related components of the measures to each of the modes. Because researchers are using these concepts and attempting to validate them empirically, further theoretic development is indicated.

Measurement of model concepts is the empiric indicator of the adequacy of the RAM. Selection of instruments congruent with the model is pivotal in testing hypotheses derived from the RAM. Measurements should reflect the framework of the model for the results of the research to contribute to the theoretic refinement of the model and, ultimately, to contribute to the knowledge base of nursing.

References

Armer, J. M. (1989). Factors influencing relocation adjustment among community-based rural elderly (Doctoral dissertation, University of Rochester, 1988). *Dissertation Abstracts International, 50*, 1321-B.

Artinian, N.T. (1989). The stress process within the Roy adaptation framework: Sources, mediators and manifestations of stress in spouses of coronary artery bypass patients during hospitalization and six weeks post discharge (Doctoral dissertation, Wayne State University, 1988). *Dissertation Abstracts International, 49*, 5225-B.

Artinian, N.T. (1991). Stress experience of spouses of patients having coronary artery bypass during hospitalization and 6 weeks after discharge. *Heart & Lung, 20*, 52-59.

Artinian, N.T. (1992). Spouse adaptation to mate's CABG surgery: 1-year follow-up. *American Journal of Critical Care, 1*(2), 36-42.

Barone, S.H. (1994). Adaptation to spinal cord injury (Doctoral dissertation, Boston College, 1993). *Dissertation Abstracts International, 54*, 3547-B.

Beck, A.T.(1978). Client affective variables: anxiety depression. *Instruments for Measuring Nursing Practice and other Health Care Variables*. DHEW Publication No. HRA 78-536.

Beck, A.T., & Beanersderfer, A. (1974). Assessment of depression: The depression inventory. *Psychological Measurement Psychopharmacology, 7*, 151-169.

Beck, A.T., Ward, C.H., Mendelson, M., Mock, J., & Erbaugh, J. (1961). An inventory for measuring depression. *Archives of General Psychiatry, 4*, 248-253.

Bergin, M.A. (1986). Psychosocial responses of marital couples experiencing primary infertility (Doctoral dissertation, Temple University, 1985). *Dissertation Abstracts International, 46*, 2197-A.

Calvert, M.M. (1989). Human-pet interaction and loneliness: A test of concepts from Roy's adaptation model. *Nursing Science Quarterly, 2*, 194-202.

Calvillo, E.R. (1992). Pain response in Mexican-American and white non-Hispanic women (Doctoral dissertation, University of California, Los Angeles, 1991). *Dissertation Abstracts International, 52*, 3524-B.

Calvillo, E.R., & Flaskerud, J.H. (1993). The adequacy and scope of Roy's adaptation model to guide cross-cultural pain research. *Nursing Science Quarterly, 6*, 118-129.

Campbell, J.M. (1992). Treating depression in well older adults: Use of diaries in cognitive therapy. *Issues in Mental Health Nursing, 13*, 19-29.

Carson, M.A. (1992). The effect of discrete muscle activity on stress response (Doctoral dissertation, Boston College, 1991). *Dissertation Abstracts International, 52*, 5757-B.

Chen, H.-L. (1994). Hearing in the elderly: Relation of hearing loss, loneliness, and self-esteem. *Journal of Gerontological Nursing, 20*(6), 22-28.

Cheng, L.C. (1991). Social support related to the sleep pattern in Southern Taiwanese hospitalized adults (Master's thesis, University of Arizona, 1990). *Masters Abstracts International, 29*, 90.

Cheng, M., & Williams, P.D. (1989). Oxygenation during chest physiotherapy of very-low-birth-weight infants: Relations among fraction of inspired oxygen levels, number of hand ventilations, and transcutaneous oxygen pressure. *Journal of Pediatric Nursing, 4*, 411-418.

Christian, A. (1993). The relationship between women's symptoms of endometriosis and self-esteem. *Journal of Obstetric, Gynecologic, & Neonatal Nursing, 22*, 370-376.

Collins, J.M. (1993). Functional health, social support, and morale of older women living along in Appalachia (Doctoral dissertation, University of Alabama at Birmingham, 1992). *Dissertation Abstracts International, 53*, 1781-B.

Cornell, D.L. (1990). Patterns of anxiety with home parenteral antibiotic theraphy (Master's thesis, University of Nevada, Reno, 1990). *Master's Abstracts International, 28*, 572.

Dobratz, M.C. (1993). Causal influences of psychological adaptation in dying. *Western Journal of Nursing Research, 15*, 708-729.

Dow, K.H.M. (1993). An analysis of the experience of surviving and having children after breast cancer (Doctoral dissertation, Boston College, 1992). *Dissertation Abstracts International, 53*, 5641-B.

Edwards, M.R. (1992). Self-esteem, sense of mastery, and adequacy of prenatal care (Doctoral dissertation, University of Alabama at Birmingham, 1991). *Dissertation Abstracts International, 53*, 768-B.

Eves, L.M. (1993). Support for parents of developmentally disabled children: Effect of adaptation (Master's thesis, D'Youville College, 1992). *Masters Abstracts International, 31*, 271.

Fahs, P.S. (1992). Effect of heparin injectate volume on pain and bruising using the Roy model (Doctoral dissertation, University of Alabama at Birmingham, 1991). *Dissertation Abstracts International, 52*, 5195-B.

Fawcett, J., Pollio, N., Tully, A., Baron, M., Henklein, J.C., & Jones, R.C. (1993). Effects of information on adaptation to cesarean birth. *Nursing Research, 42*, 49-53.

Fawcett, J., Tulman, L., & Myers, S.T. (1988). Development of the Inventory of Functional Status after Childbirth. *Journal of Nurse Midwifery, 33*, 252-260.

Fawcett, J., Tulman, L., & Spedden, J.P. (1994). Responses to vaginal birth after cesarean section. *Journal of Obstetric, Gynecologic, & Neonatal Nursing, 23*, 253-259.

Fawcett, J., & Weiss, M.E. (1993). Cross-cultural adaptation to cesarean birth. *Western Journal of Nursing Research, 15*, 282-297.

Folkman, S., Lazarus, R.S., Dunkel-Schetter, C., DeLongis, A., & Gruen, R.J. (1986). Dynamics of a stressful encounter: Cognitive appraisal, coping, and encounter outcome. *Journal of Personality and Social Psychology, 30*(5), 992-1003.

Folstein, M.F., Folstein, S.E., & McHugh, P.R. (1975). "Mini-Mental State": A practical method for grading the cognitive state of patients for the clinician. *Journal of Psychiatric Research,12,* 189-198.

Foster, P.L. (1989). The relationship between selected variables and the self-esteem in adolescent females (Doctoral dissertation, University of Alabama at Birmingham, 1989). *Dissertation Abstracts International, 50,* 3918-B.

Francis, G., Turner, J.T., & Johnson, S.B. (1985). Domestic animal visitation as therapy with adult home residents. *International Journal of Nursing Studies, 22,* 201-206.

Frederickson, K., Jackson, B.S., Strauman, T., & Strauman, J. (1991). Testing hypotheses derived from the Roy Adaptation Model. *Nursing Science Quarterly, 4,* 168-174.

Gaberson, K.B. (1991). The effect of humorous distraction on preoperative anxiety. *AORN Journal, 54,* 1258-1264.

Garcia, A.P., & White-Traut, R. (1993). Preterm infants' responses to taste/smell and tactile stimulation during an apneic episode. *Journal of Pediatric Nursing, 8,* 245-252.

Gardner, M.J. (1994). Spouse adaptation after the partner's open heart surgery. Unpublished master's thesis, Grand Valley State University.

Gilbert, C.M. (1991). A structured group nursing intervention for girls who have been sexually abused utilizing Roy's theory of the person as an adaptive system (Doctoral dissertation, University of South Carolina, 1990). *Dissertation Abstracts International, 52,* 1350-B.

Grey, M., Cameron, M.E., & Thurber, F.W. (1991). Coping and adaptation in children with diabetes. *Nursing Research, 40,* 144-149.

Gujol, M.C. (1994). A survey of pain assessment and management practices among critical care nurses. *American Journal of Critical Care, 3*(2), 123-128

Guzzetta, C.E. (1979). Relationship between stress and learning. *Advances in Nursing Science, 1*(4), 35-39.

Harrison, L.L., Leeper, J.D., & Yoon, M. (1990). Effects of early parent touch on preterm infants' heart rates and arterial oxygen saturation levels. *Journal of Advanced Nursing, 15,* 877-885.

Holcombe, J.K. (1986). Social support, perception of illness, and self-esteem of women with gynecologic cancer (Doctoral dissertation, The University of Alabama in Birmingham, 1985). *Dissertation Abstracts International, 47,* 1928-B.

House, J.S. (1981). *Workstress and social support.* Reading, MA.: Addison-Wesley.

House, J.S. (1978). *Occupational stress, social support and health.* In A. McLeon, G. Black, and M. Colligan (Eds.), Reducing Occupational Stress. Proceedings of a Conference, DHEW-NIOSH Publication No. 78-146, pp.8-29. Washington, D.C.: U.S. Government Printing Office.

Houston, K.A. (1993). An investigation of rocking as relaxation for the elderly. *Geriatric Nursing, 14,* 186-189.

Huber, P.M., Medhat, A., & Carter, M. C. (1988). Prosthetic Problem Inventory Scale. *Rehabilitation Nursing, 13,* 326-329.

Hunter, L.P. (1991). Measurement of axillary temperatures in neonates. *Western Journal of Nursing Research, 13,* 324-335.

Jackson, B.S., Strauman, J., Frederickson, K., & Strauman, T. (1991). Long-term biopsychosocial effects of interleukin-2 therapy. *Oncology Nursing Forum, 18,* 683-690.

Joseph, A.C. (1994). Content validity of the Joseph Continence Assessment Tool. Unpublished master's thesis, San Diego State University, San Diego.

Kelly, M. (1994). Visual impairment in the elderly and its impact on their daily lives (Doctoral dissertation, Texas Women's University, 1993). *Dissertation Abstracts International, 54,* 5093-B.

Khanobdee, C., Sukratanachaiyakul, V., & Gay, J.T. (1993). Couvade syndrome in expectant Thai father. *International Journal of Nursing Studies, 30,* 125-131.

Kiker, P.M. (1983). Role adequacy of pediatric outpatients undergoing surgery (Doctoral dissertation, Texas Women's University, 1983). *Dissertation Abstracts International, 44,* 1782 -B.

Komara, C.A. (1992). Effects of music on fetal response (Master's thesis, Bellarmine College, 1991). *Masters Abstracts International, 30,* 300.

Komelasky, A.L. (1990). The effect of home nursing visits on parental anxiety and CPR knowledge retention of parents of apnea-monitored infants. *Journal of Pediatric Nursing, 5,* 387-392.

Lamb, M.A. (1991). Sexual adaptation of women treated for endometrial cancer (Doctoral dissertation, Boston College, 1991). *Dissertation Abstracts International, 52,* 2994-B.

Lavender, M.G. (1989). The relationship between maternal self-esteem, work status, and sociodemographic characteristics and self-esteem of the kindergarten child (Doctoral dissertation, The University of Alabama in Birmingham, 1988). *Dissertation Abstracts International, 49,* 5229-B.

Leech, J.L. (1982). Psychosocial and physiologic needs of patients with arterial occlusive disease during the preoperative phase of hospitalization. *Heart & Lung, 11,* 442-449.

Limandri, B.J. (1986). Research and practice with abused women: Use of the Roy Adaptation Model as an explanatory framework. *Advances in Nursing Science, 8*(4), 52-61.

Lorig, K., Chastain, R., Ung, E., Shoor, S., & Holmon, H. (1989). Development and evaluation of a scale to measure perceived self-efficacy in people with arthritis. *Arthritis and Rheumatism, 32* (1) 37-44.

McGill, J.S. (1992). Functional status as it relates to hope in elders with and without cancer (Doctoral dissertation, The University of Alabama in Birmingham, 1991). *Dissertation Abstracts International, 53*, 771-B.

McGill, J.S., & Paul, P.B. (1993). Functional status and hope in elderly people with and without cancer. *Oncology Nursing Forum, 20*, 1207-1213.

McRae, M.G. (1991). Adaptation to pregnancy and motherhood: Personality characteristics of primiparas age 30 years and older (Doctoral dissertation, Boston University, 1990). *Dissertation Abstracts International, 51*, 3326-B.

Medhat, A., Huber, P.M., & Medhat, M.A. (1990). Factors that influence the level of activities in persons with lower extremity amputation. *Rehabilitation Nursing, 15*, 13-18.

Meek, Sr. S. (1993). Effects of slow stroke back massage on relaxation in hospice clients. *Image: Journal of Nursing Scholarship, 25*, 17-21.

Mock, V.L. (1987). Body image in women treated for breast cancer. (Doctoral dissertation. The Catholic University of America. *Dissertation Abstracts International.*

Modrcin-McCarthy, M.A.J. (1993). The physiological and behavioral effects of a gentle human touch nursing intervention on preterm infants (Doctoral dissertation, The University of Tennessee, 1992). *Dissertation Abstracts International, 54*, 1336-B.

Morris, B.C. (1992). Relationship between symptom distress and life quality in women with breast cancer undergoing adjuvant treatment (Master's Thesis, The University of Arizona, 1992). *Masters Abstracts International, 30*, 300.

Neiterman, E.W. (1988). Assessment of parent's presence during anesthesia induction of children (Master's thesis, University of Lowell, 1987). *Masters Abstracts International, 26*, 109.

Newman, A.M. (1991). The effect of the arthritis self-help course on arthritis self-efficacy, perceived social support, purpose and meaning in life, and arthritis impact in people with arthritis (Doctoral dissertation, University of Alabama at Birmingham, 1991). *Dissertation Abstracts International, 52*, 2995-B.

Norris, S., Campbell, L. A., & Brenhert, S. (1982). Nursing procedures and alteration in transcutaneous oxygen tension in premature infants. *Nursing Research, 31*, 330-336.

O'Leary, P.A. (1991). Family caregivers' log reports of sleep and activity behaviors of persons with Alzheimer's disease (Doctoral dissertation, University of Alabama at Birmingham, 1990). *Dissertation Abstracts International, 51*, 4780-B.

O'Leary, P.A., Haley, W.E., & Paul, P.B. (1993). Behavioral assessment in Alzheimer's disease: Use of a 24-hour log. *Psychology and Aging, 8*, 139-143.

Paier, G.S. (1994). Development and testing of an instrument to assess functional status in the elderly (Doctoral dissertation, University of Pennsylvania, 1994), *Dissertation Abstracts International, 55*, 1806-B.

Parlin, C.A. (1990). Physiological manifestations of human/animal interaction in the adult population over 55 (Master's thesis, University of Nevada, Reno, 1988). *Masters Abstracts International, 28*, 113.

Perkins, I. (1988). An analysis of relationships among interdependence in family caregivers and the elderly, caregiver burden, and adaptation of the homebound frail elderly (Doctoral dissertation, The Catholic University of America, 1987). *Dissertation Abstracts International, 48*, 3250-3251-B.

Phillips, J. A. (1991). Adaptation and injury status of industrial workers on a rotating shift pattern (Doctoral dissertation, University of Alabama at Birmingham, 1991). *Dissertation Abstracts International, 52*, 2995-B.

Phillips, J.A., & Brown, K. C. (1992). Industrial workers on rotating shift pattern: Adaptation and injury status. *AAOHN Journal, 40*, 468-476.

Pollock, S.E. (1986). Human responses to chronic illness: Physiologic and psychosocial adaptation. *Nursing Research, 35*, 90-95.

Pollock, S.E. (1989). Adaptive responses to diabetes mellitus. *Western Journal of Nursing Research, 11*, 265-280.

Pontious, S., Kennedy, A. H., Shelly, S., & Mittrucker, C. (1994). Accuracy and reliability of temperature measurement by instrument and site. *Journal of Pediatric Nursing, 9*, 114-123.

Prelewicz, T.N. (1993). The effects of animal-assisted therapy on lonliness in elderly residents of a long-term care facility using Roy's adaptation model (Master's thesis, D'Youville College, 1993). *Masters Abstracts International, 31*, 1749.

Pruden, E.P.S. (1992). Roy adaptation model testing: Dyadic adaptation, social support, and lonliness in COPD dyads (Doctoral dissertation, University of South Carolina, 1991). *Dissertation Abstracts Internatonal, 52*, 6320-B.

Razmus, I.S.(1994). Maternal adjustments to premature birth: Utilizing the Roy Adaptation Model as a theoretical framework. (Masters thesis, Grand Valley State University, 1993) *Masters Abstract International, 32*,1375.

Rich, V. L. (1992). The use of personal, organizational, and coping resources in the prevention of staff nurse burnout: A test of a model (Doctoral dissertation, University of Pittsburgh, 1991). *Dissertation Abstracts International, 52,* 3532-B.

Riegel, B., Heywood, G., Jackson, W., & Kennedy, A. (1988). Effect of nitroglycerin ointment placement on the severity of headache and flushing in patients with cardiac disease. *Heart & Lung, 17,* 426-431.

Roberson, E.L.M. (1987). Changes in oral temperature after small nebulizer inhalation treatment in adult clients. Unpublished master's thesis, Northwestern State University, Shreveport.

Robinson, J.H. (1992). A descriptive study of widows' grief responses, coping processes and social support within Roy's adaptation model (Doctoral dissertation, Wayne State University, 1991). *Dissertation Abstracts International, 52,* 6320-B.

Robinson, R.B. (1991). The relation between self-esteem and pregnancy in adolescent males and females. Unpublished master's thesis, Florida State University, Tallahassee.

Robinson, R.B., & Frank, D.I. (1994). The relation between self-esteem, sexual activity, and pregnancy. *Adolescence, 29*(113), 27-35.

Roy, C. (1977). Decision-making by the physically ill and adaptation during illness (Doctoral dissertation, University of California, Los Angeles, 1977). *Dissertation Abstracts International, 38,* 5060-A.

Roy, C. & Andrews, H.A. (1991). *The Roy Adaptation Model: The definitive statement.* Norwalk, CT: Appleton & Lange.

Scherubel, J.C.M. (1986). Description of adaptation patterns following an acute cardiac event (Doctoral dissertation, University of Illinois at Chicago, Health Sciences Center, 1985). *Dissertation Abstracts International, 46,* 2627-B.

Selman, S.W. (1989). Impact of total hip replacement on quality of life. *Orthopaedic Nursing, 8*(5), 43-49.

Shogan, M.G., & Schumann, L. L. (1993). The effect of environmental lighting on oxygen saturation of preterm infants in the NICU. *Neonatal Network Journal of Neonatal Nursing, 12*(5), 7-13.

Short, J.D. (1994). Interdependence needs and nursing care of the new family. *Issues in Comprehensive Pediatric Nursing, 17,* 1-14.

Shrubsole, J.L. (1992). Mutual aid: Promoting adaptation in women with premenstrual syndrome (Master's thesis, D'Youville College, 1992). *Masters Abstracts International, 30,* 1301.

Smith, B.J.A. (1990). Caregiver burden and adaptation in middle-aged daughters of dependent, elderly parents: A test of Roy's model (Doctoral dissertation, University of Pittsburgh, 1984). *Dissertation Abstracts International, 51,* 2290-B.

Smith, C.E., Garvis, M. S., & Martinson, I. M. (1983). Content analysis of interviews using a nursing model: A look at parents adapting to the impact of childhood cancer. *Cancer Nursing, 6*, 269-275.

Smith, C.E., Mayer, L. S., Parkhurst, C., Perkins, S.B., & Pingleton, S. K. (1991). Adaptation in families with a member requiring mechanical ventilation at home. *Heart & Lung, 20*, 349-356.

Smith, C.E., Moushey, L, Ross, J.A., Gieffer, C. (1993). Responsibilities and reactions of family caregivers of patients dependent on total parenteral nutrition at home. *Public Health Nursing, 10*, 122-128.

Smith, C.J. (1989). Cardiovascular responses in healthy males during basin bath, tub bath, and shower (Master's thesis, Texas Woman's University, 1987). *Masters Abstracts International, 27*, 103.

Stein, P.R. (1992). Life events, self-esteem, and powerlessness among adolescents (Doctoral dissertation, Texas Woman's University, 1991). *Dissertation Abstracts International, 52*, 5195-B.

Strohmyer, L.L., Noroian, E.L., Patterson, L.M., & Carlin, B.P. (1993). Adaptation six months after multiple trauma: A pilot study. *Journal of Neuroscience Nursing, 25*, 30-37.

Tulman, L., & Fawcett, J. (1990). Maternal employment following childbirth. *Research in Nursing & Health, 13,* 181-188.

Tulman, L., Fawcett, J., Groblewski, L., & Silverman, L. (1990). Changes in functional status after childbirth. *Nursing Research, 39,* 70-75.

Tulman, L., Fawcett, J., McEvoy, M. D. (1991). Development of the Inventory of Functional Status—Cancer. *Cancer Nursing, 14,* 254-260.

Tulman, L., Fawcett, J., & Weiss, M. (1993). The Inventory of Functional Status—Fathers: Development and psychometric testing. *Journal of Nurse Midwifery, 38,* 276-282.

Tulman, L., Higgins, K., Fawcett, J., Nunno, C., Vansickel, C., Haas, M. B., & Speca, M.M. (1991). The Inventory of Functional Status—Antepartum Period: Development and testing. *Journal of Nurse Midwifery, 36,* 117-123.

Varvaro, F.F. (1991). Women with coronary heart disease: An application of Roy's adaptation model. *Cardiovascular Nursing, 27*(6), 31-35.

Weiss, M.E. (1991). The relationship between marital independence and adaptation to parenthood in primiparous couples (Doctoral dissertation, University of San Diego, 1990). *Dissertation Abstracts International, 51*, 3783-B.

Zonca, B.J. (1980). The effects of a formal in-hospital patient education program on anxiety in postmyocardial infarction patients (Doctoral dissertation, Wayne State University, 1980). *Dissertation Abstracts International, 41*, 1418-A.

Bibliography

Abidin, R.R. (1983). Parenting Stress Index (PSI). Unpublished Instrument.

Achenback, T.M. (1988). *Youth self-report for ages 11-18*. Burlington, VT: University of Vermont Department of Psychiatry.

Aitken, R.C.B. (1969). Measurement of feelings using visual analogue scales. *Proceedings of the Royal Society of Medicine, 62*, 989-992.

Anthony, J.C., Le Resche, L., Niaz, U., Von Korff, M.R., & Folstein, M.F. (1982). Limits of the mini-mental state, a screening test for dementia and delirium among hospital patients. *Psychological Medicine, 12*, 397- 408.

Barjas, J.D. (1971). Sensory deprivation in geriatric patients in a nursing home. Unpublished Master's thesis, University of Arizona, as developed from Hanigfield, G. and Klett, J. (1965). The nurses' observation scale for inpatient evaluation. *Journal of Clinical Psychology, 65.*

Bergner, M., Bobbitt H.R., Pollard, W., Martin C. & Gibson, B. (1971). The sickness impact profile: Validation of a health status measurement. *Medical Care, 14*, 57-67.

Bergner, M., Bobbitt, R., Pollard, W., Martin, C., & Gibson, B. (1981). The sickness impact profile: Development and final revision of a health status measure. *Medical Care, 19*, (8), 787-805.

Billings, A.G., & Moos, R.H. (1981). The role of the coping responses and social resources in attenuating the stress of life events. *Journal of Behavioral Medicine, 4*, 139-157.

Brandt, P.A., & Weinert, C. (1981). The PRQ: A social support measure. *Nursing Research, 30*, 277-280.

Brazleton, T.B. (1984). *Clinical Development Medicine, 88*, 1-125.

Converse, P., & Robinson, J. (1973). Life satisfaction. In J. Robinson and P. Shaver (Eds). *Measures of social psychological attitudes,* (p.13).University of Michigan Institute for Social Research. Ann Arbor, MI.

Coopersmith, S. (1967). *The antecedents of self-esteem.* New York: Freeman.

Coopersmith, S. (1981). *Coopersmith self-esteem manual.* Palo Alto, Ca: Consulting Psychologists Press.

Coopersmith S. (1987). *Coopersmith self-esteem manual* (2nd ed.). Palo Alto, Ca: Consulting Psychologist Press.

Cronin-Stubbs, D.C. & Rooks, C. (1985). The stress, social support and burnout of critical care nurses: The results of research. *Heart & Lung, 14*, 31-39.

Crumbaugh, J. (1968). Cross validation of Purpose in Life Test based on Frankl's concepts. *Journal of Individual Psychology, 24.* 74-81.

Cyr, L. (1989). Sequelae of spinal cord injury after discharge from the initial rehabilitation program. *Rehabilitation Nursing, 14* (6), 326-329.

Derogatis, L.R. (1975). *Affects balance scale.* Baltimore, MD: Clinical Psychometric Research.

Derogatis, L.R.(1986). The psychosocial adjustment to illness scale. *Journal of Psychosomatic Research, 30,* (1), 77-91.

Derogatis, L.R., & Spencer, P.M. (1982). *The brief symptom inventory (BI): Administration scoring and procedure manual.* Johns Hopkins University School of Medicine.

Ferrans, C., & Powers, M. (1985). Quality of life index: Development and psychometric properties. *Advances in Nursing Science, 8*(1), 15-24.

Fitts, W.H. (1965). *Tennessee self concept scale: Manual.* Nashville, TN: Counselor Recordings and Tests.

Folkard, S., & Monk, T.H. (1979). Shiftwork and performance. *Human Factors, 21,* 483-492.

Fortinsky, R.H., Granger, C.V., & Seltzer, G.G. (1981). The use of functional assessment in understanding home care needs. *Medical Care, 14*(5), 489-497.

Frederickson, K., & Pollock, S.E. (1994). *Adaptation and quality of life in cardiac patients.* Grant funded by American Heart Association.

Gast, H. (1988). Child Mental Health Self Care Inventory. Unpublished instrument. College of Nursing, Wayne State University, Detroit, MI.

Guerney, B.J., Jr. (1977). *Relationship enhancement.* San Francisco: Jossey-Bass.

Halbreich, U., Endicott, J. & Sschact, S. (1982). The diversity of premenstrual changes as reflected in the premenstrual assessment form. *Acta Psychiatrica Scandinavia, 65,* 46-65.

Harter, A. (1985). *Manual: Social support scale for children.* Denver, CO: University of Colorado.

Harrison, L., & Woods, S. (1991). Early parental touch and preterm infants. *Journal of Obstetric, Gynecologic, & Neonatal Nursing, 20,* 229-306.

Hillard, R., Gjerde, C., & Porker, L. (1986).Validity of two psychological screening measures in family practice: Personal inventory and family APGAR. *Journal of Family Practice, 23,* 345-349.

Holmes, T., & Rahe, R. (1967). The social readjustment rating scale. *Journal of Psychosomatic Research, 11,* 213-218.

Hymovich, D.P. (1984). Development of the Chronicity Impact and Coping Instrument: Parent Questionnaire. (CICL:PQ). *Nursing Research, 33*(4), 218-222.

Jacox, A., & Stewart, M. (1973). *Psychosocial contingencies of pain experience.* Grant NUOO38, Iowa City, University of Iowa, as developed from Cornell Medical Index.

Jalowiec, A. (1979). *Jalowiec Coping Scale.* Chicago: University of Illinois.

Janis, I. & Mann, L. (1977). *Decision making: A psychological analysis of conflict, choice, and commitment.* NY: Free Press.

Johnson, J.E. (1984). Coping with elective surgery. In H.H. Werley & J.J. Fitzpatrick (Eds.), *Annual review of nursing research* (Vol.2, pp. 107-132). New York: Springer.

Jones, T.W. (1980). *Preliminary test manual: The staff burnout scale for heath professionals.* Park Ridge, IL: London House Management.

Katz, M.H., & Peotrkowski, C.S. (1983). Correlates of role strain among employed black women. *Family Relations, 32*(3), 331-339.

Keene, A., & Cullen, D. (1983). Therapeutic Intervention Scoring System (TISS): Update. *Critical Care Medicine, 11,*(1), 1-3.

Knaus,W., Zimmerman, J., Wagner, G., Draper, L., & Lawrence, P. (1983). APACHE - Acute physiology and chronic health evaluation scale: A physiologically based classification. *Critical Care Medicine, 9*(8), 591-597.

Lawton, M.P. (1975). The Philadelphia geriatric center morale scale: A revision. *Journal of Gerontology, 30,* 85-89.

Lawton, M.P., & Brody, E.M. (1969). Assessment of older people: Self-maintaining and instrumental activities of daily living. *The Gerontologist, 9,* 179-186.

Lawton, M.P., Moss, M., Fulcomer, M. & Kleban, M.H. (1982). A research and service oriented multilevel assessment instrument. *Journal of Gerontology, 37,* 91-98.

Lazarus, R., & Folkman, S. (1989). *Manual for the Hassles and Uplifts Scales.* Palo Alto, CA: Consulting Psychologists Press.

Lederman, R.P., Weingarten, C.T., & Lederman, E. (1981). Post-partum self evaluation questionnaire: Measures of maternal adaptation. In R. P. Lederman (Ed.), *Perinatal parental behavior: Nursing research and implications for newborn health.* (pp. 165-180). New York: Alan Liss. (March of Dimes Birth Defects Foundation Original Article Series, Vol. 17, No.6).

Lefebvre, R.C., & Sandford, S.L. (1985). A multi-modal questionnaire for stress. *Journal of Human Stress, 11,* 60-75.

Leiffer, M.O. (1977). Psychological changes accompanying pregnancy and motherhood. *Genetic Psychology Monographs, 95,* 55-96.

Levenson, H. (1974). Activism and powerful others: Distinctions within the concept of internal-external control. *Journal of Personality Assessment, 38,* 377-383.

Maddi, S.R., Kobasa, S.C. & Hoover, M. (1979). An Alienation Test. *Journal of Humanistic Psychology*, 19, 73-76.

Marut, J.S. & Mercer, R.T. (1979). Comparison of primiparas perceptions of vaginal and cesarean births. *Nursing Research, 28*, 260-266.

McCorkle, R., & Quint-Bendiel, J. (1983) Symptom distress, current concerns and mood after diagnosis of life threatening disease. *Social Science Medicine, 17*, 431-438.

McCubbin, H.I., McCubbin, M.A., Patterson, J.M., Cauble, A.E., Wilson, L.R., & Warwick, W. (1983). CHIP-Coping Health Inventory for Parents: An assessment of parental coping patterns in the care of the chronically ill child. *Journal of Marriage and the Family, 45*(2), 359-370.

McCubbin, H.I., & Thompatz,, A.I. (1986). *Family assessment inventories for research and practice.* Madison, WI: University of Wisconsin-Madison.

McNair, D., Lorr, M., & Droppleman, L.F. (1971). *Profile of mood states.* San Diego, CA: Educational and Industrial Training Service.

Meenan, R., Gertman, P., & Mason, J. (1980). Measuring health status in arthritis: The arthritis measurement scales. *Arthritis and Rheumatism, 23*(2), 146-152.

Mehrabian, A., & Epstein, N. (1972). A measure of emotional empathy. *Journal of Personality*, 40, 525-543.

Melzack, R. (1975).The McGill Pain Questionnaire: Major properties and scoring methods. *Pain, 1*(3), 277-299.

Melzack, R. (1983). The McGill Pain Questionnaire. In R. Melzack (Ed.). *Pain measurement and assessment.* New York: Raven Press.

Miller, J.F., (1988). Development of an instrument to measure hope. *Dissertation Abstracts International, 47*, 44-6BB. (University Microfilms No. 87-05, 572).

Montgomery, R.J.V., & Borgatta, E.E. (1985). *Family support project: Final report to the Administration on Aging* (Grant No. 90AM0046). Seattle, WA: Institute on Aging and Long Term Care, University of Washington.

Moos, R.H. (1974). *Family Environment Scale.* Palo Alto, CA: Consulting Psychologists Press.

Moos, R.H., Cronkite, R.C., Billings, A.G., & Finney, I.W. (1986). *Health and Daily Living Form manual.* Palo Alto, CA: Social Ecology Laboratory, Department of Psychiatry and Behavioral Sciences. Veterans Administration and Stanford University.

Norbeck, J.S. (1981). Social support: A model for clinical research and application. *Advances in Nursing Science,3*(4), 43-59.

Norbeck, J.S. (1984). *The Norbeck social support questionnaire.* In K.E. Barnard, P.A. Brandt, B.S. Raf, & P. Carroll (Eds.) Social support and families of vulnerable infants. White Plains, NY: March of Dimes Birth Defects Foundation, Birth Defects, Original Article Series, 20(5), 45-57.

Olson, D.H., McCubbin, H., Barnes, H., Larsen, A., Muzen, M., & Wilson, M. (1982). *Family inventories: Inventories used in a national survey of families across the family life cycle.* St. Paul, MN: University of Minnesota.

Pfeiffer E. (1985). *Functional assessment inventory.* In B. Burton, R. Cairl, D. Keller, & E. Pfeiffer. Functional assessment inventory training manual (Revised ed.) pp.124-147). Tampa, FL: Suncoast Gerontology Center, University of South Florida.

Pollock, S.E. (1982). Level of adaptation: An analysis of stress factors that affect health status (Doctoral dissertation, The University of Texas at Austin, 1981). *Dissertation Abstracts International, 42,*4364-B.

Pollock, S.E. (1984). Adaptation to Stress. *Texas Nursing, 58* (10), 12-13

Radloff, L. (1977). The CES-D scale: A self-report depression scale for research in the general population. *Journal of Applied Psychological Measurement, 1,* 385-401.

Robbins, R. (1981). A study of the relationship between adolescent pregnancy and life-change events. *Issues in Mental Health Nursing,3,* 219-236.

Rosenberg, M. (1965). *Society and the adolescent self-image.* Princeton, NJ: Princeton University Press.

Rosenberg, M. (1979). *Conceiving the self.* New York: Basic Books.

Russell, D. (1982). The measurement of loneliness. In L.A. Peplau & D. Perlman, (Eds.) *Loneliness: A sourcebook of current theory, research, and therapy,* (pp. 81-104). NY: Wiley.

Sanders, C.M., Mauger, P.A., & Strong, P.N. (1985). A *manual for the Grief Experience Inventory.* Palo Alto, CA: Consulting Psychologists Press.

Secord, P., & Jourard, S. (1953). The appraisal of body cathexis and the self. *Journal of Consulting Psychology, 17,* 343-356.

Smith, P., Hamilton, B., Granger, C. (1990). *Functional independence measure decision tree.* The Fone FIM. Research Foundation of the State University of NY. Buffalo, NY.

Spanier, G.B. (1976). Measuring dyadic adjustment: New scales for assessing the quality of marriage and similar dyads. *Journal of Marriage and the Family, 38*(1), 15-28.

Spielberger, C.D., Gorsuch, R.L. Lushene, R., Vagg, P.R., & Jacobs, G.A. (1970). *Manual for the State-Trait Anxiety Inventory.* Palo Alto, CA: Consulting Psychologists Press.

Spielberger, C.D., Gorsuch, R.L., Lushene, R., Vagg, P.R., & Jacobs, G.A. (1983). *Manual for the State-Trait Anxiety Inventory.* Palo Alto, CA: Consulting Psychologists Press.

Tasto, D., Colligan, M., Skjel, E., & Polly, W. (1978). *Health consequences of shift work.* National Technical Information Service (No. 210-75-0072). Cincinnati, OH: National Institute for Occupational Safety and Health.

Tulman, L., Fawcett, J., & Weiss, M. (1993). The Inventory of Functional Status—Fathers: Development and psychometric testing. *Journal of Nurse Midwifery, 38,* 276-282.

Varvaro, F. (1986). Sexual concerns and family functioning in women with coronary artery disease. In J. Wang (Ed.) *Creating the future through research: Proceedings of the West Virginia Nurses Association Research Group,* 7-10.

Verran, J.A., & Snyder-Halpern, R. (1988). Do patients sleep in the hospital? *Applied Nursing Research, 1*(2), 95.

Walston, K., Brown, G., Stein, M., & Dobbins, C. (1989). Comparing the short and long versions of the Arthritis Impact Measurement Scales. *Journal of Rheumatology, 16*(8), 1005-1109.

Weisman, A., & Worden, J. (1977). *Coping and vulnerability in cancer patients.* Project Omega. Cambridge, MA: Harvard Medical School.

Yeaworth, R., York, J., Hussey, S., Ingle, M.B., & Goodwin, T. (1980). The development of an Adolescent Life Change Event Scale. *Adolescence, 15,* 91-97..

Zarit, S.H., Reever, K.E., & Bach-Peterson, J. (1980). Relatives of the impaired elderly: Correlates of feelings of burden. *The Gerontologist, 23,*(6), 649-655.

Ziemer, M.M. (1983). Effects of information on postsurgical coping. *Nursing Research, 32,* 282-287.

Zuckerman, M., & Lubin, B. (1965). *Manual for the Affect Adjective Checklist.* San Diego, CA: Educational and Industrial Testing Service.

Zung, W. (1965). A self-rating depression scale. *Archives of General Psychiatry, 12,* 63-70.

Chapter 11

Contributions to Knowledge: Testing Model Propositions

One way to view nursing science is through the published writings of nurse theorists. Theories are derived from a given conceptual model and represent a systematic way of viewing the world. By deriving propositions from the model, researchable hypotheses can be developed and tested. Researchers seek to validate these views about the individual, the environment, health, and nursing. Propositions are statements that explain relationships between concepts integral to the model or explain one concept. Researchers who explicate the nature of the model as well as theories that confirm or support the structure of the model add to the knowledge base of the model as well as to nursing science (Frederickson, Jackson, Strauman, & Strauman, 1991). Conversely, lack of support for the propositions would be an appropriate conclusion when the empiric data do not conform to hypothesized expectations. For developing knowledge based on the RAM, studies had to meet both criteria for linkages to the model and criteria for scientific soundness. Out of 163 studies, 116 met the criteria established for testing propositions from the model.

Selection of Propositions

Propositions identified from studies based on the RAM were reported in the seven content chapters which were focused on physiologic, self concept, role-function, and interdependence modes, adaptive modes and processes, stimuli, and interventions.

Twelve propositions were selected for inclusiveness and for emphasis on the holistic nature of the person (See Chapter 2, Table 2.5). In addition, they were selected by the members of BBARNS as relevant for all research in this monograph. Roy and Roberts (1981) derived 97 sample propositions from the model which were based on the major concepts: theory of the person as an adaptive system and theories of the four adaptive modes. For the purpose of this work, BBARNS members analyzed and synthesized the existing body of propositions and formulated propositions for the metaparadigm concepts, adaptation processes of the person, and stimuli.

Results of Analysis and Synthesis of Propositions

Each of the generic propositions from the research review was examined for conceptual clarity and frequency in its use in deriving ancillary propositions. Ancillary propositions are defined as subsidiary or special instances of the generic propositions that the BBARNS investigators derived from the research findings of the studies reviewed. Some of these are also referred to as practice propositions because they are stated in ways directly relevant to practice. It was noted whether the generic proposition was supported by ancillary propositions tested in the reported research. The results of deriving and testing the ancillary propositions from generic propositions are discussed and related to the metaparadigm concepts, adaptive processes of the person or group, stimuli, and nursing interventions.

Metaparadigm Propositions

The metaparadigm concepts recognize the person or group as an integrated whole that has innate and acquired ways of adapting. Propositions derived from the metaparadigm concepts integrate the four main concepts in the metaparadigm of nursing: person, environment, health and nursing. By addressing the concepts in this manner, health becomes an outcome of adaptive processes that reflects patterns of being and becoming whole and being integrated with the self and the environment.

Four generic propositions were identified as specific to the metaparadigm concepts of person, environment, health, and nursing. The first proposition, "At the individual level, regulator and cognator processes affect innate and acquired ways of adapting," is focused on the concept of person. The fifth proposition, "The adequacy of cognator and regulator processes will affect adaptive responses," is specific to the concept of health. Proposition eight, "Adaptation is influenced by the integration of the person with the environment," is focused on the environment. The 12th proposition, "The goal of nursing interventions is to enhance adaptation by managing input to adaptive systems," is specific to the concept of nursing.

Concept of person. The first proposition is focused on the metaparadigm concept of person as viewed by the RAM. The theory about the adapting person reflects the unique role of the regulator and cognator in adaptation. Adaptation through regulator or cognator processes can affect a person negatively or positively producing a challenge to the adaptive system in maintaining and enhancing the well being of the self. Adaptation is the core of the RAM theoretic framework. Cognator and regulator processes are the active forces of adaptation.

Thirty-five ancillary propositional statements derived from the first proposition were tested (see Table 11.1). Of these, 33 supported and 2 did not support the proposition. The large number of propositional statements implies that the proposition which was derived from Roy's concept of person is clear enough for utilization in many studies. As a proposition derived from the metaparadigm concepts, the support of the theoretic

Table 11.1 – Results of Testing RAM Propositions: Metaparadigm Concepts

Chapter Numbers	3	4	5	6	7	8	9	Total
Proposition 1								
Total	5	1	0	11	14	1	3	35
Support/Non Support	5/0	1/0		11/0	13/1	1/0	2/1	33/2
Proposition 5								
Total	0	0	0	0	19	0	1	20
Support/Non Support					16/3		1/0	17/3
Proposition 8								
Total	0	0	0	0	1	4	3	8
Support/Non Support					1/0	4/0	3/0	8/0
Proposition 12								
Total	0	0	3	0	0	3	5	11
Support/Non Support			2/1			3/0	3/2	8/3

underpinnings of these concepts is validated. Because most of the ancillary propositions supported this first generic proposition, there is support for the way in which Roy has defined person at the conceptual level. In Chapter 7, investigators of studies on the adaptive modes and processes reported 14 ancillary propositional statements, of which 13 were supported and 1 was not supported. Investigators for five studies supported the ancillary proposition that "Cognitive processing affects self concept and self concept may affect cognitive processing." On the other hand, Roy (1977) did not support this ancillary proposition. The failure of her work to support this proposition may be indicative of the early stages of measurement of the model concepts.

Concept of health. The fifth proposition is that the adequacy of cognator and regulator processes will affect adaptive responses. This proposition implies the concept of health from the metaparadigm. Cognator and regulator subsystems help to process stimuli with the goal of adaptation, which in turn promotes health. When cognator and regulator processes contribute to the goals of adaptation, the results lead to adaptive responses. On the other hand, when cognator and regulator processes do not contribute to the goals of adaptation, ineffective responses result. The adequacy of cognator or regulator processes has the greatest effect on adaptation and health.

Twenty ancillary statements were derived and tested from the fifth generic proposition. Of these, investigators of 17 studies supported and 3 did not support the ancillary proposition. The ancillary proposition that adaptive processes relate to health was tested by investigators of six studies. Investigators in three of the studies supported the ancillary proposition and in the other three, did not. Frederickson and colleagues (1991) found that perceived physical and psychosocial well-being among cancer patients was related to longevity. However, Phillips and Brown (1992) found no relationship between mill workers' adaptation to shift work and injuries on the job. Further testing should focus on adaptation related to health in other specific populations.

Concept of environment. Adaptation as influenced by the integration of the person with the environment is the focus of the eighth proposition. The mutual interaction of people and their environment is inherent in the metaparadigm concept of environment. Conceptually, the relationship is based on the processes of synthesizing the person's internal and external environments. The goal of the interaction is to maintain integrity and growth for both the self and environment. The quality of integration determines adaptation level.

Eight ancillary propositions were derived and tested from the eighth proposition on the environment, all of which were supported. Chapter 8 was focused on studies related to stimuli, and four ancillary propositions were reported, all of which were supported. Armer (1988/1989) found that "relocation adaptation is influenced by a sense of prediction and control" among the elderly moving to congregate living. (See section below on propositions related to stimuli as further evidence concerning concept of environment.)

Responses to environmental stimuli such as relocation, eye surgery, or the use of a birth chair indicate that adaptation is facilitated by a person's integrating new stimuli as part of the self and one's environment. Future studies should address the integration of environment as promoting adaptation.

Concept of nursing. The emphasis of the 12th proposition is on the central focus of the RAM—that the goal of nursing interventions is to enhance adaptation by managing input to adaptive systems. Derived from the metaparadigm concept of nursing, model based nursing assessments and interventions were focused on managing the focal or contextual stimuli. Nurses enter the client system by using the nursing process and managing incoming stimuli to promote adaptation. Nurses, therefore, recognize the role of identification and management of stimuli, developing theories of intervention and their effect on patient outcomes. In this context, nursing interventions become a powerful force for managing focal or contextual stimuli to produce integrity and growth, thus increasing adaptation level.

In the research reported on proposition 12, eleven ancillary propositions were derived. Researchers in eight studies supported the proposition and researchers in three did not. In Chapter 9, testing of five ancillary propositions related to interventions were described. Three were supported, and two were not. Guzetta (1979), Meek (1993), and Parlin (1988/1990) supported the ancillary proposition that the goal of nursing interventions is to enhance adaptation and manage input to adaptive systems. Prelewicz as well as Meek and Parlin (1993) studied the effects of pets on the elderly. Prelewicz found that animal-assisted therapy did not decrease loneliness among the elderly in a nursing home. However, results were statistically significant in the direction of promoting adaptation in most studies related to the effects of pets. Investigators used pets as novel stimuli and the interventions were effective while posing few risks.

In summary, almost half of the ancillary propositions tested in the category of nursing's metaparadigm concepts were related to the concept of person, of which 94% were supported. Theoretically and empirically there is support for Roy's conceptualization of the person as an adaptive system. Almost 25% of the ancillary propositions tested were related to the concept of health of which most were supported. Theoretically and empirically, there is support for Roy's conceptualization of health as an outcome of adaptation. Approximately 75% of the propositions tested were related to concepts of person or health. Of these, only 5 out of 55 propositions were not supported, or fewer than 10%. Less than 13% of the propositions tested were focused on the metaparadigm concepts of environment or nursing. Of these, 15% were not supported. Researchers have provided support for Roy's conceptualization of the metaparadigm concepts of person and health. Future research should be directed toward testing propositions derived from the RAM concepts of nursing and environment.

Propositions on Adaptive Processes of Person or Group

Adaptation processes of the person involve the integration of cognator and regulator subsystems through perception. The outcomes of further information processing; learning; judgment; and emotion, or neural chemical, and endocrine coping are viewed as holistic adaptation.

The following propositions were derived from the theory of adaptive processes of person or group: (a) proposition two, at the group level, stabilizer and innovator processes affect adaptation; (b) proposition four, the characteristics of the internal and external stimuli influences the adequacy of cognitive and emotional processes; (c) proposition six, adaptation in one mode is affected by adaptation in other modes through cognator and regulator connectives; (d) proposition nine, the variable of time influences the process of adaptation; (e) proposition 10, the variable of perception influences the process of adaptation; and (f) proposition 11, perception influences adaptation through linking the regulator and cognator subsystems.

Proposition two is that at the group level, stabilizer and innovator processes affect adaptation. The stabilizer-innovator is the group-level equivalent of the cognator-regulator for the individual. The stabilizer-innovator is the core of adaptive group processing and facilitates transition for groups during environmental changes. Researchers reported (see Table 11.2) five derived propositional statements; four were supported and one was not. In Chapter 9, intervention studies, two ancillary propositional statements were reported, one of which was supported. Campbell (1992) supported the derived proposition that nurses are able to accurately identify patients who are depressed. On the other hand, Fahs (1991/1992) did not support the ancillary proposition that nurses can affect costs of injections by using low-dose injectate volume. Further development and testing of the second proposition is warranted. Publication of research results for applying the model to groups is more recent and less extensive than are reports about individual adaptation. Therefore, propositions and methods related to group adaptation require further refinement.

The fourth proposition is that the characteristics of internal and external stimuli influence the adequacy of cognitive and emotional processes. A stimulus affects the learned strategies used for adaptation and is derived from the theory of the adapting person. The magnitude and characteristics of the stimulus affect homeostasis and growth. There were 17 ancillary propositional statements, of which 16 were supported and 1 was not supported. In Chapter 7, covering research on the adaptation modes and processes, nine ancillary propositional statements were tested. Of these, researchers supported eight propositions and did not support one. An ancillary proposition, "Nurses' judgments about nursing problems and actions are affected by experience and education" was both supported and not supported by Trentini (1985/1986). Trentini found that nurses' levels of education were related to the number of nursing actions for solving problems for patients with end-stage renal disease. In contrast, Trentini reported that nurses' judgments about the number of problems were not affected by type of education or experience. With investigators from only nine studies testing this proposition, further study is warranted on the effect of stimuli on the integration of thinking and emotion and on subsequent adaptation.

The sixth proposition—that adaptation in one mode is affected by adaptation in other modes through cognator and regulator connectives–was derived from the theory of the adaptive person. Recognizing that the person or group is an integrated whole, it is through interaction among the modes that wholeness is manifested. Because adaptation is a response from the whole person, adaptive responses are relevant for all modes. Twenty-two ancillary propositional statements were tested, of which 17 were supported and 5 were not supported. In Chapter 4, about studies related to self-concept mode research, four ancillary propositions were reported—

Table 11.2 –Results of Testing RAM Propositions: Adaptive Processes of Person or Group

Chapter numbers	3	4	5	6	7	8	9	Total
Proposition 2								
Total	0	0	0	0	3	0	2	5
Support/ Non Support					3/0		1/1	4/1
Proposition 4								
Total	0	0	1	2	9	1	4	17
Support/Non Support			1/0	2/0	8/1	1/0	4/0	16/1
Proposition 6								
Total	0	4	3	3	3	1	8	22
Support/Non Support		4/0	3/0	3/0	2/1	1/0	4/4	17/5
Proposition 9								
Total	3	3	2	6	3	4	2	23
Support/Non Support	3/0	3/0	1/1	4/2	3/0	4/0	2/0	20/3
Proposition 10								
Total	0	0	0	0	0	3	1	4
Support/Non Support						3/0	0/1	3/1
Proposition 11								
Total	0	0	0	0	0	1	2	3
Support/Non Support						1/0	2/0	3/0

all of which were tested and supported. Chen (1994) reported that levels of loneliness (interdependence mode) and self esteem (self concept mode) were associated with levels of hearing loss (physiologic mode). Further testing is warranted to quantify levels of adaptation in each mode and the subsequent effect on adaptation level of the other modes.

The variable of time influencing the process of adaptation is the focus of the ninth proposition. Time is central to understanding the process of adaptation. Factors such as age of the person, progression of the illness and changing severity of the alteration affect adaptation level. Strengthening of existing coping strategies and developing new ones also affect adaptation level. Passage of time provides the opportunity for the processes to evolve.

As the number of nursing interventions increase over time, the cognator and regulator subsystems are available to process the effect of incoming stimuli and thereby facilitate adaptation. Twenty-three ancillary propositional statements were tested that were related to this generic proposition; 20 were supported. In Chapter 6, which was about studies related to the interdependence mode, information was given about six ancillary propositions that were tested. Four were supported; two were not. Artinian (1988/1989, 1991, 1992) supported the ancillary proposition that spouses adapt to their partners' conditions over time. Conversely, Grinspun (1991) found that spouses of head-injured patients did not adapt to their partner's condition over time. Proposition nine addresses time as a factor in adaptive processes, but it is very generally stated. A determining factor of the studies that did not support the proposition, may be the nature of the physiologic deficits (inability to communicate) and the degree of permanence of an injury or physiologic change in the spouse. In other words, the intensity of the stimulus might be a factor in changing predictions about adaptation over time.

The 10th proposition is that the variable of perception influences the process of adaptation. Derived from the theory of adaptation processes of the person, regulatory behaviors associated with perception have an effect on the adaptation process. Individuals possess afferent sources that determine the level and quality of perception. Perceptions are fundamental aspects of the person and greatly influence adaptation. In the research reported, three of the four derived ancillary propositions were supported; one was not. In Chapter 7, which was about studies focused on stimuli, Armer (1988/1989) and Dahlen (1980) supported the proposition that perception of an event is a stronger predictor of adaptation than is the focal stimulus. Armer also reported that perception of an event and contextual stimuli are stronger combined predictors of an event than is the focal stimulus.

The 11th proposition—that perception influences adaptation through linking the regulator and cognator subsystems—was derived from the theory of adaptation processes of the person. Biologic stimuli and behavioral stimuli are connected through the process of perception. The process of perception influences adaptation through linking the regulator and cognator subsystems. The person's perceptions of a dysfunction have a profound effect on the person's response and adaptation. In the reported studies, three ancillary propositional statements were tested and all were supported. In Chapter 9, which was about studies focused on interventions, Hjelm-Karlsson (1989) supported the ancillary proposition that patient education related to a medical procedure reduces pain and discomfort. This is a more complex proposition, in that it incorporates analysis and synthesis of timing as well as the relationship between biologic and behavioral processes in a complex design that includes interventions and comparisons.

Of the six propositions tested in the category of adaptive processes of person or group, 84% of the ancillary propositions tested were from just three propositions: four, six, and nine. These three generic propositions were focused on the characteristics of the stimuli and the adequacy of cognitive and emotional processes. For example, adaptation in one mode being affected by adaptation in the other modes through cognator-regulator connectives and the variable of time influencing the process of adaptation. Of the 62 ancillary propositions tested, 85% were supported. In summary, strong support exists for the effects of time, the adequacy of the cognator-regulator, and of the stimuli on adaptation.

Propositions 2, 10, and 11 accounted for only 16% of the ancillary propositions tested in the category of adaptive processes of person or group. Of these, 17% were not supported. The three generic propositions focused on the effect of the stabilizer-innovator on adaptation in groups, the effect of perception on adaptation, and the role of perception on adaptation through linking the cognator-regulator. The paucity of studies on the role of perception and adaptation provides clear direction that future research is needed. Although some investigators strongly support the effects of perception on adaptation, further research is indicated. In the area of groups and the role of stabilizer-innovator processes, additional conceptualization and research are needed.

Propositions Related to Stimuli

The concept of stimuli includes incoming information—both internal and external—and their effects on the cognator and regulator. In this context, the effect of the focal stimulus becomes a major determinant of adaptation level of the whole and integrated self. Two propositions were derived from the concept of stimuli: numbers three and seven (see Table 11.3).

The third proposition is that the characteristics of the internal and external stimuli influence adaptive responses. The nature and magnitude

Table 11.3 – Results of Testing RAM Propositions: Stimuli

Chapter numbers	3	4	5	6	7	8	9	Total
Proposition 3								
Total	20	5	4	33	16	9	15	102
Support/Non Support	15/5	2/3	4/0	32/1	15/1	9/0	8/7	85/17
Proposition 7								
Total	2	5	4	0	7	4	3	25
Support/ Non Support	1/1	5/0	3/1		7/0	4/0	2/1	22/3

of all inputs into the system, or person, alter the nature and magnitude of the outputs or behaviors. Behavioral responses are determined by the magnitude of exposure to the stimuli and adaptation level. Therefore, changes in the stimuli result in changes in adaptive responses. In the research reviewed, 102 propositional statements related to stimuli were tested; 85 were supported and 17 were not. In Chapter 3 about physiologic adaptive mode research, an ancillary propositional statement was reported that stimuli can be identified that predict adaptive and ineffective responses in the physiologic mode. Gervasini (1994) supported the statement by generating a statistically significant list of variables predictive of sepsis or nonsepsis in critically ill trauma patients. On the other hand, Rustic (1993) did not find a relationship between the effects of relocation and the development of physical symptoms of international graduate students. It is interesting to observe the number of research questions that tested this proposition. This phenomena in part may be because of the empiric nature of the proposition. The effect of stimuli on adaptation appears to be one of the best demonstrated theoretic building blocks of the model.

The seventh proposition indicates that the pooled effect of focal, contextual, and residual stimuli determines adaptation level. Adaptation is viewed as a process and characteristic of the person in interaction with the environment. As an information-processing system, the person takes in and responds to the combined effect of focal, contextual, and residual stimuli. The effect of the three types of stimuli was discussed in Chapter 1. Of 25 ancillary propositional statements derived from the research, 22 supported the generic proposition and 3 did not. In Chapter 5 about role function research findings, three of the four ancillary propositions were tested and supported. Fawcett and Weiss (1993) found that preparation for cesarean birth influences adaptation. However, when Fawcett and Weiss studied the influence of cultural differences on adaptation to cesarean birth they found no support for the ancillary proposition. A relatively even distribution was evident among the chapters regarding investigators testing the seventh proposition. The findings from the research on the combined effects of stimuli on adaptation have added to the knowledge base of the model and have provided direction for future research. The magnitude and characteristics of the focal stimuli should help determine the effects of the contextual and residual stimuli on adaptation.

From the two propositions related to stimuli, 127 ancillary propositions were tested. A total of 275 ancillary propositions were tested from all of the content chapters. Of these, 39% were tested for proposition three, which was related to the characteristics of the stimuli influencing adaptive responses, and 10% were tested for proposition seven which proposes that the combined effect of all three levels of stimuli determine the adaptation level. Forty-nine per cent of all ancillary propositions tested were related to the concept of stimuli, of which 94% were supported. There is then, theoretic and empiric support for Roy's conceptualization of stimuli. Both the numbers of studies and the support of the ancillary propositions provide evidence that the concept of stimuli in the RAM has validity and reliability. By synthesizing propositions three and seven, there is confirmation of a theory about stimuli: The characteristics and pooled effect of the stimuli determine adaptation level and influence adaptive responses.

Summary

This chapter was focused on contributions to knowledge through the testing of propositions. Of the 163 studies included in this monograph, 116 studies were identified for inclusion in this chapter. Twelve generic propositions were identified and ancillary propositions derived from the reported research. The generic propositions were categorized according to their relationship to nursing's metaparadigm concepts, the adaptive processes of person or group, and stimuli. An overwhelming majority of the ancillary propositions were supported, thus providing theoretic and empiric support for selected concepts of the model. Knowledge development through research and testing of propositions based on the RAM has contributed to nursing science.

References

Armer, J.M. (1989). Factors influencing relocation adjustment among community-based rural elderly (Doctoral dissertation, University of Rochester, 1988). *Dissertation Abstracts International, 50,* 1321-B.

Artinian, N.T. (1989). The stress process within the Roy adaptation framework: Sources, mediators and manifestations of stress in spouses of coronary artery bypass patients during hospitalization and six weeks post discharge (Doctoral dissertation, Wayne State University, 1988). *Dissertation Abstracts International, 49,* 5225-B.

Artinian, N.T. (1991). Stress experience of spouses of patients having coronary artery bypass during hospitalization and six weeks after discharge. *Heart & Lung, 20,* 52-59.

Artinian, N T. (1992). Spouse adaptation to mate's CABG surgery: 1-year follow-up. *American Journal of Critical Care 1*(2), 36-42.

Campbell, J.M. (1992). Treating depression in well older adults: Use of diaries in cognitive therapy. *Issues in Mental Health Nursing, 13,* 19-29.

Chen, H.L. (1994). Hearing in the elderly: Relation of hearing loss, loneliness, and self-esteem. *Journal of Gerontological Nursing, 20*(6), 22-28.

Dahlen, R.A. (1980). Analysis of selected factor related to the elderly person's ability to adapt to visual prostheses following senile cataract surgery (Doctoral dissertation, The Catholic University of America, 1980). *Dissertation Abstracts International, 41,* 389-B.

Fahs, P. (1992). Effect of heparin injectate volume on pain and bruising using the Roy Model (Doctoral dissertation, University of Alabama, 1991). *Dissertation Abstracts International, 52,* 5195-B.

Fawcett, J. & Weiss, M.E. (1993). Cross-cultural adaptation to cesarean birth. *Western Journal of Nursing Research, 15,* 282-297.

Frederickson, K., Jackson, B., Strauman, T. & Strauman, J. (1991). Testing hypotheses derived from the Roy Adaptation Model. *Nursing Science Quarterly,* 4, 168-174.

Gervasini, A.A. (1994). Classification of trauma patients with a septic profile utilizing a predictor model. Unpublished doctoral dissertation, Boston College, Boston.

Grinspun, D. (1991). Factors influencing adaptation of spouses of head trauma patients. Unpublished master's thesis, University of Michigan, Ann Arbor.

Guzetta, C.E. (1979). Relationship between stress and learning. *Advances in Nursing Science, 1* (4), 35-39.

Hjelm-Karlsson, K. (1989). Effects of information to patients undergoing intravenous pyelography: An intervention study. *Journal of Advanced Nursing,* 14, 853-62.

Meek, Sr. S. (1993). Effects of slow stroke back massage on relaxation in hospice clients. *Image: Journal of Nursing Scholarship, 25,* 17-21.

Parlin, C.A. (1990). Physiological manifestations of human/animal interaction in adult population over fifty-five (Master's thesis, University of Nevada, Reno, 1988). *Masters Abstracts International, 28,* 113.

Phillips, J.A., & Brown, K. C. (1992). Industrial workers on rotating shift pattern: Adaptation and injury status. *AAOHN Journal, 40,* 468-476.

Prelewicz, T.N. (1993). The effects of animal-assisted therapy on loneliness in elderly residents of a long-term care facility utilizing Roy's adaptation model (Master's thesis, D'Youville College, 1993). *Masters Abstracts International, 31,* 1749.

Roy, C. (1977). Decision-making by the physically ill and adaptation during illness (Doctoral dissertation, University of California, Los Angeles, 1977). *Dissertation Abstracts International, 38,* 5060-A.

Roy, C., & Roberts, S. (1981). *Theory construction in nursing: An adaptation model.* Englewood Cliffs, NJ: Prentice Hall, Inc.

Rustic, D.L. (1993). A study of somatic symptomatology: Occurrence and severity as reported by international graduate students at Michigan State University. (Master's thesis, Michigan State University, 1992). *Masters Abstracts International, 31,* 282.

Trentini, M. (1986). Nurses' decisions in dialysis patient care: An application of the Roy Adaptation Model (Doctoral dissertation, The University of Alabama in Birmingham, 1985). *Dissertation Abstracts International, 47,* 575-B.

Chapter 12

Applications to Nursing Practice

In this chapter information from research reports are included which focused on key concepts of the Roy Adaptation Model (RAM) identified in Chapters 3 through 9. Of the 163 studies included in this monograph, 116 met the established criteria for methodologic and theoretic adequacy discussed in Chapter 2. These 116 studies were reviewed and examined for their applications to nursing practice based on three categories: (a) high potential for implementation, (b) further clinial evaluation before implementation, and (c) further research indicated before implementation.

Purpose

The purpose of this chapter is to synthesize findings of research from the RAM that can be implemented in the practice setting. Although it is generally not warranted to recommend the implementaton of any study without replication, the studies we recommend for implementation are those that had empiric support concerning effectiveness and did not pose harmful risks to subjects. Consequently, studies evaluated to have a high potential for implementation (*n*=60) will be presented. Studies evaluated as needing further clinical evaluation before implementation or needing further testing before implementation will not be included in this chapter. Studies in these two categories require further refinement before contributions to nursing practice can be synthesized.

Background

Nursing practice based on the RAM involves a distinctive use of the nursing process. Nursing process is a problem-solving approach that enables nurses to identify levels of adaptation and coping abilities, to identify difficulties, and to intervene to promote adaptation. As described in the model (Roy & Andrews, 1991; 1999), nursing process relates to the view of a person or group as an adaptive system. Six steps have been identified in the nursing process utilizing the RAM. The six steps are: (a) assessment of behavior, (b) assessment of stimuli, (c) nursing diagnosis, (d) goal setting, (e) intervention, and (f) evaluation.

Using the model-based nursing process, nurses assess the person's behavior and the focal and contextual stimuli influencing the behavior. Goals establishing behavioral outcomes for the person are formulated and interventions designed to manage stimuli are planned and implemented. Evaluation involves judging the effectiveness of the interventions in relation to the established goals. The nursing process is ongoing and steps occur simultaneously—even though each step is separated for discussion. Nurses may be assessing and intervening concurrently.

The nursing process according to the model will serve as the framework for this chapter. Applications for nursing practice from the 60 studies will be synthesized using the steps of the nursing process. Several studies had implications for practice in more than one phase of the nursing process. Consequently, findings from some studies will appear in more than one section.

Assessment of Behavior

According to Roy, behavior indicates how a person is managing to cope with or adapt to changes in health status (Roy & Andrews, 1991). Behavior is defined as internal or external actions and reactions under specific circumstances. Nurses are primarily concerned with behavior that requires further adaptive responses as a result of environmental changes challenging the person's coping ability. Findings from three studies indicated environmental changes or behavioral responses which require in depth nursing assessment.

Preston and Dellasega (1990) found that older married women had the poorest health status and the highest stress levels as compared to older single women and single or married men. This finding in conjunction with the finding from Gardner (1994), who also studied older women, that the highest percentage of ineffective adaptation and perceived problems occurred in the interdependence mode, indicates that older married women are at high risk for ineffective adaptation. Results from these two studies also indicate that nurses should assess the general state of the marital relationship, especially in older married women to identify behaviors associated with ineffective adaptation.

The third study that identified the need for increased behavioral assessment was by Foster (1989/1990). Findings from this study indicated that nurses can perform in-depth assessments to discern pregnant adolescents' self concepts and value of self as well as identifying adaptive and ineffective behaviors. This assessment increases in importance when nurses are working with adolescents whose siblings or mothers had a child during adolescence. These adolescents are at higher risk for pregnancy and poor self-concept.

Assessment of Stimuli

The second step of the nursing process according to the model is identification of internal and external stimuli that are influencing behavior. These stimuli include all conditions, circumstances, and influences surrounding or affecting behavior. Findings from nine studies indicated stimuli which require in-depth nursing assessments.

As a result of studies conducted by Gagliardi (1991) and Dow (1992/ 1993), nurses who work with families having a child with Duchenne muscular dystrophy or with women surviving breast cancer need guidelines for assessing the array of losses experienced by these people and their families. Gagliardi included useful descriptions to facilitate assessment of families with chronically ill children. Dow developed the Adaptation After Surviving Cancer Profile. Guidelines from both of these researchers can be used to assess adaptation outcomes with specific populations.

Findings from several studies indicated that nurses should actively assess important contextual stimuli that influence the adaptive process. These contextual stimuli include the hardships and demands experienced by spouses of patients undergoing coronary artery bypass (CABG) surgery (Artinian, 1988/1989, 1991,1992) and the effects of caregiver burden on the needs of the caregiver (Perkins, 1987/1988). Assessing the needs of caregivers becomes increasingly important in situations where the person receiving care has poor mental health or impaired cognitive status (Grinspun, 1991).

Nurses who work with adolescents can obtain assessment data related to recent significant life events that have been perceived negatively or as uncontrollable according to Stein (1991/1992). Such adolescents are at risk for feelings of powerlessness and low self-esteem. Nurses assessing adolescents should actively seek this information because adolescents may not be inclined to share feelings with adults without being prompted to do so.

Lavender (1988/1989) examined self-esteem in kindergarten children and found no significant differences in the self-esteem scores between children of working mothers and those whose mothers did not work. Additionally, the families' socioeconomic status was not related to self-esteem in the kindergarten child. The children at risk for low self-esteem may be the children of single-parent families. Consequently, nurses who work with young children should be attuned to assessing self-esteem in young children from single-parent households.

Results from two studies indicate that the time needed for adaptation after severe stressors may be longer than is recognized by many health providers. Artinian (1992) and Robinson (1991/1992) indicated that the effects of stress continued for at least 1 year after open-heart surgery and the experience of bereavement, respectively. The effects of severe stressors may be present in other populations as well and nurses should seek information regarding stressful events.

Nursing Diagnosis

Nursing diagnosis is a judgment resulting in a statement conveying the person's adaptation status according to the model. One investigator derived implications for nursing practice using the nursing diagnoses typology of the model. DeRuvo (1992/1993) identified and described nursing diagnoses and their defining characteristics using the RAM and Gordon's Functional Health Patterns. Findings from the study indicated that a universal set of nursing diagnoses existed for clients receiving outpatient radiation therapy for head and neck or digestive system cancers. Although only one author used a nursing diagnosis approach, the typology was used frequently by many authors to describe research problems under investigation.

Goal Setting

The general goal of nursing intervention has been defined as maintaining and enhancing adaptive behaviors (Roy & Andrews, 1991). In order to facilitate goal attainment, nurses will identify factors that affect the process of adaptation. These factors are taken into account in planning nursing care. Implications for practice related to the planning phase of the nursing process were derived from 20 studies. Knowledge synthesized from these studies was divided into planning for families and patients throughout the life cycle and planning for patients in acute care settings.

Planning for Families and Individuals Throughout the Life Cycle

Planning for families and individuals throughout the life cycle includes knowledge needed by nurses to effectively plan nursing care for families, children, pregnant women, and the elderly. Findings from 16 studies contributed knowledge to plan nursing interventions for individuals or families throughout the life cycle.

Findings from three studies focused on family structure. Scherubel (1985/1986) found that family characteristics of cohesion, achievement orientation, and strong religious values were associated with positive adaptive responses in patients following CABG surgery. Similarly, positive adaptation responses were enhanced when parents recognized that they could identify what would meet their ill child's needs (Smith, Garvis, & Martinson, 1983). Although strong family values and the recognition by parents that they are capable of identifying the needs of the ill child enhanced adaptation, the diagnosis and treatment of cancer in a child clearly causes stress in families (Wright, 1993).

Artinian (1988/1989; 1991; 1992) and Grinspun (1991) emphasized the importance of planning by nurses to provide emotional support to meet the needs of significant others and to incorporate these needs into the total plan of care. A planned approach could increase the possibility that the support needs of significant others would be identified and adequately assessed. Three investigators (Bean, 1987/1988; DeRuvo, 1992/1993; Leech, 1982) found that support from nurses and family members should be planned based upon the assessment and timing of the stimuli experienced by clients. As the clients' conditions change, so do the needs for support from nurses and family members.

One study had implications for the planning of nursing care for children. Grey, Cameron, and Thurber's (1991) study results indicated that nurses who care for children with diabetes need to plan their care with the knowledge that age and secondary sexual development can be explanatory concerning a large variation in psychosexual adaptation and the metabolic control of diabetes. Although nurses cannot change the factors of age nor the development of secondary sexual development, they can modify perception of these stimuli and assist children to express their fears and concerns.

Legault (1990/1991) and Edwards (1991/1992) identified the necessity of planning nursing interventions to support effective adaptation to pregnancy. Legault addressed the importance of helping women develop realistic expectations of pregnancy and motherhood, and Edwards addressed the necessity of supporting the self concept of women from low income families. Both authors emphasized the importance of planning to prevent nurses from missing the subtle cues associated with unrealistic expectations or low-income status.

When nurses are planning interventions for the elderly, they should consider the contextual stimuli of socioeconomic status and its effect on health and adaptation (McGill 1991/1992; McGill & Paul, 1993). These researchers suggest that if there is no possibility of improving socioeconomic status, nurses should help clients identify other positive stimuli in their lives to promote adaptation. The results from a study by Chen (1994) indicated that adaptation of the elderly to hearing loss requires planning by the nurse to encourage successful adjustment to the use of hearing aids. The elderly with hearing losses may need to be reminded frequently by nurses to wear the hearing aid and may require support to adjust successfully. Additional results from this study indicate that elderly women who have hearing handicaps were more at risk for ineffective adaptation than were elderly men.

Planning for Patients in the Acute Care Setting

Four studies contributed knowledge needed by nurses when planning interventions for patients in acute care settings. Adults were subjects in three studies; children in an isolation unit were subjects in a fourth study.

Results of studies by Barone (1993/1994) and Strohmyer, Noroian, Patterson, and Carlin (1993) indicated the necessity of planning nursing interventions which assist patients to achieve desired outcomes. Strohmyer and colleagues found that adaptation could be facilitated in multiple trauma patients if patients could anticipate and plan for the post trauma problems. The problems included self-devaluation, guilt, depression, hostility, body-image distortions, and anxiety. Barone indicated that integration of spinal cord injured patients' use of escape/avoidance coping strategies and maintenance of hope into the plan of care were important in encouraging adaptation immediately following injury. Nurses need to know that more time is required for psychosocial adaptation for older people than for younger people with spinal cord injury. Realistic planning by nurses may be a key factor in adaptation.

The planning of patient teaching was emphasized by the results from a study by Guzzetta (1979). The study findings revealed that psychological anxiety and learning are inversely related in adult cardiac patients. Therefore, the timing of teaching is critical in planning optimum learning outcomes. Nurses need to be aware of the relationship between learning and anxiety so that both formal and informal teaching may be timed to increase adaptation.

Broeder (1985) described the reactions of children to illustrations of a nurse in isolation attire and identified that procedures were the most stressful events experienced by children. Nurses working with children in isolation units can recognize the fear precipitated by isolation attire and modify procedures to reduce the stress experienced by children.

Interventions

According to the RAM, the focus of nursing interventions is to alter the stimuli that influence behaviors in an effort to increase adaptation (Roy & Andrews, 1991). Whenever possible, the focus of nursing interventions is the focal stimulus. However, when management of a focal stimulus is not possible, the contextual stimuli are managed and at times interventions are focused on cognator or regulator processes. For clarity of presentation of the findings from the research, nursing interventions have been categorized according to the RAM concepts of (a) cognator, (b) physiologic, (c) self-concept, (d) role function, and (e) interdependence. The cognator and interdependence components of the model have been further classified into subgroups of interventions.

Cognator Interventions

According to the model, the cognator subsystem includes perceptual/information processing, learning, judgment, and emotion. The majority of studies that used interventions focued on cognator processes were related to processes associated with learning. The processes associated with learning include imitation, reinforcement, and insight. Cognator interventions were divided into perceptual processing, patient education, parent education, community education, and nursing education.

Perceptual processing. Results from two studies involved perceptual processing. Campbell (1992) used cognitive therapy techniques to enhance adaptation in depressed elderly patients, and Gaberson (1991) used music and humor audiotapes to enhance adaptation in patients undergoing medical or surgical procedures. Nurses' use of these techniques to enhance adaptation has wide ranging implications, because the practicing nurse can use cognitive therapy or music and humor audiotapes with a variety of patients in multiple settings.

Patient education. The need for increased patient and significant other information was a recurring theme through most of the 60 studies included in this chapter. Patients and significant others need additional information about cesarean births (Fawcett & Weiss, 1993), open-heart surgery (Artinian 1988/1989, 1991, 1992; Silva, 1987), grief (Robinson, 1991/1992), potentially painful medical procedures (Hjelm-Karlsson, 1989) and technology (Campbell-Heider, 1988, 1993; Smith, Mayer, Parkhurst, Perkins, & Pingleton, 1991). Several authors specified the depth and breadth of knowledge needed by patients and significant others to increase adaptive capabilities. Bean (1987/1988), DeRuvo (1992/1993), and Leech (1982) indicated that adaptation could be enhanced by providing ill patients with additional information regarding their conditions. Patients become more aware of the presence and progression of their illness during procedures and treatments. In addition to information about their conditions, patients need to know details about their therapy, such as what it is, what it does including side effects, and how long they will be receiving it (Cornell, 1990; Dahlen, 1980, Leuze & McKenzie, 1987). Patients may also need counseling about the anxiety they experience and what can be done to decrease anxiety. The knowledge that many therapies and procedures will be time limited encourages adaptation (Campbell-Heider, 1988,1993).

According to results from a study by Artinian (1991), nurses should share expectations with significant others. Nurses can educate significant others so that they are able to distinguish between normal and abnormal symptoms. Knowing what to expect and knowing what is common or what is deviant could provide significant others with more of a sense of control over the situation. Nurses should also educate significant others to become aware of the effects of the focal stimulus on their own adaptation.

Investigators for two studies identified specific populations that could benefit from counseling, and investigators for two additional studies identified benefits of counseling about the effects of stress. Dow (1992/1993) maintained that nurses can tentatively counsel women considering having children after having treatment for breast cancer—that they are not at greater risk for developing recurrent or metastatic disease. Selman (1989) stated that nurses can counsel people considering total hip replacement surgery regarding the success of the surgery. It is helpful for patients considering total hip replacement surgery to know that after the surgery there is typically an increase in the quality of life and that surgery restores the person to a more normal life. Both studies that addressed the effects of stress (Pollock, 1981/1982; Preston & Dellasega, 1990), indicated the importance of counseling clients about stress as a way to enhance adaptation. Nurses could benefit from additional studies that develop practical knowledge to counsel patients regarding the outcomes of specific procedures or treatments.

Parent, family education. Results from four studies indicated the importance of perinatal education to facilitate adaptation to parental roles. Fawcett and Burritt (1985) developed a cesarean delivery education pamphlet. The authors emphasized the importance of a follow-up telephone call or home visit to reinforce the pamphlet's content and to emphasize the need to prepare for a cesarean birth. Fawcett and Weiss (1993) reemphasized the importance of providing information about the cesarean birth process, and Legault (1990/1991) noted the importance of assisting women enrolled in prenatal classes to use resources to facilitate role transition. Legault also identified the need to include information in prenatal classes about postpartum depression and other commonly occurring postpartum conditions. Education during the birth process was encouraged by Reichert, Baron, and Fawcett (1993). Results from this study indicated that adaptation was enhanced when nurses provided information about the birth process during labor and delivery.

Findings from a study by Hart (1988/1989) identified the misconceptions held by rural parents when treating fever in children. Parents need instruction about the principles of fever management including accurate methods of measuring temperature, correct medications to use, and other appropriate methods for reducing temperature. Nurses working with parents and children should be aware of misconceptions commonly held by parents and should routinely include instructions about fever management.

Nursing education. Results from two studies indicated the necessity of educating nurses about temperature measurement and the development of sepsis in trauma patients. Pontious, Kennedy, Shelly, and Mittrucker (1994) found that the level of inservice education significantly affected all temperature readings obtained at any site by any measurement instrument. Results from this study pose multiple questions regarding the quality control of many nursing procedures. Because the measurement of temperature varied by the level of inservice education, reasonable doubt exists regarding the accuracy of other routine measurements.

Gervasini (1994) found that patients who experienced a longer lag time between injury and treatment and had higher injury scores had more sepsis. Nurses should be taught to decrease lag time between injury and treatment to promote adaptation.

Community. In addition to teaching nurses about the importance of decreasing lag time, the public should be taught so that injured people seek treatment as soon as possible (Gervasini, 1994). The public also should be taught that people with disabilities are sometimes stigmatized (Gagliardi, 1991). Gagliardi recommended that nurses implement programs that increase contact between disabled and nondisabled children as an appropriate strategy to decrease stigma.

Physiologic Mode Interventions

Researchers in four studies indicated nursing interventions related to clients' physiologic status. Hunter (1991) and Pontious and colleagues (1994) examined methods of temperature measurement. According to Pontious and colleagues, Tempa-DOT was the most clinically useful method of temperature measurement, and the oral site was the most accurate when measuring temperature in children in an acute-care setting. The authors indicated that with younger children the axillary site should be used rather than the oral site. Findings from the Hunter study indicated that 3 minutes is the clinically appropriate time for measuring axillary temperature in newborns, because stabilization occurred in 100% of the sample using two different thermometers.

Dobratz (1993) found that pain management in hospice patients increased physiologic adaptation, and Carson (1991/1992) identified a specific activity that contributed to psychological adaptation for well adults. The specific activity used by Carson in a laboratory setting was lifting a small barbell to decrease stress. Lifting a small barbell demonstrated a positive effect on psychological adaptation to stress. This intervention may serve as a distraction and, therefore, increase adaptive capabilities.

Self-Concept Mode Interventions

The RAM indicates the self-concept mode as consisting of the physical self and the personal self. This mode is a composite of beliefs and feelings that one holds about oneself at a given point in time. Investigators of two studies using adolescents as subjects, indicated interventions related to the self-concept mode. Stein (1991/1992) and Foster (1989/1990) found that adolescents may be at risk for feeling powerless and low self-esteem. The investigators recommended that nurses may be able to help adolescents to identify choices and options that decrease the feelings of powerlessness and enhance self-esteem. Ill or pregnant adolescents are at particular risk for feelings of powerlessness. Nurses can provide opportunities for choosing the timing and sequencing of procedures, which may decrease feelings of powerlessness, thereby increasing self-esteem. Nurses need to be aware that youth from lower socioeconomic classes are more likely than are youth from middle and upper socioeconomic classes to experience feelings of powerlessness and low self-esteem.

Role Function Mode Interventions

According to the RAM, the role function mode is focused on roles a person fulfills in society. This mode is concerned with social integrity, the need to know who one is in relation to others, so that one can act appropriately. The results from one study (Nyqvist & Sjoden, 1993) were focused on interventions related to the role function mode. Nyqvist and Sjoden recommended that nurses should encourage persistence and confidence in the new mother's ability to breastfeed. Nurses should facilitate early extensive physical contact with the newborn and should supply structured information on breastfeeding. Facilitation of private, undisturbed parent and infant contact with active participation in the infant's care and feeding were found to be very important.

Interdependence Mode Interventions

As identified in the model, the interdependence mode is focused on interactions related to giving and receiving love, value, and respect. These interactions center upon significant others and support systems. For ease of presentation, interdependence nursing interventions will be divided into support systems—including significant others and nurses, support programs, and advocacy.

Support systems. Several researchers indicated that providing emotional support, a traditional nursing activity, should be expanded (Artinian, 1992; Campbell-Heider, 1988, 1993; Gardner, 1994; Gibson, 1993/1994; Grinspun, 1991). Fawcett and Weiss (1993) recommended that nurses not only provide support, but also convey a feeling of caring and concern, as well as technical expertise. In addition, health care professionals should be sensitive to cultural differences without preconceived expectations. Gibson (1993/1994) expanded the ideas of caring and concern indicated by Fawcett and Weiss to include understanding mothers' needs for hypervigilance and nurses' needs to provide guidance for families with ill children. Gibson also recommended that families with a chronically ill child be assigned a nurse who can visit on a long-term basis for affirmation, encouragement, information, and guidance.

Enlisting the support of family and friends to promote adaptation to stimuli was recommended by several investigators. The presence of partners during the delivery process (Reichert et al., 1993), the support of family and friends during the movement of elderly people into congregate living facilities (Armer, 1989), and the presence of loved ones surrounding the hospice patient (Dobratz, 1993) all were found to promote adaptation. Results of these three studies indicate that nurses should encourage visits from friends and family as frequently as possible.

One study (Rich, 1991/1992) examined the support provided to nurses by the employing institutions. Study findings revealed a significant negative correlation between organizational resources and burnout in nurses. To decrease burnout in nurses, the institution's administrators can support nurses by increasing organizational resources.

Support programs. Stress management programs were encouraged for elderly married women (Preston & Dellasega, 1990) and for women with spouses who had undergone CABG surgery (Artinian, 1992). The researchers in these two studies demonstrated that married women, especially elderly married women, may need increased nursing support for adaptation.

Gibson (1993/1994) and Grinspun (1991) recommended support groups for parents and significant others to share their feelings, learn new coping skills, and identify positive contextual stimuli in their lives. Nurses can be instrumental in developing support groups and providing support group information to parents and significant others.

The development of specific types of support programs was endorsed by Calvert (1989), Gervasini (1994), and Newman (1991). Calvert recommended that nurses organize pet programs in institutions and other settings where loneliness can occur, such as adult day-care centers. Calvert also suggested that nurses, employed in institutions with pet programs, encourage pet rounds so that pet interaction can occur throughout the resident population. Development of trauma-prevention programs as recommended by Gervasini should focus not only on decreasing the incidence of trauma but also on identifying high-risk behaviors and modifying these behaviors to reflect a protective pattern. Newman found that an arthritis self-help group facilitated arthritis self-efficacy for managing pain and other symptoms. Nurses are uniquely qualified to establish these types of groups which enhance adaptation.

Advocacy. The results from three studies indicate the need for nurses to be advocates for family caregivers (Gibson, 1993/1994; Perkins, 1987/1988; Smith et al., 1991). Traditional nursing activity of patient advocacy should be modified to include family caregivers because the well-being of clients frequently depends on the well-being of the caregivers. Meeting the needs of caregivers includes more than giving support in their caregiver role and may include helping them get time for themselves for meeting their own physical and psychosocial needs. Perkins (1987/1988) indicated that nurses can prevent early or inappropriate admission of the elderly to long-term care facilities by encouraging caregivers to maintain their own quality of life and encouraging supportive family relationships.

Artinian (1991), Silva (1987), and Reichert and colleagues (1993) stated that the nursing role includes acting as a change agent to remove both personal and institutional barriers to meet the needs of patients and significant others. Changing policies that interfere with meeting the needs of patients and significant others becomes necessary to enhance adaptation. Institutions and patients should benefit from changes that make the institution more family oriented.

Evaluation

The last phase of the nursing process is evaluation. According to the RAM, evaluation involves judging the effectiveness of nursing interventions. Many studies included in this chapter in the intervention category also incorporated evaluation as a component of the study and will not be repeated in this section. Four studies were focused on evaluation, one on the evaluation of nursing interventions. Investigators in this study and three others evaluated the usefulness of the RAM and are included in this section.

Kiikkala and Peitsi (1991) evaluated the change in nursing assessment and documentation when the model was implemented in practice. The authors concluded that the use of the RAM in practice improved nursing assessments by helping to focus nursing attention on self-concept, role function, and interdependence needs of patients—not just on physiologic needs. Nursing documentation reflected the improved assessments, and the researchers concluded that the use of the model improved nursing practice.

Three researchers identified the RAM as being useful for ongoing nursing assessments in a variety of settings. Leuze and McKenzie (1987) concluded that the RAM improved preoperative assessments, and Dahlen (1980) concluded that the model was beneficial as a guide in measuring adaptation in the elderly following cataract surgery. According to Cornell (1990), use of the model helped to identify patterns of anxiety. The three investigators measured and evaluated focal and contextual stimuli according to the RAM, and agreed that the model successfully guided their studies.

Summary

In this chapter, we have focused on research reports identified in Chapters 3 through 9 that were evaluated to have a high potential for implementation in nursing practice. Of the 163 reports of studies included in this monograph, 60 were identified for inclusion in this chapter based on the established criteria. Findings from these studies were synthesized using the phases of the nursing process to identify implications for nursing practice. This synthesis indicates that the RAM can help guide research-based nursing practice and strengthen the relationship between theory, research, and practice.

References

Armer, J.M. (1989). Factors influencing relocation adjustment among community-based rural elderly (Doctoral dissertation, University of Rochester, 1988). *Dissertation Abstracts International, 50,* 1321-B.

Artinian, N.T. (1989). The stress process within the Roy adaptation framework: Sources, mediators and manifestations of stress in spouses of coronary artery bypass patients during hospitalization and six weeks post discharge (Doctoral dissertation, Wayne State University, (1988). *Dissertation Abstracts International, 49,* 5225-B.

Artinian, N.T. (1991). Stress experience of spouses of patients having coronary artery bypass during hospitalization and 6 weeks after discharge. *Heart & Lung, 20,* 52-59.

Artinian, N.T. (1992). Spouse adaptation to mate's CABG surgery: 1-year follow-up. *American Journal of Critical Care, 1* (2), 36-42.

Barone, S.H. (1994). Adaptation to spinal cord injury (Doctoral dissertation, Boston College, 1993). *Dissertation Abstracts International, 54,* 3547-B.

Bean, C.A. (1988). Needs and stimuli influencing needs of adult cancer patients (Doctoral dissertation, University of Alabama in Birmingham, 1987). *Dissertation Abstracts International, 48,* 2259-B.

Broeder, J.L. (1985). School-age children's perceptions of isolation after hospital discharge. *Maternal Child Nursing Journal, 14,* 153-174.

Calvert, M.M. (1989). Human-pet interaction and loneliness: A test of concepts from Roy's adaptation model. *Nursing Science Quarterly, 2,* 194-202.

Campbell, J. M. (1992). Treating depression in well older adults: Use of aries in cognitive therapy. *Issues in Mental Health Nursing, 13,* 19-29.

Campbell-Heider, N. (1988) Patient adaptation to the hospital technological environment (Doctoral dissertation, The University of Rochester, 1988). *Dissertation Abstracts International, 49,* 1618-B.

Campbell-Heider, N. (1993). Patient adaptation to technology: An application of the Roy model to nursing research. *Journal of the New York State Nurses Association 24*(2), 22-27.

Carson, M.A. (1992). The effect of discrete muscle activity on stress response (Doctoral dissertation, Boston College, 1991), *Dissertation Abstracts International, 52,* 5757-B.

Chen, H.L. (1994). Hearing in the elderly: Relation of hearing loss, loneliness, and self-esteem. *Journal of Gerontological Nursing, 20*(6), 22-28.

Cornell, D.L. (1990). Patterns of anxiety with home parenteral antibiotic therapy (Master's thesis, University of Nevada, Reno, 1990). *Masters Abstracts International, 28,* 572.

Dahlen, R.A. (1980). Analysis of selected factors related to the elderly person's ability to adapt to visual prostheses following senile cataract surgery (Doctoral dissertation, The Catholic University of America, 1980). *Dissertation Abstracts International, 41,* 389-B.

DeRuvo, S.L.S. (1993). Nursing diagnoses using Roy's adaptation model for persons with cancer receiving external beam radiation (Master's thesis, The University Arizona, 1992). *Masters Abstracts International, 31,* 270.

Dobratz, M.C. (1993). Causal influence of psychological adaptation on dying. *Western Journal of Nursing Research, 15,* 708-729.

Dow, K.H. (1993). An analysis of the experience of surviving and having children after breast cancer (Doctoral dissertation, Boston College, 1992). *Dissertation Abstracts International, 53,* 5641-B.

Edwards, M.R. (1992). Self-esteem, sense of mastery, and adequacy of prenatal care (Doctoral dissertation, University of Alabama in Birmingham, 1991). *Dissertation Abstracts International, 53,* 768-B.

Fawcett, J., & Burritt, J. (1985). An exploratory study of antenatal preparation for cesarean birth. *Journal of Obstetric, Gynecologic, & Neonatal Nursing, 14,* 224-230.

Fawcett, J., & Weiss, M.E. (1993). Cross-cultural adaptation to cesarean birth. *Western Journal of Nursing Research, 15,* 282-297.

Foster, P.L. (1990). The relationship between selected variables and the self-esteem in adolescent females (Doctoral dissertation, University of Alabama in Birmingham, 1989). *Dissertation Abstracts International, 50,* 3918-B.

Gaberson, K.B. (1991). The effect of humorous distraction on preoperative anxiety. *AORN Journal, 54,* 1258-1264.

Gagliardi, B.A. (1991). The impact of Duchenne muscular dystrophy on families. *Orthopaedic Nursing, 10*(5), 41-49.

Gardner, M.J. (1994). Spouse adaptation after the partner's open heart surgery, Unpublished master's thesis, Grand Valley State University.

Gervasini, A. A. (1994). Classification of trauma patients with a septic profile utilizing a predictor model. Unpublished doctoral dissertation, Boston College, Boston.

Gibson, C.H. (1994). A study of empowerment in mothers of chronically ill children (Doctoral dissertation, Boston College, 1993). *Dissertation Abstracts International, 54,* 4078-B.

Grey, M., Cameron, M. E., & Thurber, F. W. (1991). Coping and adaption in children with diabetes. *Nursing Research, 40,* 144-149.

Grinspun, D. (1991). Factors influencing adaptation of spouses of head trauma patients. Unpublished master's thesis, University of Michigan, Ann Arbor.

Guzzetta, C.E. (1979). Relationship between stress and learning. *Advances in Nursing Science, 1*(4), 35-39.

Hart, M.A. (1989). Rural parents' perception and management of fever in their school-age children. (Masters thesis, University of Florida, 1988). *Masters Abstracts International, 27,* 376.

Hjelm-Karlsson, K. (1989). Effects of information to patients undergoing intravenous pyelography: An intervention study. *Journal of Advanced Nursing, 14,* 853-62.

Hunter, L.P. (1991). Measurement of axillary temperatures in neonates. *Western Journal of Nursing Research, 13,* 324-335.

Kiikkala, I., & Peitsi, T. (1991). The care of children with minimal brain dysfunction: A Roy adaptation analysis. *Journal of Pediatric Nursing, 6,* 290-292.

Lavender, M.G. (1989). The relationship between maternal self-esteem, work status, and sociodemographic characteristics and self-esteem of the kindergarten child (Doctoral dissertation, The University of Alabama in Birmingham, 1988). *Dissertation Abstracts International, 49,* 5229-B.

Leech, J.L. (1982). Psychosocial and physiologic needs of patients with arterial occlusive disease during the preoperative phase of hospitalization. *Heart & Lung, 11,* 442-449.

Legault, F.M. (1991). Adaptation within the role function and self-concept modes among women during the postpartum period (Master's thesis, D'Youville College, 1990). *Masters Abstracts International, 29,* 439.

Leuze, M. & McKenzie, J. (1987). Preoperative assessment using the Roy Adaptation Model. *AORN Journal, 46,* 1122-1134.

McGill, J.S. (1992). Functional status as it relates to hope in elders with and without cancer (Doctoral dissertation, The University of Alabama in Birmingham, 1991). *Dissertation Abstracts International, 53,* 771-B.

McGill, J.S., & Paul, P.B. (1993). Functional status and hope in elderly people with an without cancer. *Oncology Nursing Forum, 20,* 1207-1213.

Newman, A.M. (1991). The effect of the arthritis self-help course on arthritis self-efficacy, perceived social support, purpose and meaning in life, and arthritis impact in people with arthritis (Doctoral dissertation, University of Alabama at Birmingham, 1991). *Dissertation Abstracts International, 52,* 2995-B.

Nyqvist, K.H., & Sjoden, P.O. (1993). Advice concerning breast-feeding from mothers of infants admitted to a neonatal intensive care unit: The Roy Adaptation Model as a conceptual structure. *Journal of Advanced Nursing, 18,* 54-63.

Perkins, I. (1988). An analysis of relationships among interdependence in family care givers and the elderly, care giver burden, and adaptation of the homebound frail elderly (Doctoral dissertation, The Catholic University of America, 1987). *Dissertation Abstracts International, 48,* 3250-3251-B.

Pollock, S.E. (1982). Level of adaptation: An analysis of stress factors that affect health status (Doctoral dissertation, The University of Texas at Austin, 1981). *Dissertation Abstracts International, 42,* 436-B.

Pontious, S., Kennedy, A.H., Shelly, S., & Mittrucker, C. (1994). Accuracy and reliability of temperature measurement by instrument and site. *Journal of Pediatric Nursing, 9*(2), 114-123.

Preston, D.B. & Dellasega, C. (1990). Elderly women and stress: Does marriage make a difference? *Journal of Gerontological Nursing, 16*(4), 26-31.

Reichert, J.A., Baron, M., & Fawcett, J. (1993). Changes in attitudes toward cesarean birth. *Journal of Obstetric, Gynecologic, and Neonatal Nursing, 22,* 159-167.

Rich, V.L. (1992). The use of personal, organizational, and coping resources in the prevention of staff nurse burnout: A test of a model (Doctoral dissertation, University of Pittsburg, 1991). *Dissertation Abstracts International, 52,* 3532-B.

Robinson, J.H. (1992). A descriptive study of widows' grief responses, coping processes and social support within Roy's adaptation (Doctoral dissertation, Wayne State University, 1991). *Dissertation Abstracts International, 52,* 6320-B.

Roy, C., & Andrews, H. (1991). *The Roy adaptation model: The definitive statement.* Norwalk, CT: Appleton & Lange.

Roy, C., & Andrews, H. (1999). *The Roy adaptation model.* Stamford, CT: Appleton & Lange.

Scherubel, J.C.M. (1986). Description of adaptation patterns following an acute cardiac event (Doctoral dissertation, University of Illinois at Chicago, Health Sciences Center, 1985). *Dissertation Abstracts International, 46,* 2627-B.

Selman, S.W. (1989). Impact of total hip replacement of quality of life. *Orthopaedic Nursing, 8*(5), 43-49.

Silva, M.C. (1987). Needs of spouses of surgical patients: A conceptualization within the Roy Adaptation Model. *Scholarly Inquiry for Nursing Practice, 1,* 29-44.

Smith, C.E., Garvis, M. S., & Martinson, I. M. (1983). Content analysis of interviews using a nursing model: A look at parents adapting to the impact of childhood cancer. *Cancer Nursing, 6,* 269-275.

Smith, C.E., Mayer, L. S., Parkhurst, C., Perkins, S. B., & Pingleton, S. K.

(1991). Adaptation in families with a member requiring mechanical ventilation at home. *Heart & Lung, 20,* 349-356.

Stein, P.R. (1992). Life events, self-esteem, and powerlessness among adolescents (Doctoral dissertation, Texas Woman's University, 1991). *Dissertation Abstracts International, 52,* 5195-B.

Strohmyer, L.L., Noroian, E.L., Patterson, L.M., & Carlin, B.P. (1993). Adaptation six months after multiple trauma: A pilot study. *Journal of Neuroscience Nursing, 25,* 30-37.

Wright, P.S. (1993). Parents' perceptions of their quality of life. *Journal of Pediatric Oncology Nursing, 10,* 139-145.

Chapter 13

Directions for Future Theory Development and Research

The review of published research based on the Roy Adaptation Model (RAM) from 1970 through 1994 has indicated evidence both for the contributions of the model to nursing science and for identifying areas that need further work. Information in this chapter will set directions for future theory development and research using conclusions from the analyses described earlier. Questions to be addressed are: (a) How has the literature addressed Roy's structure for knowledge based on the RAM (Roy & Andrews, 1991) and what new areas for investigation have been revealed by the composite analysis? (b) Is there a need for additions, deletions, or changes to the key concepts of the model? (c) What recommendations can be made about measuring model concepts and are other directions related to methodology suggested from reviewing the first 25 years of published research? (d) What directions for theorizing and for research will be given highest priority, based on this integrated review project?

Research Directions Based on Structure of Knowledge

Chapter 10 contains a summary of how concepts from the RAM have been measured. Chapters 11 and 12 include an integration of the findings of RAM-based research to describe contributions to nursing knowledge and applications to nursing practice.

Progress is encouraging in that the model has proved useful to investigators for deriving propositions and testing research questions. The view that conceptual models are useful in the scientific enterprise has had both proponents (Fawcett, 1995) and opponents (Bullough & Bullough, 1994). The analysis, evaluation, and synthesis of studies presented by the authors of this monograph support the value of a conceptual model in providing a structure for developing knowledge for nursing. The findings of the studies taken as a whole contribute to nursing science and provide the basis for improving practice.

The BBARNS members noted the substantial contributions of nurse researchers to the understanding of nursing science and to the advancement of the RAM. However, it is also recognized that, just as each researcher reporting a given study noted limitations of the research and provided recommendations for further scientific development, so too, each BBARNS member identified areas for further development within the content areas reviewed. One way of bringing together these diverse observations and the summaries of the last three chapters is to compare the findings of the project with the structure for knowledge proposed by Roy (Roy & Andrews, 1991; see Table 13.1) and to identify which areas have substantial research and which have not yet received attention.

Basic Nursing Science

Basic nursing science, according to Roy (Roy & Andrews, 1991) involves looking at people and groups as adaptive systems. Focusing on human processes and patterns, basic knowledge for nursing includes understanding humans in their environments as related to health. In the basic science of nursing, then, adaptive processes are described and explained—both cognator-regulator activity for individuals and stabilizer-innovator activity for groups. Basic nursing scientists—following the model—strive to understand the stability of adaptive patterns and the dynamics of evolving adaptive patterns. Those who follow the model are provided direction for exploring adaptive modes, their development and interrelatedness, and factors that influence adaptive modes including culture. Nursing knowl-

---

Table 13.1 – Structure of Knowledge Based on the RAM

Basic Nursing Science

Person and group as adaptive systems
- Adaptive Processes
    Cognator-regulator activities
    Stabilizer-innovator activities
    Stability of adaptive patterns
    Dynamics of evaluating adaptive patterns
- Adaptive modes
    Development
    Interrelatedness
    Cultural and other influences
- Adaptation Related to Health
    Person and environment interaction
    Integration of adaptive modes

Clinical Nursing Science

- Changes in cognator-regulator or stabilizer-innovator effectiveness
- Changes within and among adaptive modes
- Nursing care to promote adaptive processes
    in times of transition; during environmental changes; during acute and chronic illness, injury, treatment, and technologic threats

---

edge based on the model allows nurses to relate adaptation to health by exploring person and environment interactions and understanding the integration of adaptive modes.

The research reviewed all stemmed from the RAM as a conceptual framework. However, each researcher, or team of researchers, posed their own questions for research. Thus it cannot be expected that the results represent an integrated program of research. Rather, the testing of propositions based on the findings of studies by other researchers was an exercise of analysis, evaluation, and synthesis by the BBARNS members to prepare an integrated review.

Areas of strength related to basic nursing science in the composite review include confirmation of the usefulness of key metapardigm concepts, of the theory of adaptive systems, and of the role of stimuli in adaptation, as described in the testing of generic propositions in Chapter 11. Selected nursing phenomena based on the RAM have been studied. Of particular note, the concepts of person and health and the effects of levels of stimuli on adaptation have been well supported and validated. Notably, approximately 75% of the ancillary propositions tested were related to the concepts of person or health.

Cognator and regulator activity has been described in adults and children, healthy people, and those with chronic and acute health conditions. Adaptive modes and processes have been studied in key populations of interest to nursing, such as preterm infants, the elderly, abuse victims, care givers, adults with AIDS, and the dying. Similarly, there is new literature on viewing groups as adaptive systems, though in the studies reviewed, research with samples of individuals or members of families outnumbered research with groups as adaptive systems 159 to 4. The limited use of published work on groups as adaptive systems has implications for further theoretic work and for publication in texts that are more readily available than the Roy and Anway publication, which has been out of print for several years.

The extensive support for propositions related to stimuli was an unexpected finding. In many cases, the researchers clarified the nature and effect of stimuli in given situations. However, the review left in doubt the relative importance of such common stimuli as age and gender. The stimuli variables will be best understood when they are considered part of the pooled effect on adaptation, rather than simply demographic variables. The importance of adaptation level as a major stimulus has been addressed in the most recent conceptual clarifications of the model. Roy described three levels of adaptation—integrated, compensatory, and compromised (Roy & Andrews, 1999).

Study has begun on the dynamics of evolving adaptive patterns. Some clear descriptions of the stages of adaptation in dying patients were reported by Dobratz, in women having children after breast cancer by Dow, and in families with chronically ill children by Gibson and Gagliardi. In each study, some of the influencing factors were identified. However, it will take complex research designs, most likely triangulating qualitative and quantitative approaches, in diverse populations to reach a purposeful and imaginative understanding of the dynamics of evolving adaptive patterns.

Of particular value for understanding the basic nursing science based on the RAM was the repeated finding of a reciprocal relationship between adaptive processes and adaptive modes. For example, cognator activity affects self concept, and self concept affects cognator activity. In their early work on developing propositions, Roy and Roberts (1981) noted that the adaptation model implies multivariate and nonlinear configurations. A simple linear, unidirectional, bivariate relationship will not capture the essence of the dynamics of evolving adaptation. Use of advanced statistical techniques of multivariate and structural equation models will be required to test these relationships further.

Relative to understanding the four adaptive modes, reviews of studies in the relevant chapters provide insights into adaptive mode behavior in a variety of situations. Among these are self-concept changes during teen pregnancy and role function adaptation to cesarean birth, changes in oxygenation during nursing procedures, and predicting sepsis in trauma patients. Furthermore, investigators of 15 studies demonstrated the interrelatedness of adaptive modes. Areas in basic nursing science that need study are factors that influence development of the adaptive modes. In particular, the effects of culture on adaptive mode development and behavior is an important area for future investigation. Research across the life span was not complete. No studies related to the interdependence adaptive mode in children were found in the current review. All major concepts of the model need to be studied in all age groups and in commonly occurring situations of health and illness.

Although evidence was provided to validate the usefulness of metaparadigm concepts of person and health as defined by the RAM, much work remains in delineating how promoting adaptation contributes to health. Great potential lies in explicating relationships between and among adaptive processes, by integrating new developments in related fields such as psychoneuroimmunology. Also, the role of perception in the integration of the adaptive modes should be further defined on a conceptual and theoretic basis and then tested empirically.

Clinical Nursing Science

According to Roy (Roy & Andrews, 1991), the clinical science based on the RAM is divided into changes in cognator-regulator and stabilizer-innovator effectiveness, changes within and among the adaptive modes, and nursing care to promote adaptive processes. Research in the latter category focuses particularly on transition during environmental change, acute and chronic illness, injury, treatment, and technologic threats. Areas of strength in the composite research review that relate to clinical nursing science were identified in Chapter 12. Nursing practice applications included findings related to assessment of behavior, assessment of stimuli, nursing diagnosis, goal setting, and interventions. Predictable findings of the effectiveness of teaching and providing support were noted and use of the model allowed for further specificity concerning these variables. Evidence was provided that pivotal variables in clinical nursing science are perception and time. The importance of patients' perceptions was established, and direction was given for ways in which nurses assess patients' perceptions. It would be useful to have nurses in advanced practice develop protocols that identify patient and family perceptions in commonly occurring clinical situations in their fields of practice.

Time was repeatedly identified as important to changes in adaptive effectiveness. Pilot studies are needed in order to specify the appropriate time for effective intervention and the interval for measuring adaptation. Given the constellation of stimuli, and particularly the magnitude and characteristics of the focal stimulus, adaptation may occur instantaneously, as in oxygen saturation during suctioning, or over years, as in adaptation to spinal cord injury. The interventions of teaching health and providing support can be made more effective by further understanding the role of perception and time in a given clinical situation. Further, the clarification of stimuli in basic nursing science will have direct relevance for clinical nursing science because the management of stimuli is a primary focus for nursing interventions.

Another strength of the research review in relation to clinical nursing science was that several studies dealt with describing transitions, such as elderly people changing their type of residence. Many studies related to adaptation to acute or chronic illness, injury, and response to treatment and technologic threats. Studies were conducted during hospitalizations for illness or injury, and they included samples of people dealing with cancer as a chronic condition, as well as other long-term conditions such as spinal cord injury, arthritis, and diabetes. Childrens' responses to isolation and adults' responses to invasive and noninvasive technology were also described. In general, the studies had correlational designs and investigators described the adaptive outcomes and some of the factors associated with adaptation.

Researchers should design and test nursing interventions to promote adaptive processes in times of transition and during acute and chronic illness, injury, and response to treatment and technologic threats. Intervention studies can be focused both on managing stimuli and on ways that nurses can directly deal with cognator and regulator processes, as noted in Chapter 9. The need for knowledge development related to the clinical science of nursing implies having programs of research that deal with given patient populations. An example was provided by the work of Fawcett and colleagues in the studies related to cesarean birth (see Chapter 5).

Examining the research analyzed and synthesized in this monograph according to Roy's structure of knowledge was useful in summarizing recommendations for future research based on the RAM. Two types of recommendations were identified: (a) areas of knowledge that have received little attention in the studies from 1970 to 1994, and (b) further specifications of topics for research within the structure of knowledge. Table 13.2 shows the recommended foci for further research based on the RAM, as identified in this review.

Table 13.2 Recommended Foci for Nursing Research Based on the RAM

Basic Nursing Science

1. Groups as Adaptive Systems.
2. Age and gender as part of pooled effect on adaptation.
3. Levels of adaptation as integrated, compensatory, and compromised.
4. Dynamics of evolving adaptive patterns.
5. Reciprocal relationships of adaptive modes and processes.
6. Factors influencing adaptive mode development, particularly the effect of culture.
7. Extension of major concepts to all age groups and commonly occurring situations of health and illness.
8. Interdependence mode adaptation in children.
9. Relationship of adaptation to health.
10. Conceptual, theoretic, and empiric basis of perception in integrating the adaptive modes.

Clinical Nursing Science

11. Protocols to identify patient and family perceptions in commonly occurring clinical situations.
12. Appropriate timing for effectiveness of given nursing interventions.
13. Appropriate time interval to measure adaptation as an outcome in differing situations.
14. Specific stimuli to manage the effectiveness of given nursing interventions.
15. Programs of research to design and test interventions to promote adaptive processes in given patient populations.
16. Intervention studies that deal directly with cognator and regulator processes.

Recommendations for Model Development

The major recommendations for model development lie in expansion and clarification of concepts. The usefulness of major concepts of the model was supported by the testing of propositions embedded in the research projects reviewed. The concept of stimuli as a useful description of the metaparadigm concept of environment was worthy of consideration by Roy. Roy (1997) recently published a redefinition of the concept of adaptation implying that Helson's (1964) categories of stimuli may have served their purpose. Roy has responded to the outcome of the research review by providing definitions of three levels of adaptation (Roy & Andrews, 1999). The intent is to clarify this key internal stimulus and to make it more amenable to clinical research. In particular, the updated conceptual definitions should be helpful for those doing intervention research.

Two concepts emerged that need further conceptual and theoretic development. Time, as it relates to adaptive processing, and thus to the design of nursing interventions, should be examined fully and integrated into the RAM. Also perceptions as connectives between regulator and cognator processing should be analyzed and synthesized.

The research reviewers revealed no clear indication for changing or deleting any major model concept. However, studies of the concept of a group as an adaptive system were limited. As a result, Roy has reconsidered the theoretic work and maintained the stabilizer-innovator processes, but simplified the concept concerning adaptive modes for groups (Roy & Andrews, 1999). The adaptive modes for both individuals and groups are now named physiologic/physical, self concept/group identity, role function, and interdependence. Updated definitions of each and the related theory base should be useful in future research.

Finally, BBARNS members recognize that confirmation of propositions from research of 25 years is at best tentative. Reviews such as the one reported in this monograph, and integrated research reviews for studies in languages other than English, can be helpful in further development of the RAM.

Recommendations for Research Methods

Chapter 10 contains a summary of the ways concepts of the model were measured in the studies reviewed. The early development of instruments specific for the model's concepts was noted. Strengths in measuring physiologic and self-concept adaptive mode variables, functional status of the role function mode, and social support of the interdependence adaptive mode were described. Additional work is needed to develop instruments in all four modes, to measure the magnitude and characteristics of stimuli; and especially, to develop measurement approaches for adaptation as a process and outcome. A major area for research method development using the RAM is measurement of cognator-regulator and stabilizer-innovator effectiveness.

Variability of measures such as heart rate and blood pressure support the need to use people as their own controls in measuring adaptation over time and the usefulness of repeated measures designs. Further, given that the model has specific theoretic bases for the major conceptual definitions, researchers should develop instruments that are valid measures of specific concepts. Researchers need to meet the same rigorous standards for psychometric properties expected of instruments already in use when developing instruments to measure concepts of the RAM. Successful use of the same tool by many investigators is a sign of its usefulness. In some cases, tools available in the general domain used in studies reviewed in this monograph were evaluated by BBARNS members for the best match with the model's concepts. Continued examination of relevance of tools will increase validity of the measurement strategies.

The need for triangulated and multivariate methods was identified above. In addition, the current development of nursing as a young science, and in particular the short history of RAM-based research (25 years), emphasize the need for replication of studies where findings are promising and the redesign of studies where findings were equivocal. Individual investigators identified design issues that could be improved in future studies. Particular issues in nursing intervention studies include attention to power analysis and adequate sampling. Another issue is the need for prospective research designs, both qualitative and quantitative, to supplement the correlational and post hoc studies that were prevalent in this review.

Summary of Research Priorities for the Future

Priorities for future theory development and research were derived from the integrated review of research based on the RAM. Numerous implications for future research were noted in the previous chapters. Key priorities for future research based on analysis and synthesis of the 163 studies are summarized. Priorities for theory development are to develop middle-range theories related to cognator and regulator processes to strengthen basic nursing science based on the model. Theories related to the four adaptive modes and their relationships with the adaptive subsystems can make a substantial contribution to understanding theories of the adapting person. Further, continued conceptual development of focal, contextual, and residual stimuli is warranted for developing the clinical science of nursing based on the RAM. Adaptation level as an internal stimulus, using updated conceptual definitions and adaptation levels as they relate to adaptive outcomes can be studied. Group-level theories for families, communities, and nursing care systems is recommended for basic and clinical nursing science.

Priorities for research include the recommended foci for research identified earlier. In addition, a high priority is replication of studies that could not be recommended for practice either because of the limited support or the risk involved. Finally, intervention studies, particularly those that include the potential of cognator effectiveness to promote patient adaptation, have high priority. Diversified and targeted prospective research designs are recommended.

References

Bullough, B., & Bullough, V. (Eds.). (1994). *Nursing theory: History and critique*. In Nursing issues for the nineties and beyond pp. 64-82) NY: Springer.

Fawcett, J. (1995). *Analysis and evaluation of conceptual models of nursing* (3rd ed.). Philadelphia: Davis.

Helson, A (1964). *Adaptation-level theory*. New York: Harper & Row.

Roy, C. (1997). Future of the Roy Model: Challenge to redefine adaptation. *Nursing Science Quarterly, 10*, 42-48.

Roy, C., & Andrews, H. (1991). *The Roy adaptation model: The definitive statement* E. Norwalk, CT: Appleton & Lange.

Roy, C., & Andrews, H. (1999). *The Roy adaptation model: The definitive statement* (2nd ed.) E. Norwalk, CT: Appleton & Lange.

Roy, C., & Anway, J. (1989). Roy's adaptation model: Theories and propositions for administration. In B. Henry, C. Arndt, M. DiVicenti, & G. Marriner-Toomy, (Eds.) *Dimensions and issues in nursing administration*. St. Louis, MO: Mosby.

Roy, C., & Roberts, S. (1981). *Theory construction in nursing: An adaptation model*. Englewood Cliffs, NJ: Prentice Hall.